PRINCIPLES AND PRACTICE
OF RELAPSE PREVENTION

PRINCIPLES AND PRACTICE OF RELAPSE PREVENTION

EDITED BY
PETER H. WILSON

FOREWORD BY
G. TERENCE WILSON

THE GUILFORD PRESS
NEW YORK   LONDON

© 1992 The Guilford Press
A Division of Guilford Publications, Inc.
72 Spring Street, New York, NY 10012

Printed in the United States of America

This book is printed on acid-free paper.

Last digit is print number: 9 8 7 6 5 4 3 2 1

Library of Congress Cataloging-in-Publication Data

Principles and practice of relapse prevention / Peter H. Wilson,
   editor.
       p.   cm.
   Includes bibliographical references and indexes.
   ISBN 0-89862-891-1
   1. Mental illness—Relapse—Prevention. 2. Compulsive behavior—
Relapse—Prevention. 3. Psychotherapy. 4. Mental Disorders—
rehabilitation. I. Wilson, Peter H.
   [DNLM: 1. Behavior, Addictive—rehabilitation. 2. Behavior
Therapy—methods. WM 425 P957]
RC489.R44P75 1992
616/89'03—dc20
DNLM/DLC
for Library of Congress   92-1558
                                                              CIP

CONTRIBUTORS

Gavin Andrews, M.D. Clinical Research Unit for Anxiety Disorders, School of Psychiatry, The University of New South Wales, Darlinghurst, New South Wales, Australia

Sandra T. Azar, Ph.D. Department of Psychology, Clark University, Worcester, Massachusetts

David H. Barlow, Ph.D. Center for Stress and Anxiety Disorders, State University of New York at Albany, Albany, New York

Eric Blaauw, M.A. Department of Clinical Psychology, University of Groningen, Groningen, The Netherlands

Timothy A. Brown, Psy.D. Center for Stress and Anxiety Disorders, State University of New York at Albany, Albany, New York

Diana Damer, Ph.D. Department of Psychology, West Virginia University, Morgantown, West Virginia

Paul M. G. Emmelkamp, Ph.D. Department of Psychology, University of Groningen, Groningen, The Netherlands

Elizabeth S. Ferguson, M.A. Department of Psychology, Clark University, Worcester, Massachusetts

William Fremouw, Ph.D. Department of Psychology, West Virginia University, Morgantown, West Virginia

S. M. Hudson, Ph.D. Department of Psychology, University of Canterbury, Christchurch, New Zealand

Neil Jacobson, Ph.D. Department of Psychology, University of Washington, Seattle, Washington

Tracy Karnatz, M.A. Department of Psychology, The University of Illinois at Chicago, Chicago, Illinois

David J. Kavanagh, Ph.D. Department of Psychology, University of Sydney, Sydney, New South Wales, Australia

Jan Kloek, M.A. Department of Clinical Psychology, University of Groningen, The Netherlands

G. Alan Marlatt, Ph.D. Department of Psychology, University of Washington, Seattle, Washington

W. L. Marshall, Ph.D. Department of Psychology, Queen's University, Kingston, Ontario, Canada

Robin J. Mermelstein, Ph.D. Department of Psychology, The University of Illinois at Chicago, Chicago, Illinois

Michael K. Nicholas, Ph.D. School of Psychology, University of New South Wales, Sydney, Australia

Lisa Orimoto, M.A. Department of Psychology, University of Hawaii, Honolulu, Hawaii

Simona Reichmann, M.A. Department of Psychology, The University of Illinois at Chicago, Chicago, Illinois

Julian M. Somers, M.S. Department of Psychology, University of Washington, Seattle, Washington

Paula Truax, M.S. Department of Psychology, University of Washington, Seattle, Washington.

Craig T. Twentyman, Ph.D. Social Science Research Institute, University of Hawaii at Manoa, Manoa, Hawaii

Kelly Bemis Vitousek, Ph.D. Department of Psychology, University of Hawaii, Honolulu, Hawaii

T. Ward, M.A. Kia Marama Treatment Unit, Rolleston Prison, Rolleston, New Zealand

Peter H. Wilson, Ph.D. School of Psychology, The Flinders University of South Australia, Adelaide, Australia

FOREWORD

In 1985 Marlatt and Gordon published what has become a landmark text on the principles and procedures of relapse prevention in the treatment of addictive disorders. The approach was controversial then, and remains so today in some quarters. The reason is that it challenges the hegemony that the addiction-as-a-disease model has had over the conceptualization and treatment of addictive disorders. Nevertheless, perhaps because it provided a more flexible alternative for treating addictive disorders, relapse prevention has been widely embraced by practitioners. Moreover, consistent with the thinking behind the approach, it has been extended to an ever-expanding range of nonaddictive clinical disorders. Clinical practice has outpaced rigorous research, however, and there is a need to take stock of what has been learned and what challenges remain. The present text does precisely this in an admirable fashion.

One of the major contributions of this edited collection is that it brings together in one volume, with one overall perspective, the diverse applications of relapse prevention to very different clinical disorders. Too often in the past there has been no communication between researchers across different disorders even though their interventions have been very similar. The present text makes it is easier to identify the commonalities and differences among disorders, and to consider what implications these comparisons have for the application of relapse prevention strategies. For example, Fremouw and Damer in their chapter on obesity make the important observation that obesity is a biological condition that is inherently different from behavioral disorders such as cigarette smoking and alcohol abuse. As such, eating behavior per se is typically not the problem and cannot be the target of relapse prevention in the manner that consuming alcohol might be. This important distinction is not always appreciated in the treatment of obesity.

Another major strength of this volume is the impressive list of contributors. The editor is to be commended for securing contributions from experts in their respective fields who combine clinical know-how with scholarly analysis of the literature. It is the scientist-practitioner approach, which this book as a whole embodies, that is best calculated to advance our understanding of the problems involved in producing lasting treatment change.

This text provides the best review to date of what has been done to improve maintenance of treatment-induced change. What I found particularly helpful was the critical focus on the conceptual and methodological limitations of existing approaches to relapse prevention, as well as the balanced appraisal of its clinical utility. In his thoughtful reflections on the directions for future research in relapse prevention, Peter H. Wilson (the editor) highlights some of the more pressing methodological and conceptual problems. None is more striking than the persisting paucity of rigorous research on long-term outcome. Moreover, as Wilson points out, in most of the studies on relapse and its prevention the follow-up assessments have typically not gone beyond one year. Given the obvious need for long-term follow-up studies of clinical effectiveness, and given the theoretical and practical importance of critically evaluating the relapse prevention approach, it really is remarkable that so little has been done. The hope is that this scholarly volume will spur more investigators to meet this challenge.

I have already emphasized the scientist-practitioner bent of this volume. As the most up-to-date and comprehensive analysis of current research on relapse prevention, the book is a must for clinical researchers. As a rich source of pragmatic suggestions about how to facilitate lasting therapeutic change, it can enhance practitioners' clinical effectiveness. For example, Orimoto and Vitousek, in an unusually incisive analysis of the treatment of eating disorders, provide detailed clinical recommendations for enhancing maintenance of change. Similarly, in his chapter on depression, Wilson offers a number of practical suggestions that should find their way into informed clinical practice. Last, and hardly least, this book should prove to be an invaluable reference for students in clinical psychology and psychiatry.

G. Terence Wilson, Ph.D.
Rutgers University

CONTENTS

PRINCIPLES AND PRACTICE
OF RELAPSE PREVENTION

CHAPTER 1

RELAPSE PREVENTION: CONCEPTUAL AND METHODOLOGICAL ISSUES

Peter H. Wilson

THE FLINDERS UNIVERSITY OF SOUTH AUSTRALIA

RELAPSE: PSYCHOLOGICAL SEISMOLOGY

A great challenge for science has been the prediction of certain future events: eclipses of the sun, the arrival of comets, tomorrow's weather, volcanic erruptions, and earthquakes are examples of such phenomena. In the case of some of these natural events, such as earthquakes, an even more fundamental goal is to prevent their occurrence, or, at least, to minimize the ensuing damage and destruction. These cataclysmic events strike with great devastation at seemingly random intervals in selected parts of the world. The great challenge for seismologists is to be able to predict such events with the ease with which we can predict the return of Halley's comet or an eclipse of the sun. To do so will require great leaps in our knowledge about the nature of the earth's crust, the factors that trigger the event, and the processes involved in the actual occurrence of an earthquake. These tasks seem sufficiently daunting without even considering the further difficulties involved in taking steps to prevent earthquakes. The task confronting the researcher who is interested in relapse bears some resemblance to that of the seismologist. As earthquakes are more likely to occur in certain zones, so too are relapses more likely to occur in people with certain types of problems such as depression, addictions, and schizophrenia. We can predict the types of disorders in which the relapse is more likely to occur and, to some extent, identify those individuals who are most prone to experience a relapse, but, as with earthquakes, we have great difficulty in predicting the timing of the relapse or its severity.

This book provides an overview of the research conducted to date on relapse and its prevention following behavioral and cognitive interventions for a variety of problems. To some extent, it is a reflection of the development of the field of cognitive and behavioral therapies that such a book now appears timely. Clearly, there is an implication in the use of the term "relapse prevention" that behavioral and cognitive therapies are successful in the short term in many problem areas. While one cannot speak with equal confidence about the efficacy of treatment in all problem areas, and there are many gaps in our knowledge of the processes that underlie successful intervention, the last three decades have witnessed an unprecedented research effort directed at the understanding and modification of psychological problems. It is testimony to that work that we can now begin to address seriously the question of relapse and its prevention and to explore the issues that surround the long-term maintenance of behavioral change.

Amidst the burgeoning research on the treatment of psychological problems there has always been a need to consider the long-term effects of interventions (e.g., Eysenck, 1963; Hersen, 1979). Marlatt and Gordon's seminal work in the area (Marlatt & Gordon, 1985) has sparked a great deal of research on relapse and its prevention in the addictions, and some of that influence is now being felt in other areas. Many cognitive and behavioral techniques appear to have short-term benefits, but, by comparison, little is known about the long-term effects. How long do effects endure after successful intervention? What proportion of people relapse and what distinguishes them from those who maintain their treatment gains? What causes relapse? How can relapse be prevented or minimized? This book attempts to delineate the current knowledge base concerning these questions. The answers to these questions have important implications for our conception of various problem ·domains and for the provision of the most effective and economical treatment.

Interest in the subject of relapse, or its obverse, maintenance, is indicated by the number of significant papers that have appeared on this topic in recent years. Apart from the book by Marlatt and Gordon (1985), another book has appeared recently that is devoted to relapse in sexual deviations (Laws, 1989). Two miniseries have appeared in the journal *Behavior Therapy,* one of which is on maintenance in behavioral medicine, with papers on smoking (Glasgow & Lichtenstein, 1987), hypertension (Jacob, Wing, & Shapiro, 1987), weight loss (Brownell & Jeffery, 1987), chronic headache (Blanchard, 1987), and Raynaud disease (Freedman, 1987). The second miniseries in *Behavior Therapy* included a review of social learning-based marital therapy (Jacobson, 1989) and other papers on more general topics in the area of maintenance of behavioral change and generalization (Edelstein, 1989; Kendall, 1989; Stokes & Osnes, 1989). Other reviews have appeared on specific problem areas such as depression (Belsher & Costello, 1988; Wilson, 1989), obesity (Westover & Lanyon, 1990), and smoking (Brandon, Zelman, & Baker, 1987). Furthermore, a number of research papers have appeared that include relatively long follow-up periods, such as 5- to 6-year follow-ups of alcohol abuse (Rychtarik, Foy, Scott, Lokey, & Prue, 1987), a 2½-year follow-up of smoking cessation (Glasgow, Klesges, Klesges, Vasey, & Gunnarson, 1985), an 8-year follow-up of agoraphobia (Burns, Thorpe, & Cavallaro, 1986), a 4- and 6-year follow-up of headache sufferers (Blanchard, Andrasik, Guarnieri, Neff, & Rodichok, 1987; Lisspers & Öst, 1990), and a 2¼-year follow-up of depression (McLean & Hakstian, 1990). These examples provide a clear sign that the field is beginning to embrace maintenance as an important research and clinical issue.

WHAT IS RELAPSE?

At the most general level, relapse is the return of problem behavior following some problem-free period. The main difficulties lie in determining what constitutes a return of problem behavior or symptoms: How can we define a problem-free period, and how long should the problem-free period last before we regard any return of difficulties as a relapse? Brownell, Marlatt, Lichtenstein, and Wilson (1986) and Marlatt and Gordon (1985) point out that the definition of "relapse" provided in *Webster's New Collegiate Dictionary* refers both to an outcome and to a process. The outcome is reflected in the use of the term "relapse" to denote "a recurrence of symptoms of a disease after a period of improvement," and the process is captured in the phrase "the act or instance of backsliding, worsening, or subsiding." Others (e.g., Klerman, 1978) have sought to distinguish between relapse and recurrence on the grounds of continuity of the original "episode" (relapse) versus instigation of a new "episode" (recurrence). In addition, Marlatt and Gordon (1985) distinguish between "lapse" and relapse, arguing that a lapse implies a temporary state of affairs that might, under some circumstances, lead to a relapse. The main difficulty in the definition of relapse is drawing clear distinctions between these various terms (lapse, recurrence, relapse) and clarifying their usage in relation to different types of problems or disorders. In the chapters that follow, many authors address the definition of "relapse" as it relates to the behavioral problem or disorder under discussion, highlight the main conceptual difficulties as they relate to each problem area, and offer some heuristic solutions.

WHY STUDY RELAPSE?

A major reason for studying relapse is the need to improve the efficacy of treatments. Many problems in patients who attend clinics and hospitals are widely recognized to be chronic or recurrent in nature, such as depression (Keller, Shapiro, Lavori, & Wolfe, 1982), schizophrenia (Breier, Schreiber, Dyer, & Pickar, 1991), and the addictions (Hunt, Barnett, & Branch, 1971). Treatments that are effective in the short term but fail to provide long-term maintenance of gains may lead the individual to utilize health services at a greater rate than would otherwise be the case. Clearly, continued or recurrent psychopathology may have an effect on employment levels, engagement in antisocial behavior, and the use of social services. Thus, the long-term effects of treatment may have implications for the general economic and social welfare of society. Importantly, the continuance of behavioral problems may reduce a person's quality of life and place limitations on his/her successful pursuit of personal goals. The study of predictors and precipitants of relapse will, it is hoped, lead to a better understanding of the processes involved in relapse and to the development of interventions with greater long-term effectiveness, with an overall gain for the individual and society.

A second important reason for the study of relapse is the light that such work might shed on the causes of problem behaviors or disorders. For example, if it were found that a return of depressive symptoms was preceded in many cases by high levels of life stresses and a particular cognitive style, one might be tempted to look more closely at these factors as causes of depression. However, the relationship between causes of relapse and causes of the disorder is not necessarily clear-cut. One has to ask the question: Are factors that promote relapse similar to or identical to those that initiate the disorder? For example, high levels of expressed emotion (critism overprotection, etc.) have been implicated as factors that have a high predictive value for relapse in schizophrenia (see Kavanagh, Chapter 7, this volume), but the separate question remains as to whether similar patterns of communication are responsible, in some part, for the initiation of the disorder. Certain psychological and biological processes may cause the disorder to occur, but other processes may promote relapses. Of course, there may be variation from one problem to another in the extent to which the triggers of relapse and the original causal processes are similar. Nevertheless, the study of relapse may be a useful guide in generating testable hypotheses about basic causes. A sample of treated individuals certainly provides a convenient and economical means for accelerating the search for such hypotheses, and any hypothesized causal factors can then be tested using other research methods.

Thus, there are several reasons for studying all the facets of relapse, including both its prediction and prevention as well as the processes that promote relapse. A number of researchers have already begun to develop and evaluate relapse prevention (RP) strategies, and much of this work forms the subject of subsequent chapters. The types of approaches to RP have varied quite considerably. Some of these techniques are described in the following section.

TYPES OF RP STRATEGIES

Several different types of RP strategies have been developed and evaluated to varying degrees with different types of problem behaviors. These techniques have included (1) booster sessions; (2) treatment programs with RP strategies integrated into the initial treatment; and (3) procedures that require minimal therapist contact such as periodic reminder letters, telephone calls, or the provision of therapy-related materials.

Booster Sessions

The most common form of RP strategy is the implementation of some form of booster sessions, that is, the inclusion of additional therapy sessions that occur at some point in time after the termination of the initial treatment program. The effectiveness of booster sessions has now been evaluated with a wide range of problems, including assertiveness (Baggs & Spence, 1990; Riedel, Fenwick, & Jillings, 1986), depression (Baker & Wilson, 1985; Kavanagh & Wilson, 1987), headache (Andrasik, Blanchard, Neff, & Rodichok, 1984), hypertension (Blanchard et al. 1987), smoking (Brandon et al., 1987), and obesity (Perri et al., 1987). The scheduling, timing, and content of these booster sessions have varied considerably across studies. Booster sessions may commence immediately after the conclusion of treatment or after some considerable lapse of time from termination. When booster sessions occur immediately after the conclusion of the initial treatment, the distinction between treatment and maintenance is likely to become blurred. The content of the booster sessions may be linked directly to the content of the original treatment or may involve new techniques that are more specifically designed to prevent relapse. As Whisman (1990) points out in his review of booster sessions, despite these procedural variations, little research has been conducted on the importance of the scheduling and content of such programs.

In most instances, booster sessions are scheduled to occur on certain predetermined dates. Prior scheduling may have the advantage that the person does not need to wait until he/she has detected any difficulties before recontacting the therapist, which may often be only after a significant reemergence of the original problem. When a problem has reemerged, the therapy sessions may be more likely to involve some implementation of the original techniques, perhaps with some modifications in light of the recent experiences by the client. The reemergence of the problem may have several negative consequences for the client, such as reduced expectations about his/her efficacy to perform the behaviors necessary to maintain improvement (i.e., reduced self-efficacy) or lowered beliefs that the therapy techniques or therapist will be effective in alleviating the problem. Prior scheduling may result in the early detection by the therapist of alterations in the person's vulnerability to relapse brought about by changes in life circumstances, slight reemergence of the problem, or the development of new problems. Additional sessions could then be scheduled to deal with these matters without necessarily resulting in lowered self-efficacy and reduced expectations about success. One problem with this approach is that scheduling is essentially random unless it is informed by data that enable the therapist to predict the timing of relapse. We are a long way from predicting the timing of relapse in most problem areas. Thus, an important goal of research is to collect data not only on the overall occurrence of relapse but also on the timing of relapse. The therapist would then be in a position to know what proportion of people with a given type of problem relapse at certain points in time after the termination of treatment. Such information might result in more rational decisions being made about the most beneficial period for the scheduling of RP sessions. Nevertheless, even the best data are unlikely to result in highly specific predictions about the likely timing of relapse for certain individuals. Relapse may be expected to vary not only in relation to potentially knowable factors such as posttreatment severity or pretreatment history and symptomatology, but also in relation to factors that are inherently *not* knowable at the end of treatment such as the occurrence of future life events. Inevitably, clinicians will still need to base decisions about the timing of booster sessions partly on information about the individual person. Similar points could be made about the decision to terminate the booster program itself.

The content of booster sessions has also varied considerably in the existing literature. Booster sessions can differ on a number of dimensions, including (1) quantity of therapist contact and support, (2) amount of support from others with similar problems, such as the "Buddy system" (e.g., Abrams & Rollick, 1983), (3) inclusion of other family members, (4) reimplementation of the original treatment aims and procedures, (5) addition of mail and telephone contact, (6) relocation of the treatment to a new site such as the natural environment (e.g., home or workplace), (7) use of procedures designed to maintain adherence to certain procedures, and (8) introduction of new, specific maintenance procedures. The variation in content in the existing literature makes it difficult to reach general conclusions about the efficacy of booster sessions. In addition, it is possible that booster sessions have different levels of effectiveness for different types of problems. Brownell et al. (1986) conclude that "booster sessions have been used most extensively in the obesity and smoking areas and have been consistently ineffective" (p. 772). It has also been argued, in the treatment of smoking, that booster sessions might serve simply to delay an eventual relapse (Brandon et al., 1987). In reviewing 26 studies designed to evaluate the effectiveness of booster sessions across a wide range of problems, Whisman (1990) concludes that such sessions "were found to be modestly successful" and that "maintenance sessions were found to significantly enhance behavior change (on at least some treatment outcome measures for at least some of the subjects) in 15 (58%) of the studies" (p. 165). Thus, some types of booster sessions may be of some value. Nevertheless, it is difficult not to agree with Whisman that a great deal of the research has suffered both from methodological problems, especially low statistical power, and conceptual difficulties, such as a poorly established rationale for the selection of components and the timing of procedures.

Integrated Therapy and RP

Apart from booster sessions, the other major RP technique involves the provision of specific anti-relapse sessions prior to termination of therapy in which quite specific skills designed to prevent relapse are introduced. In a sense, one can argue that RP ought to commence from the first moment of therapy. The most highly developed version of an approach in which this combination of treatment and RP is integrated is advanced by Marlatt and Gordon (1985). In broad terms, these strategies might involve (1) identification of high-risk situations, (2) development of specific ways to cope with selected high-risk situations, (3) early identification of the return of symptoms, (4) identification and modification of certain vulnerability factors, (5) generalization training, and (6) adaptation of original treatment techniques for future requirements. Details of this approach are provided later in this chapter and in other chapters on addictive problems.

Minimal Contact Procedures

Other approaches to RP can include the provision of tape recordings or printed material. This material may be used by the client on a regular basis, as in the case of relaxation tapes for anxiety disorders, insomnia, headaches, or hypertension. Printed material, such as a self-guide to *in vivo* exposure for phobias or stimulus control instructions for smoking cessation, may help to remind people of the major techniques to use when they anticipate some return of the original difficulty. Of course, some individually tailored materials that are specifically related to the content of the client's treatment sessions are likely to be particularly useful. The identification of high-risk situations in Marlatt and Gordon's RP program for alcohol consumption represents one such technique. Using this approach, a list of situations would be generated by the person that is highly related to the elicitation of the drinking behavior, such as "going to a party," or "having an argument at work," and strategies would be identified that are likely to minimize problem drinking upon the occurrence of each of these high-risk situations. The high-risk situations and the relevant strategies would be listed on a special page of the materials and given to the client upon treatment termination. Similar techniques can be used in the treatment of depression and other problems. For example, in depression, situations that often lead to a reduction in mood can be identified, and strategies for dealing with such situations can be listed. The main advantage of such techniques is that clients can be readily reminded about what to do during periods of stress, when they may find great difficulty in remembering the therapy techniques that had been previously suggested or used.

Surprisingly little reference is made in the literature to any of the minimal intervention techniques. In general, there appears to be an underutilization of audio and video techniques. Relaxation tapes are probably the most common minimal RP technique in use. Of course, there are many self-help books for the treatment of various problems, such as depression, obesity, or smoking, and some of these materials can be adapted for use in an RP program. Some other forms of RP exist that require only minimal intervention on the part of the therapist. Included here are periodic telephone calls, letters, or referral to self-help groups. Overall, there is considerable scope for the development of materials that are specifically designed to assist people to maintain gains following treatment. Although there have been some evaluations of such procedures, particularly in the smoking-cessation programs (e.g., Kottke, Battista, DeFriesse, & Brekke, 1988), more research on the efficacy of these minimal approaches to RP is badly needed.

In the subsequent chapters, information on the effectiveness of booster sessions, pretermination sessions, and therapy materials is provided. For some problems, such as addictions, this information is relatively rich. For others, such as depression or the anxiety disorders, it is very sparse indeed. However, in all areas of the study of RP and prediction, there are methodological issues that need to be addressed. The main methodological problems in the conduct of this research are outlined in the following section.

METHODOLOGICAL PROBLEMS IN THE STUDY OF RELAPSE

The Index of Relapse

An important decision that needs to be made by the researcher concerns the selection of the best indicator of relapse. Many researchers merely report means and standard deviations without indicating the proportion of subjects who have met some clinical criterion for successful maintenance. Mean scores on dependent variables at selected points in time can be rather misleading as a guide to the maintenance of treatment effects in some problem areas due to the cyclic or intermittent nature of some disorders. Individuals can be symptom free at the time selected by the researchers for the assessment but may have experienced significant problems in the intervening period. Relapse rates can be underestimated by reliance on a single point in time without obtaining information on the intervening period. Thus, there is a need either for some continuous measure of severity that can be utilized over a long period of time or for some retrospective method of assessment that can be conducted by the researcher at one or more specific points in time. The use of significant others to provide additional material may also be helpful. The methods of assessment used in the studies of relapse and its prevention also vary considerably in intensity. The main choice for the researcher is between relatively economical approaches such as mail-return testing or telephone contact or more time-consuming and expensive approaches such as personal interviews, behavioral observations, and clinical ratings. Each of these techniques has certain advantages and disadvantages, and the ultimate choice will be partly determined by the nature of the problem and budgetary constraints.

The proportion of subjects who seek further treatment may also need to be considered as an index of relapse. This variable has been used as a criterion in some studies but not in others. However, this criterion poses some problems since return to treatment can be affected by factors other than the reemergence of the original problem, such as the extent to which help-seeking behaviors are either discouraged or encouraged by the content of the initial treatment. Receipt of additional treatment may also overestimate relapse since some people may be seeking treatment for problems other than the original one. Nevertheless, details of further treatment may be very helpful in the interpretation of follow-up data, especially if sufficient information is collected that enables the researcher to know the reasons for the additional treatment, its quantity and content, and other details.

Whatever method of assessment is chosen, the researcher must also define the criteria for relapse. At the present time, the use of different criteria for relapse within the same problem domain presents considerable difficulties in making comparisons between studies. As will be seen in subsequent chapters, there is a need for a more uniform approach to the definition of relapse, employing a number of replicable, standardized criteria for each problem area.

Length of Follow-Up Period

There are considerable variations in the length and intensity of follow-up assessments. Follow-up periods in many studies of cognitive–behavioral therapy are relatively short, usually with an assessment at a single point in time. The duration of follow-up periods in the literature reviewed in this book has varied from a few weeks to many years after the termination of treatment. Clearly, there needs to be some rationale for the selection of specific follow-up periods for different types of problems. Information that comes from the study of the natural course of disorders after treatment could be used to make judgments about the length of follow-up for a given problem area. For example, the rate of relapse per month might be used to indicate the point at which further relapse is markedly unlikely to occur. These data could be used to define the minimum and maximum follow-up period that would be needed to study relapse in that disorder.

Role of Initial Treatment Response

A common problem in the study of relapse is the failure to separate initial treatment responders from nonresponders. It makes little sense to combine data from subjects who respond well to an initial intervention with data from those who respond poorly or not at all. If all data are combined in this manner, relapse will be confused with failure of the initial treatment. Thus, it is important to examine the course of subjects who have successfully responded to treatment separately from those who responded less well. Of course, if responders are separated from nonresponders in the investigation, the researcher has the additional difficulty of determining the criteria for defining an initial treatment response in the different studies, although Jacobson, Follette, and Revenstorf (1984) have suggested a number of possible solutions to this problem.

Sample Size

The power of statistical tests to detect potentially important differences depends, in part, on the size of the sample. Special problems occur in the study of RP because of the need to study the same group of subjects over long periods of time. One of the major difficulties in this type of research is subject attrition over time. This attrition may occur because of failure to keep appointments or simply through loss of contact with subjects who change residence in the course of the study. Researchers need to ensure that there are sufficient subjects in the initial treatment phase so that such losses can be sustained without too much degradation of power. Apart from power considerations, subject attrition might also result in the operation of selection biases, which may lead to difficulties in making inferences from the results. Kendall (1991) has suggested that loss of contact may be reduced by requesting subjects to provide telephone numbers and addresses for two friends or relatives who can be expected to know their whereabouts in the years ahead. Such a procedure might greatly increase the sample size that is available at longer-term follow-up assessments of 5 years or more. Hughes and Hatsukami (1984) suggest that offers of free reprints of the published article might increase the return rate of follow-up questionnaires, although they report negative findings for the effect of this inducement in their study of smoking. Monetary deposits have also been used to improve completion of follow-up procedures (e.g., Eufemia & Weslowski, 1985). Clearly, more research on the factors that increase compliance with follow-up contact is needed in order to indicate likely solutions to this problem.

Investigations of Predictors of Relapse

Certain methodological problems exist in the investigation of predictors of initial treatment response and relapse that do not seem to have been given sufficient recognition in the literature to date. As mentioned above, relatively large sample sizes are needed in order to provide sufficient statistical power to detect potentially important differences. A related issue is the importance of ensuring that there is a sufficient range of values for any particular prognostic variable in a given study. In many predictive studies, there appear to be problems of restricted range in some variables such as IQ, socioeconomic status, age, and duration of the disorder. Such variables may become significant predictors of response or relapse only when the potential range of variation in the population is covered adequately in the sample. To use a hypothetical example, if the researcher is interested in IQ as a predictor of response to cognitive therapy, the range of IQ scores represented in the sample will be an important determinant of the likelihood of detecting an effect. Within a limited range of IQ (such as 105–125), a certain effect may not be evident, but over a broader range (e.g., 80–130), the effect of IQ as a predictor of response to cognitive therapy may indeed be evident. Thus, in studies of the prediction of relapse, large samples are needed with adequate coverage of the range of scores to which one might wish to generalize.

In the prediction of relapse, an important question arises concerning the selection of the point in time from which the prediction is to be made. The researcher may select from one or more of at least five different temporal points. Prediction can be made from variables that reflect (1) the person's known history, personal characteristics, and other background variables that are generally available at pretreatment; (2) the person's status at pretreatment itself; (3) measures obtained during treatment; (4) the person's status at posttreatment; or (5) measures obtained during the follow-up period itself. Some examples of the types of variables that can be utilized within each category are provided here:

1. *History and other background variables:* Number and type of previous life events, duration of the disorder, number of episodes of the disorder, coexistence of other disorders, age, gender, and socioeconomic status.
2. *Status at pretreatment:* Severity of problem, types of symptomatology, cognitive style, subclassification of type of disorder if relevant (e.g., dysthymia vs. major depressive episode; social phobia vs. small animal phobia).
3. *Measures obtained during treatment:* Compliance with treatment, speed of recovery, course of disorder during treatment, quality of therapy.
4. *Status at posttreatment:* Degree of improvement, level of severity on posttest measures, theory-related dependent variables.
5. *Measures obtained during the follow-up period:* Occurrence and reaction to life events, social support, adherence to continued use of procedures.

While not intended to be exhaustive, the above list provides a summary of the types of measures that might be of interest in the prediction of relapse. However, it will be noted that these variables fall into several different classes. Some variables reflect enduring characteristics of the person (e.g., gender); some are a result of the process of therapy itself (e.g., compliance, quality); others are indicative of the initial treatment outcome (e.g., posttreatment severity); and a fourth group is possibly based on some theoretical rationale (e.g., classification, cognitive style). The ways in which these types of variables contribute to the prediction of relapse have not been incorporated into a general model of relapse, nor have many of these variables been subjected to systematic empirical study. There is clearly a need for the development of either a general model of relapse or a model of relapse with respect to each individual disorder. In any case, researchers need to be aware of the levels of information that they are gathering at the outset of the design of the treatment evaluation. Hierarchical multiple regression equations can be utilized to good effect in the analysis of this type of data, but the techniques have been underutilized to date. An additional point that seems to have been overlooked is the time frame over which the researcher suspects that a certain prognostic variable is likely to operate. It is possible that short- and long-term relapse may well be predicted by different sets of variables. Although there are a number of problems in the prediction of relapse, this area of study represents one of the most important areas for the development of theories of relapse on which successful prevention programs can be based.

WHY PEOPLE RELAPSE:
IN SEARCH OF A CONCEPTUAL FRAMEWORK

As mentioned above, only some prognostic variables seem to be derived from a theory about the disorder and the processes responsible for relapse. Of course, some variables that might have attained no prior theoretical interest, such as age, might lead the researcher to develop hypotheses to account for effects that are empirically obtained. However, if research is to progress in this area, there is a need to consider relapse within some general framework. Marlatt and Gordon (1985), in their influential book *Relapse Prevention: Maintenance Strategies in the Treatment of Addictive Behaviors,* presented a theoretical account of relapse and methods for RP in problems such as alcohol abuse, smoking, and weight control. Because of its importance in the development of much of the subsequent work on RP, this model needs to be discussed in some detail. In the model, addictions are explained as acquired habit patterns that are on a continuum from normal to excessive and are governed by similar cognitive and experiential processes in which antecedent events, beliefs, and expectations, prior learning history, and behavioral consequences play important roles in the continued use of the particular substance.

The conceptual model of relapse proposed by Marlatt and Gordon in the addictive disorders may be instructive in our efforts to deal with in other areas. Stated in its most general terms, an effective treatment

results in enhanced perception of control (high self-efficacy) over important events that are likely to reinstate problem behavior. Through effective treatment, the person learns to recognize and respond to situations
that place him/her at high risk for reinstatement of the problem behavior,
and he/she acquires positive outcome expectancies about the use of
coping responses in such situations. As the person uses such coping
strategies in future situations his/her sense of mastery increases, facilitating the maintenance of effective coping strategies.

Marlatt and Gordon point out that most previous treatments for
addictions have emphasized securing an initial response to therapy.
However, it is well documented that the addictive problems are highly
susceptible to recurrence following successful intervention. They state
that previous approaches to RP have tended to involve increasing the
number of initial treatment components in the belief that at least one of
the components may have some enduring effect for each individual. In
contrast, Marlatt and Gordon suggest that the maintenance stage ought to
be considered a period in which there is the "opportunity for new learning to occur" (p. 25) as the person is faced with situations, events, moods,
and beliefs that might increase the risk of reinstatement of addictive
behaviors. They contrast the view of reemergence of the problem as a
series of individual "lapses" with the "all-or-none model" that is implicit in
popular views and about relapse (p. 31).

Relapse may occur because of a failure at any one of a number of
points in the chain of events from initial treatment to maintenance: An
effective treatment may not necessarily lead to perceived control or
enhanced self-efficacy; the person may fail to recognize and respond
appropriately to high-risk situations; he/she may fail to develop adequate
coping responses or, if he/she does develop such responses, he/she may
still have negative outcome expectancies about the use of such strategies
in future situations; clients may use ineffective responses or they may
have positive expectancies about the effects of old coping strategies that,
in reality, have failed in the past; the person may make incorrect attributions about the cause of lapses. It is possible that relapse could result from
a breakdown in any of these areas. Stated in this most general way,
Marlatt and Gordon's approach provides a set of variables that can be
subjected to empirical scrutiny in studies of relapse in virtually any
problem area. A major influence on the work conducted by Marlatt and
others in the addictive area has been the careful study and analysis of
relapse as a phenomenon in its own right. It is also evident that the work
of Bandura (1977) has led a number of researchers to focus their attention
on the role of self-efficacy as a predictor of long-term outcome (e.g.,
Bernier & Avard, 1986; Condiotte & Lichtenstein, 1981; DiClemente,
1981; Godding & Glasgow, 1985; Kavanagh & Wilson, 1987; McIntyre,
Lichtenstein, & Mermelstein, 1983; Sitharthan & Kavanagh, 1990).

MARLATT AND GORDON'S RP APPROACH

A number of techniques were described in the Marlatt and Gordon book that are collectively known as "relapse prevention." These techniques are designed to maximize maintenance within the framework espoused above. RP is a self-management approach based on social-learning theory in which the goal is "to teach individuals who are trying to change their behavior how to anticipate and cope with the problem of relapse" (p. 3). Although the following list is not exhaustive, the principal techniques include:

1. Identification of high-risk situations.
2. Coping with negative emotional states.
3. Coping with interpersonal conflict.
4. Coping with social pressure.
5. Coping skills training (relaxation training, stress management, decision-making skills).
6. Preparation for high-risk situations.
7. Slip recovery and relapse crisis debriefing.
8. Life-style interventions.
9. Programmed relapse, relapse rehearsal.
10. Education about the effects of drugs.

Marlatt and Gordon suggest that the components of an ideal RP program are those which:

1. Are effective for clinically significant periods.
2. Enhance and maintain compliance and adherence.
3. Involve a mixture of techniques, including both behavioral and cognitive techniques.
4. Develop motivation and decision-making skills.
5. Involve both verbal and nonverbal components.
6. Replace maladaptive habits with alternative behaviors and skills.
7. Help people to cope with new problem situations.
8. Help people to cope with failure experiences.
9. Make use of client support systems.

A major component of the RP program is the identification of high-risk situations through self-monitoring, self-efficacy ratings, and detailed analysis of past relapse episodes. The aim of these techniques is to increase the therapist's knowledge of the factors that might lead to relapse and to increase the client's awareness of the operation of these factors. Self-efficacy ratings might also be made in which the person is asked to list situations in which he/she may use the substance in question, rate the degree of temptation that he/she would experience, and rate how confident he/she feels that he/she will be able to cope effectively in these situations without engaging in excessive consumption. A considerable amount of attention is given both to environmental cues and to the role of cognitive factors (attributions, expectations) in this analysis. Clients are encouraged to view the maintenance period as an opportunity for new learning to occur, so that they can develop new strategies for dealing with high-risk situations. Clients are taught skills that might help them in coping with negative emotional states such as anger, anxiety and depression, interpersonal conflict, and social pressure to consume the substance. Other general coping skills training might also be introduced such as self-instructional skills training, relaxation training, stress management, and assertiveness training.

A key element of the RP approach is the preparation for high-risk situations. Essentially, this preparation involves the development of skills that may help the person to recognize when he/she is about to enter a high-risk situation and skills with which he/she can respond to that situation. Clients are asked to provide written accounts of what they actually would do in each risk situation, and this information, together with self-monitoring exercises, can be utilized to develop more effective strategies. Programmed relapse and high-risk rehearsal are techniques in which the person is taught to cope with high-risk situations through role play or in live situations under the guidance of the therapist. Thus, the client might be required to have an alcoholic drink or smoke a cigarette and to engage in self-control behaviors that are designed to maintain control over drinking or smoking. Role play or covert modeling of situations requiring assertive responses to social pressure from peers might also be conducted.

One aim of therapy is to enhance self-efficacy concerning ability to cope with high-risk situations. Clients are asked to rate their confidence in handling the situations on specially constructed questionnaires such as the Situational Confidence Questionnaire (Annis, 1982), which requires subjects to rate their confidence to be able to not drink heavily "if I would see an advertisement for my favorite booze" or "if I were depressed about things in general," etc. A similar scale for smoking has been developed by Condiotte and Lichtenstein (1981), which calls for ratings of the probability of resisting the urge to smoke in various situations. Individually tailored techniques can be developed to help clients to deal with urges and cravings they might experience in these situations.

An important aspect RP is the use of particular procedures to deal with the occurrence of a reinstatement of the problem behavior. In advance of such an event, counterstatements that are designed to correct potentially negative constructions of the "lapse" are written down. Relapse crisis debriefing might also occur in which cognitive restructuring is undertaken in relation to attributions regarding failure. One key concept discussed by Marlatt and Gordon is referred to as the "abstinence violation effect." This term is used to refer to the cognitions that are frequently experienced by clients following engagement in a behavior they have been attempting to control, such as smoking one cigarette or consuming one drink. When the goal is abstinence, a person may quickly regard him- or herself as having failed and can justify continued high-level consumption on the grounds that the abstinence rule has already been violated. The abstinence violation effect might be avoided by adequate preparation of the client through cognitive methods and high-risk rehearsal. Alternatively, the client might choose another treatment goal rather than abstinence, such as controlled drinking, smoking, or gambling.

Life-style modification is also employed in the Marlatt and Gordon program. Part of this approach involves the assessment of daily activities, which are rated for enjoyment and desirability. The therapist looks for sources of stress arising from work, family, friends, and external demands. An attempt is made to increase the level of engagement in pleasant activities, physical activities, and sources of relaxation. Another aspect of the RP program involves the presentation of educational material about the nature of drugs and their effects. Thus, Marlatt and Gordon's RP program contains a number of specific components that are designed to provide people with the appropriate skills to minimize relapse. While the above description is expected to be sufficiently detailed to enable the reader to assimilate other material in the present text, those readers who wish to gain more comprehensive information are referred to Marlatt and Gordon (1985) for a fuller description of the procedures.

Marlatt and Gordon are writing within an avowedly cognitive–behavioral framework. Thus, they incorporate cognitive concepts such as self-efficacy, attributions, and expectations into their model of relapse and its prevention. On the other hand, Sulzer-Azaroff and Mayer (1991) discuss relapse and maintenance within a more strictly behavioral tradition. Their approaches are more obviously centered within an operant program. As they point out, behavior may be modified by changes in reinforcement schedules or alterations in the properties of discriminative stimuli. They suggest that common sources of relapse include abrupt cessation of reinforcement, continued reinforcement for the previous unwanted behavior, punishment of the modified behavior, and the presence of discriminative stimuli that elicit either unwanted behavior or behavior that interferes with the occurrence of the desired behavior (p. 518). Sulzer-Azaroff and Mayer (1991) describe a number of approaches that may help to maintain behavior once it has been established, including the gradual transition from artificial to natural reinforcers, alteration of specific characteristics of the reinforcement program, or the introduction of "self-reinforcement" techniques (pp. 517–535). Methods such as overlearning have frequently been recommended as an approach to RP and have been utilized successfully in the treatment of enuresis (e.g., Houts, Peterson, & Whelan, 1986; Young & Morgan, 1972). Errorless learning, in which an acquisition phase is constructed in such a way that errors are minimized, has also been suggested by Sulzer-Azaroff and Mayer as an approach to maintenance. It is argued that errors are unlikely to recur if such errors have rarely been made in the presence of the stimulus conditions under which the initial learning has taken place. This approach can be seen as operating in the slow-speech method for the treatment of stuttering (see Andrews, Chapter 14, this volume). Other approaches might involve the fading of antecedent stimuli during training or allowing a gradual transition to take place to the natural stimuli in the environment in which the desired behavior is expected to occur. Similarly, the fading of reinforcement or alterations from "artificial" to natural reinforcers represent important maintenance strategies in operant programs. The use of these procedures can be seen in many of the self-control programs for obesity or smoking. Changing other parameters of the reinforcement program can also be used, such as gradually increasing the length of time prior to the occurrence of the reward and increasing the demands prior to the provision of reinforcement.

It would be erroneous to view the cognitive–behavioral program espoused by Marlatt and Gordon as being incompatible with the approach of Sulzer-Azaroff and Mayer. For example, a good deal of attention can be given to the identification and use of natural contingencies within the Marlatt and Gordon RP approach. Clearly, alcohol consumption may be elicited by certain environmental stimuli that have been associated with previous drinking situations (e.g., passing a certain hotel on the way home from work), and may be subjected to a regular pattern of reinforcement (such as the approval of a set of friends or coworkers). Any successful RP program for alcohol abuse will include procedures that are designed to (1) reduce the potency of the discriminative stimuli and (2) decrease the likelihood of the occurrence of both rewards for drinking and punishments for not drinking. Marlatt and Gordon's RP program adds a set of cognitive components to other techniques that have their roots in behavioral theory and therapy. Sulzer-Azaroff and Mayer (1991, pp. 528–534) also describe procedures that are designed to show people how they can reinforce their own behavior, alter their environment, and make life-style changes in ways that parallel the suggestions made by Marlatt and Gordon. Although the techniques espoused by Sulzer-Azaroff and Mayer are more consistent with the use of operant interventions, the differences between their approach and that of Marlatt and Gordon lie more in the description of the theoretical rationale than in the procedures themselves. The main characteristic of both these approaches is the use of theoretically derived principles and empirically testable propositions about the causes and prevention of relapse.

CONCLUSION

The aim of this chapter has been to provide a general introduction to the field of relapse and its prevention in cognitive–behavioral therapy. I have attempted to delineate the major types of RP strategies, such as the provision of booster sessions, the implementation of integrated treatment/maintenance programs, and the use of minimal contact interventions. I have touched on a number of methodological and conceptual difficulties in the prediction and prevention of relapse in order to highlight the principal issues that need to be considered throughout the subsequent chapters. Research on relapse and maintenance is undoubtedly in its infancy, but it is indeed heartening to see that the topic is becoming a more significant focus of researchers in the field of cognitive and behavioral therapies. It is hoped that the remaining chapters in this book alert the reader to the principal developments in this field, promote further research in the area, and assist clinicians in their endeavors to prevent relapse following cognitive–behavioral interventions.

REFERENCES

Abrams, D. B., & Rollick, M. J. (1983). Behavioral weight-loss intervention at the worksite: Feasibility and maintenance. *Journal of Consulting and Clinical Psychology, 51*, 226–233.

Andrasik, F., Blanchard, E. B., Neff, D. F., & Rodichok, L. D. (1984). Biofeedback and relaxation training for chronic headache: A controlled comparison of booster treatments and regular contacts for long-term maintenance. *Journal of Consulting and Clinical Psychology, 52*, 609–615.

Annis, H. M. (1982). *Situational Confidence Questionnaire*. Toronto: Addiction Research Foundation.

Baggs, K., & Spence, S. H. (1990). Effectiveness of booster sessions in the maintenance and enhancement of treatment gains following assertion training. *Journal of Consulting and Clinical Psychology, 58*, 845–854.

Baker, A. L., & Wilson, P. H. (1985). Cognitive–behavior therapy for depression: The effects of booster sessions on relapse. *Behavior Therapy, 16*, 335–344.

Bandura, A. (1977). Self-efficacy: Toward a unifying theory of behavioral change. *Psychological Review, 84*, 191–215.

Belsher, G., & Costello, C. G. (1988). Relapse after recovery from unipolar depression: A critical review. *Psychological Bulletin, 104,* 84–96.

Bernier, M., & Avard, J. (1986). Self-efficacy, outcome, and attrition in a weight-reduction program. *Cognitive Therapy and Research, 10,* 319–338.

Blanchard, E. B. (1987). Long-term effects of behavioral treatment of chronic headache. *Behavior Therapy, 18,* 375–385.

Blanchard, E. B., Andrasik, F., Guarnieri, P., Neff, D. F., & Rodichok, L. D. (1987). Two-, three-, and four-year follow-up on the self-regulatory treatment of chronic headache. *Journal of Consulting and Clinical Psychology, 55,* 257–259.

Brandon, T. H., Zelman, D. C., & Baker, T. B. (1987). Effects of maintenance sessions on smoking relapse: Delaying the inevitable? *Journal of Consulting and Clinical Psychology, 55,* 780–782.

Breier, A., Schreiber, J. L., Dyer, J., & Pickar, D. (1991). National Institute of Mental Health longitudinal study of chronic schizophrenia. *Archives of General Psychiatry, 48,* 239–246.

Brownell, K. D., & Jeffery, R. W. (1987). Improving long-term weight loss: Pushing the limits of treatment. *Behavior Therapy, 18,* 375–386.

Brownell, K. D., Marlatt, G. A., Lichtenstein, E., & Wilson, G. T. (1986). Understanding and preventing relapse. *American Psychologist, 41,* 765–782.

Burns, L. E., Thorpe, G. L., & Cavallaro, L. A. (1986). Agoraphobia 8 years after behavioral treatment: A follow-up study with interview, self-report, and behavioral data. *Behavior Therapy, 17,* 580–591.

Condiotte, M. M., & Lichtenstein, E. (1981). Self-efficacy and relapse in smoking cessation programs. *Journal of Consulting and Clinical Psychology, 49,* 648–658.

DiClemente, C. (1981). Self-efficacy and smoking cessation maintenance: A preliminary report. *Cognitive Therapy and Research, 5,* 175–187.

Edelstein, B. A. (1989). Generalization: Terminological, methodological and conceptual issues. *Behavior Therapy, 20,* 311–324.

Eufemia, R. L., & Weslowski, M. D. (1985). Attrition in behavioral studies of obesity: A meta-analytic review. *The Behavior Therapist, 8,* 115–116.

Eysenck, H. J. (1963). Behavior therapy, extinction and relapse in neurosis. *British Journal of Psychiatry, 109,* 12–18.

Freedman, R. R. (1987). Long-term effectiveness of behavioral treatments for Raynaud's disease. *Behavior Therapy, 18,* 387–399.

Glasgow, R. E., Klesges, R. C., Klesges, L. M., Vasey, M. W., & Gunnarson, D. F. (1985). Long-term effects of a controlled smoking program: A 2.5 year follow-up. *Behavior Therapy, 16,* 303–307.

Glasgow, R. E., & Lichtenstein, E. (1987). Long-term effects of behavioral smoking cessation interventions. *Behavior Therapy, 18,* 297–324.

Godding, P. R., & Glasgow, R. E. (1985). Self-efficacy and outcome expectations as predictors of controlled smoking status. *Cognitive Therapy and Research, 9,* 583–590.

Hersen, M. (1979). Limitations and problems in the clinical application of behavioral techniques in psychiatric settings. *Behavior Therapy, 10,* 65–80.

Houts, A. C., Peterson, J. K., & Whelan, J. P. (1986). Prevention of relapse in full-spectrum hometraining for primary enuresis: A components analysis. *Behavior Therapy, 17,* 462–469.

Hughes, J. R., & Hatsukami, D. K. (1984). Free reprints to increase return of follow-up questionnaires. *Behavior Therapy, 15,* 557.

Hunt, W. A., Barnett, L. W., & Branch, L. G. (1971). Relapse rates in addiction programs. *Journal of Clinical Psychology, 27,* 455–456.

Jacob, R. G., Wing, R., & Shapiro, A. P. (1987). The behavioral treatment of hypertension: Long-term effects. *Behavior Therapy, 18,* 325–352.

Jacobson, N. S. (1989). The maintenance of treatment gains following social learning-based marital therapy. *Behavior Therapy, 20,* 325–336.

Jacobson, N. S., Follette, W. C., & Revenstorf, D. (1984). Psychotherapy outcome research: Methods for reporting variability and evaluating clinical significance. *Behavior Therapy, 15,* 336–352.

Kavanagh, D. J., & Wilson, P. H. (1987). Prediction of outcome with a group version of cognitive therapy for depression. *Behaviour Research and Therapy, 27,* 333–343.

Keller, M. B., Shapiro, R. W., Lavori, P. W., & Wolfe, N. (1982). Relapse in major depressive disorder: Analysis with the life table. *Archives of General Psychiatry, 39,* 911–915.

Kendall, P. C. (1989). The generalization and maintenance of behavior change: Comments, considerations, and the "no-cure" criticism. *Behavior Therapy, 20,* 357–364.

Kendall, P. C. (1991). Behavioral assessment and methodology. In C. M. Franks, G. T. Wilson, P. C. Kendall, & J. P. Foreyt (Eds.), *Review of behavior therapy: Theory and practice* (Vol. 12, pp. 44–71). New York: Guilford Press.

Klerman, G. L. (1978). Long-term treatment of affective disorders. In M. A. Lipton, A. DiMascio, & K. F. Killam (Eds.), *Psychopharmacology: A generation of progress* (pp. 1303–1311). New York: Raven Press.

Kottke, T. E., Battista, R. N., DeFriesse, G. H., & Brekke, M. L. (1988). Attributes of successful smoking cessation interventions in medical practice. *Journal of the American Medical Association, 259,* 2,883–2,889.

Laws, D. R. (Ed.). (1989). *Relapse prevention with sex offenders.* New York: Guilford Press.

Lisspers, J., & Öst, L-G. (1990). Long-term follow-up of migraine treatment: Do the effects remain up to six years? *Behaviour Research and Therapy, 28,* 313–322.

Marlatt, G. A., & Gordon, J. R. (Eds.). (1985). *Relapse prevention: Maintenance strategies in the treatment of addictive behaviors.* New York: Guilford Press.

McIntyre, K. O., Lichtenstein, E., & Mermelstein, R. J. (1983). Self-efficacy and relapse in smoking cessation: A replication and extension. *Journal of Consulting and Clinical Psychology, 51,* 632–633.

McLean, P. D., & Hakstian, A. R. (1990). Relative endurance of unipolar depression treatment effects: Longitudinal follow-up. *Journal of Consulting and Clinical Psychology, 58,* 482–488.

Perri, M. G., McAdoo, W. G., McAllister, D. A., Lauer, J. B., Jordon, R. C., Yancey, D. Z., & Nezu, A. M. (1987). Effects of peer support and therapist contact on long-term weight loss. *Journal of Consulting and Clinical Psychology, 55,* 615–617.

Riedel, H. P. R., Fenwick, C. R., & Jillings, C. R. (1986). Efficacy of booster sessions after training in assertiveness. *Perceptual and Motor Skills, 62,* 791–798.

Rychtarik, R. G., Foy, D. W., Scott, T., Lokey, L, & Prue, D. M. (1987). Five–six-year follow-up of broad-spectrum behavioral treatment for alcoholism: Effects of training controlled drinking skills. *Journal of Consulting and Clinical Psychology, 55,* 106–108.

Sitharthan, T., Kavanagh, D. J. (1990). Role of self-efficacy in predicting outcomes from a programme for controlled drinking. *Drug and Alcohol Dependence, 27,* 87–94.

Stokes, T. F., & Osnes, P. G. (1989). An operant pursuit of generalization. *Behavior Therapy, 20,* 337–355.

Sulzer-Azaroff, B., & Mayer, G. R. (1991). *Behavior analysis for lasting change.* New York: Holt, Rinehart and Winston.

Westover, S. A., & Lanyon, R. I. (1990). The maintenance of weight loss after behavioral treatment: A review. *Behavior Modification, 14,* 123–137.

Whisman, M. A. (1990). The efficacy of booster maintenance sessions in behavior therapy: Review and methodological critique. *Clinical Psychology Review, 10,* 155–170.

Wilson, P. H. (1989). Cognitive–behaviour therapy for depression: Empirical findings and methodological issues in the evaluation of outcome. *Behaviour Change, 6,* 85–95.

Young, G. C., & Morgan, R. T. T. (1972). Overlearning in the conditioning treatment of enuresis: A long term follow-up study. *Behaviour Research and Therapy, 10,* 419–420.

CHAPTER 2

ALCOHOL PROBLEMS

Julian M. Somers
G. Alan Marlatt
UNIVERSITY OF WASHINGTON

The 1980s have witnessed a major transformation in the conceptualization of relapse among alcohol researchers and clinicians. Relapse prevention (RP) may have begun as a treatment objective, but for many it has become a treatment philosophy or model. Conceptions of what this model entails, however, are no doubt diverse. In this chapter, we present an overview of the application of RP to drinking behavior, summarize some of the relevant recent literature, and discuss some possibilities for future applications and research. The theoretical glue that binds our discussion will be more often implicit than explicit in this chapter. Nonetheless, when we focus on the broader context in which relapse must be seen to occur, we draw on a public health perspective, emphasizing a stepped-care approach to treatment. Through the lens of this public health model, RP can be seen as a component of a comprehensive approach to combating drinking problems that extends from primary prevention to treatment.

A LAPSE OF "RELAPSE"

Recently several writers have developed arguments critical of the term "relapse" as applied to alcohol problems and other addictions. Grabowski (1986) has argued that relapse connotes an underlying disease process that is either absent or present, but that behavioral disorders are not similarly dichotomous. One "has" a disease but one "engages in" drug use. Extending this position, Saunders and Allsop (1989) maintain that those who subscribe to a nondisease view of addiction "should immediately and forever reject the use of the word 'relapse,' because it perpetuates disease model notions and rhetoric" (p. 252). Just as some psychologists are reluctant to use the term "relapse," other treatment professionals are reluctant to extend use of the term beyond a dichotomous framework. For example, Mermelstein and colleagues at the University of Illinois at Chicago recently studied a sample in which they noted eight distinct categories of smoking-cessation outcome (ranging from continuously abstinent to continuous smoking, with various intermediate stages). Reactions to the study were reported in the *U.S. Journal of Drug and Alcohol Dependence* (Meacham, 1991):

> Researcher Stephanie Brown, director of The Addictions Institute, Menlo Park, Calif., when told of Mermelstein's study, guessed that alcoholics trying to quit drinking probably exhibit similar patterns. "But you don't change the definition of relapse because of that," Brown said. "In chemical dependency you are either using or you're not using." . . . Brown suggested, the field would do best to "keep it simple," and confine relapse to the act of taking a drink. "Then the other issues of recovery can take their proper place." (p. 10)

A number of edifying points are raised in the process of this analysis of terminology. However, for a variety of reasons we are reluctant to jettison or replace technical terms because they appear to transcend ideological divisions. "Relapse," defined as "falling back" to a less desired state of being, adequately describes the phenomenon of returning to problematic drinking after making an attempt to change one's behavior. Disease processes, although they may be connoted by the term "relapse," are not intrinsic to it. In fact, "relapse" also carries connotations that are favorable to nondisease interpretations. For example, the component term "lapse" denotes slipping. A slip may well be an unfortunate occurrence, but as in the case of slips of the tongue *(lapsus linguae)*, they can provide important material from which to learn. When a drinker's lapse is dealt with in such a way that it provides new information that may enhance adherence to his/her alcohol-related objectives, then the original lapse may be termed a "prolapse," or a falling forward to an advanced position. Optimally, an ideal goal of eliminating problematic drinking behavior would attempt to avoid lapses altogether. But given the high likelihood that lapses will occur, it is possible to deal with these events as prolapses, and in so doing reduce the probability of relapse.

Basis in Social Learning

Based on the principles of social learning theory, the RP model considers drinking behavior (like other behavior) to be substantially learned. Within this learning perspective, relapse has been reframed from being a variable associated with outcome to one associated with the process of change. This reframing can be understood largely in pragmatic terms. The course of changing problematic drinking behavior is seldom unwavering, with relapse being the norm rather than the exception (Armor, Polich, & Stambul, 1978). Yet until recently, the goal of professional treatment has been to effect immediate abstinence from alcohol rather than to maintain changes in drinking. In some respects, this approach has been doubly unfortunate, because it sets the stage for a sense of failure in not only the client but the clinician as well.

Complementarity of RP

Behavioral scientists have played a central role in formulating criticisms of conventional treatment for alcohol problems (e.g., Litman, Eiser, Rawson, & Oppenheimer, 1977; Litman, 1980), as well as in developing alternative forms of intervention. In the area of RP, several writers have introduced techniques and strategies that are of practical benefit to clinicians and researchers (e.g., Marlatt & Gordon, 1985; Annis, 1986a; Litman, 1986; Wanigaratne, Wallace, Pullin, Keaney, & Farmer, 1990; Daley, 1991). These approaches may be viewed as complementing, rather than competing with, other forms of treatment. For example, depending on the needs of an individual client, RP strategies may be applied conjunctively with Alcoholics Anonymous (AA) participation or they may follow some form of hospital-based treatment (Gorski & Miller, 1982). A presentation of the numerous techniques now associated with RP and their clinical application is beyond the scope of this chapter. However, the above cited texts are among those resources that the interested reader could consult.

Stages of Change

The question of how to determine the appropriateness of RP techniques for a particular client may be addressed within the framework of the "stages of change" model (Prochaska & DiClemente, 1982, 1983). This model, which is based on a meta-analysis of theories of psychotherapy and behavioral change, provides a useful heuristic for those working with alcohol problems. The model posits that there is a sequence of phases that individuals pass through in the development and change of problem behaviors. Four principle phases are identified as follows: (1) precontemplation, in which the individual is not actively contemplating change in his/her behavior and does not consider his/her behavior, often correctly, to be problematic; (2) contemplation, in which the individual is, to some extent, considering changing his/her behavior but has not yet taken steps to do so; (3) action, the phase in which change is undertaken; and (4) maintenance, in which the individual attempts to sustain the changes made during the action phase. RP is most intimately concerned with the maintenance phase of change. However, circumstances in the real world tend to blur the seemingly discrete boundaries of the change process. Lapses may necessitate renewed attention to the change process. Or the commitment of clients to the process of change may wane to the extent that contemplation must be reexamined. Both the clinician and the client practicing RP must remain mindful of the reasons for contemplating change and the actions taken in the service of change throughout the maintenance process.

Contemplation and Decision

The quality of the initial decision to alter one's drinking habits may be seen as a distal factor relating to outcome. In a study involving problem drinkers as well as other drug users, Hall and Havassy (1986) found that the clarity and quality of each subject's drug use goal at the outset of treatment were predictive of their rate of return to drug use and abstinence at 3 months. Clients' initial commitment to change may enhance their degree of compliance with treatment, which has consistently been found to be related to outcome (Finney, Moos, & Chan, 1981; Westermeyer & Neider, 1984; Fawcett et al., 1987). Beyond the client's initial state of preparedness, therapists can have an impact on a client's motivation to change his/her drinking habits (Miller, 1985).

A decision matrix may be helpful as a means of prioritizing and organizing a client's motivations for changing his/her drinking (see Marlatt, 1985a). Similar to the "decisional balance sheet" developed by Janis and Mann (1977), a decision matrix distinguishes positive from negative consequences of changing one's drinking, both in the long and short term. In addition to consolidating the client's motivations for change, the decision matrix may be a diagnostic aid, revealing aspects of the change process that may be particularly difficult. A copy of the completed decision matrix should be retained by both the client and therapist, serving as a reminder of the reasons for seeking treatment and as a reference point from which to gauge subsequent progress.

Adherence to stressful decisions has previously been related to the degree of social support that one receives (Janis, 1983). For many clients, the decision to maintain alcohol-related goals may be facilitated by a caring, nondirective therapist. For example, in feedback sessions focusing on risk for alcohol problems, an empathic therapeutic style has led to better outcomes than a confrontational style (Miller & Sovereign, 1988).

By emphasizing that therapists be supportive of clients' decisions and goals, RP contrasts with more traditional forms of treatment for alcohol dependence. Many treatment programs prescribe a goal for clients (i.e., abstinence) and provide the rationale for this prescription (i.e., the presence of a disease). RP encourages clients to articulate their own reasons for change and to select their own goals regarding alcohol. This client-centered approach is cultivated in the service of long-term change. The primary goal of RP is to provide clients with self-management skills and self-knowledge concerning alcohol that will enable them to independently chart a nonproblematic course for themselves. Reflecting on this aspect of RP, Sandahl and Ronnberg (1990) noted that "relapse prevention could be regarded as training in making choices" (p. 473).

It should be emphasized that the particular goal articulated by a client at the outset of treatment is not necessarily the position he/she will wind up adopting in the long run. For example, a client may wish to attempt moderate drinking before deciding to abstain, or vice versa. Among individuals who successfully change their alcohol-dependent behavior without treatment, it is frequently noted that following a period of abstinence, moderate drinking is adopted as a long-term practice (Sobell, in press). Alternatively, individuals who initially select moderation goals often end up becoming abstainers (Miller et al., in press). These results emphasize the variability between individuals in the process of change and argue that among problematic drinkers there may be many pathways to recovery. The dogma that has previously sustained the recommendation that all "alcoholics" must abstain forever deserves to be replaced by skeptical empiricism. If the client proves able to moderate his/her drinking, fine. If experience dictates that such a goal is untenable, however, then abstinence may indeed be the preferred immediate objective.

The Therapeutic Relationship

RP places the problem drinker and the clinician in a collegial relationship. The clinician presents himself or herself not as an expert able to impart a cure. Instead, the process of change is tailored uniquely to each individual client. RP is ideographic rather than nomothetic, striving to understand the role of alcohol in the context of each client's life. The approach to this understanding proceeds at two levels: "functional" and "topographic." In functional terms clients are encouraged to appreciate the meaning of alcohol in their life: What do they gain from drinking? What do they lose? What do they avoid? This line of inquiry may lead to a variety of possibilities for change. Family and job-related issues may come to light; marital or other relationship problems may become salient. This, in turn, may illuminate important therapy goals or may suggest general life-style changes that could help the client. Topographical analyses are aimed at the form that the client's drinking behavior takes. This entails the identification of high-risk situations and familiar patterns of drinking, which may in turn suggest a role for coping skills or specific behavioral modification.

Although they are substantially interrelated, the form and function of an individual's drinking are usefully distinguished. For example, Saunders and Allsop (1987) have pointed out that although clients will report the occurrence of lapses in novel and unexpected situations, a number of lapses occur in familiar situations with which the client had previously successfully coped. Efforts to develop coping skills that are specific to a given setting may prove useful but cannot be considered apart from the client's mental "set." Ultimately, both the form of the drinking behavior and its meaning must be responded to. A variety of assessment materials is available to assist the clinician in probing these areas (Sobell, Sobell, & Nirenberg, 1988). Interventions that interrupt the client's pattern of drinking are not likely to be successfully maintained unless some alternative behaviors are introduced that address the role of drinking in the client's life.

CONDITIONING FACTORS AND RELAPSE

Conditioned stimuli may be understood as mediators of lapses. For example, lapses are known to occur with greater frequency in particular types of situations (see Cummings, Gordon, & Marlatt, 1980). These "high-risk" situations are not identified solely by the presence of alcohol-related cues, however. Physiological, affective, and cognitive factors may also be involved in the mediation of lapses (Shiffman & Wills, 1985). It has recently been proposed, however, that the RP model may misjudge the role of conditioning factors, specifically conditioned craving, in the relapse process (Heather & Stallard, 1989). These authors suggest that RP overlooks the model of conditioned tolerance developed by Siegal (1983). Despite the established importance of Siegal's work, the relevance of this model for the phenomenon of craving has not been established. It is important to recognize that Siegal's model addresses physiological processes associated with tolerance and withdrawal. The subjective response of craving has not been clearly linked to these physiological processes (see Drummond, Cooper, & Glautier, 1990).

RP considers craving to be a subjectively perceived state of motivation (Marlatt, 1978). It may be helpful clinically to distinguish cravings from urges by regarding craving as the subjective desire for the effects of alcohol whereas urges imply the motivational intent to drink. This distinction may enable clients to fine-tune their responses to the experience of craving by recognizing that the desire for drink may be dealt with in an alternative (i.e., nondrinking) manner.

Despite its potential clinical utility, craving has not been found to be a primary precipitant of lapses (e.g., Ludwig, 1972; Marlatt & Gordon, 1985; Drummond et al., 1990). Among the multiple factors that have been associated with drinking lapses, negative emotional states, interpersonal conflict, and social pressure have been found to be the most commonly reported precipitants (Marlatt & Gordon, 1980; Marlatt, 1985b). It would be misleading, however, to view any single factor as the "cause" of a lapse. In terms of a conditioning model, multiple discriminative stimuli must be considered, some of which may be outside the individual drinker, others within. In addition, events preceding the lapse, such as seemingly irrelevant decisions, should be examined.

Related to the role of conditioning factors is the efficacy of cue exposure as a treatment for problem drinking. In their recent review of the cue exposure literature, Drummond et al. (1990) found no evidence for the effectiveness of this form of treatment. Underlying this negative conclusion is the finding that "no published human study has so far demonstrated that CRs [conditioned responses] to environmental cues represent a causal factor in relapse in either drug or alcohol dependence" (p. 738). Multiple factors may be relevant to this issue. For example, the relationship between negative emotional states and lapses may be indicative of a form of state-dependent learning (Bouton & Swartzentruber, 1991). Changes in affect may significantly alter the meaning of cues to which a drinker has been exposed during treatment. In addition, indviduals who experience cue exposure may be under the impression that they will be free of urges to drink following treatment. Should urges or craving subsequently occur, the client may feel unprepared to handle the situation or might infer that treatment has failed.

The efficacy of cue exposure techniques may be enhanced in a number of ways. It has been proposed that cue exposure can be combined with RP in a comprehensive approach to treatment (Cooney, Baker, & Pomerleau, 1983; Marlatt, 1990). Toward the objective of enhancing self-efficacy in high-risk situations, RP encourages clients to practice a variety of coping skills. It follows that efficacy will increase as more challenging situations are successfully dealt with. RP may incorporate cue exposure by having clients practice drink-refusal skills or other coping tactics while in the presence of relevant drink-related stimuli, either in the therapist's office or *in situ*. Opportunities for this sort of integration may be identified with conventional assessment materials such as the Situational Competency Test (Chaney, O'Leary, & Marlatt, 1978). Clients should be made aware of the theory linking cue exposure to successful coping, so that they appreciate that subsequent temptations and craving do not represent treatment failure.

Further integration of traditional conditioning techniques and RP may be facilitated by considering the stages-of-change model outlined above. Viewed independently, cue exposure may initiate a change in drinking behavior but contributes little to the maintenance of such changes. As with other processes that focus on initiating change, cue exposure techniques may be coupled with strategies that address the maintenance phase of behavioral change. Because they focus on different phases of the behavioral change process, there may be little gained from a comparison of cue exposure with RP strategies (see Heather & Stallard, 1989). Instead, cue exposure and RP may be optimally utilized in conjunction with one another.

Self-Efficacy Training

A basic goal of RP is to provide the client with enhanced self-management skills. Solomon and Annis (1990) recently compared the power of outcome expectancies and self-efficacy ratings to predict drinking behavior following treatment. Consistent with Bandura's (1986) theory, outcome expectancies did not predict posttreatment drinking levels, while self-efficacy ratings were strongly related to drinking following treatment. Similarly, Allsop and Saunders (1989) found self-efficacy ratings to be the best available predictor of drinking outcome at 6 months posttreatment. Enhanced self-efficacy is a goal that is approached gradually, however.

The compensatory model of helping and coping (Brickman et al., 1982) is relevant to this point. RP has previously been allied with this model of the change process (Marlatt, 1985a). Applied to alcohol, the compensatory model views the individual as not being morally responsible for the development of drinking problems. By contrast, individuals are held responsible for changing their behavior. Thus, there is a transition implicit in this heuristic whereby the individual drinker comes to assume greater responsibility for his/her behavior. This shift in responsibility is experiential and corresponds to changes in self-efficacy. According to Bandura (1977), self-efficacy may be enhanced through performance accomplishments or modeling processes. Experience among alcohol researchers has confirmed the relationship between alcohol-related efficacy and actual drinking experiences (e.g., Chaney, O'Leary, & Marlatt, 1978; Allsop & Saunders, 1989). As individuals accumulate experience dealing successfully with risky situations, their self-efficacy and experience of responsibility increase. This cyclical process, which is well established within self-efficacy theory (Bandura, 1977), will proceed at its own rate for each individual.

A number of assessment materials and procedures are relevant to the enhancement of self-efficacy. High-risk situations may be identified by utilizing measures such as the *Situational Confidence Questionnaire* (Annis, 1982). Alternatively, clients may be informally asked to relate situations in which they have been particularly likely to drink, or in which previous lapses have occurred. Once identified, coping skills and response alternatives may be matched to a client's high-risk situations. A further technique that may be useful is self-monitoring. Clients may monitor their alcohol consumption for a period of 2 weeks in order to identify patterns and trends in their drinking, including time of day, setting, mood, the amount consumed, and situational factors prior to and following drinking. Self-monitoring may also be performed by clients as they change their drinking behavior. While the prospect of permanently modifying one's drinking may appear duanting, a 2- or 4-week self-monitoring period may seem manageable to clients. Clients are asked to keep track of their urges and temptations for alcohol, the situations in which these arise, and their responses. This relatively unpressured exercise may illuminate risky situations, while it provides clients with efficacy-enhancing experiences arising from those situations in which they successfully maintained adherence to their drinking goal.

RESEARCH ON RP

In an earlier discussion of alcohol RP, Donovan and Chaney (1985) pointed out that research and empirical validation are necessary to prevent RP itself from experiencing a "lapse" into the same status as its ideological predecessors in the field of alcohol research. To date, however, there have been relatively few controlled clinical trials of the efficacy of RP. In this section, we review the recent literature in this area. Subsequently, we discuss some apparent challenges to researchers interested in applying the RP model and possible avenues by which to circumvent such challenges.

In general, aftercare has been found to be strongly related to the maintenance of treatment changes (Ito & Donovan, 1986), although not all forms of aftercare have proven to be effective (e.g., Fitzgerald & Mulford, 1985). In a study involving DWI (driving while intoxicated) offenders, Rosenberg and Brian (1986) found no differences in alcohol-related outcome measures between a comparison group and two treatment groups, one of which was based on RP. Ito, Donovan, and Hall (1988) similarly found no significant differences between RP and interpersonal process groups in a variety of outcome measures including time to first drink, alcohol consumption, abstinence, drinking days, and aftercare attendance. Unfortunately, the interpretability of each of these studies is compromised by factors such as missing data (Rosenberg & Brian) and similarity in the protocols between ostensibly different groups (Ito, Donovan, & Hall). Previous research conducted by Chaney et al. (1978) demonstrated significant decreases in alcohol consumption with RP versus discussion-only and no-treatment control groups. The RP group of this study included a variety of components, including modeling, behavioral rehearsal, and verbal coaching. Subsequent research has suggested that each of these components may be effective in reducing relapse. For example, among individuals of relatively high socioeconomic status, it has been found that verbal transmission of RP principles may be as effective as behavioral rehearsal (Jones, Kanfer, & Lanyon, 1982). This result is consistent with a review of alcohol treatment literature conducted by Miller and Hester (1986), in which the authors suggested that clients with a lower conceptual ability may benefit from well-structured therapy to a greater extent than those with higher conceptual ability. The possibility that clients with higher verbal skills can uniquely benefit from discussion remains a largely untested hypothesis, however.

Utilizing RP techniques, Annis and Davis (1988) have reported reductions in drinking from 46 drinks per week (on average) to fewer than 2 drinks per week at 3 months, and fewer than 6 drinks at 6 months. Moreover, a participant's self-efficacy ratings improved alongside changes in drinking. Treatment incorporated both group and individual therapy spanning eight sessions, and focused on identifying and anticipating high-risk situations as well as self-monitoring. In a similar study, Sandahl and Ronnberg (1990) reported overall reductions in drinking at 12 months, noting that successful outcome was related to both increased self-efficacy and the quality of the client's initial decision to change his/her behavior. In addition, those who successfully changed their behavior were more likely to have selected moderate drinking as their goal rather than abstinence. The final study considered in this review resembles the two preceding ones but has a few notable differences. Allsop and Saunders (1989) utilized random assignment to compare active RP with a discussion group and a treatment-as-usual group. The results, following eight sessions, indicated that performance-based treatment led to better outcomes than verbally mediated RP. At 6 months, subjects in the discussion and treatment-as-usual groups reported twice as many heavy drinking days as the active RP group. Subjects in this study worked in pairs, in contrast to the group format more commonly utilized by researchers. Of interest, posttreatment self-efficacy was the best predictor of outcome among subjects in this study. Collectively, the studies reviewed offer support for the efficacy of RP. They also highlight components of RP that may be particularly relevant to the change process, such as enhancing the client's initial commitment to change and developing improved self-efficacy. A particularly salient finding is the association between performance-based treatment and outcome. While some clients appear to benefit from clinical advice and feedback, the process of change seems to be further facilitated by exposure to high-risk situations and the active development of skills that are responsive to the pressures of these situations.

Comments on RP Research

As illustrated by the preceding review, research on RP continues to advance along relatively conventional lines, with apparently promising and informative results. It may be important, however, to bear in mind certain limitations of this research as it informs the theory and implementation of RP. Two primary points are relevant to this issue. First, in contrast to the group designs typically employed in outcome research, RP is a highly ideographic approach to dealing with alcohol problems. Much of the success of RP is based on its clinical utility as a comprehensive approach linking case conceptualization with treatment. Unfortunately, many of the connections between diagnosis and treatment are obscured through the reporting of aggregate figures. A related concern centers on whether RP is optimally effective in an individual or a group setting. As indicated above, research has been conducted using both implementation strategies, but the differential effectiveness of these approaches has not been studied. A second point involves the comparative nature of outcome research, and particularly the selection of a relevant comparison group. What, for instance, constitutes an appropriate comparison group by which to evaluate RP? As a maintenance strategy, RP should fittingly be compared with other programs that attempt to sustain change once it has been initiated, such as AA. However, few alternative maintenance strategies are amenable and receptive to research. Beyond the foregoing issues, the existing research on relapse does not facilitate ready comparisons of the efficacy of different treatments. This is in part due to methodological differences between studies concerning the duration of follow-up intervals as well as the criteria by which the term "relapse" is operationally defined. A number of studies have focused on the role of treatment intensity and duration, finding no differences in outcome as a function of these factors (Office of Technology Assessment [OTA]), 1983; Annis, 1986b; Miller & Hester, 1986). However, these findings do not address the question whether there are differences in outcome relating to qualitatively different treatments. Moreover, global comparisons of different treatments leave unanswered the question whether certain subpopulations of clients may benefit differentially from various approaches. One comparative study (known as

Project MATCH) involving AA, motivational interviewing, and RP is currently being conducted at a number of sites in the United States and promises to answer several important questions. On a smaller scale, the prospect of matching clients to particular aspects of RP itself may also be pursued. Within RP, a great deal remains to be learned about the efficacy of different practices for various types of clients. The objective of clinical utility must clearly underlie future research efforts, and toward this goal it may be necessary to substantially reconsider current methodological practices (see, e.g., Persons, 1990).

TOWARD THE FUTURE—A SPECTRAL VIEW OF RP

The concept of "matching" has pervasive import for the field of alcohol treatment. A primary conclusion of the recently completed Institute of Medicine Report (1990) was that no single form of treatment is optimal for all forms of alcohol problems. This finding would be unremarkable in most areas of therapeutics. However, the alcohol treatment field has been slow to move beyond a nomothetic framework toward the development of case-specific strategies. With this goal in mind, it may be useful to consider the role of matching strategies within a broad-based approach to prevention. Figure 2.1 illustrates the domain of alcohol consumption habits and related problems within the population.

As illustrated, alcohol consumption and alcohol problems are not synonyms, although they clearly correlate. The distinction between the two may be drawn in order to specify the goals of intervention. For example, although the focus of RP is typically on reducing the client's consumption of alcohol, our ultimate goal is the reduction of alcohol-related problems in the client's life. This goal may be pursued at any point along the spectrum of alcohol problems. Among those whose drinking is nonproblematic, a number of primary prevention strategies may be effectively implemented. Similarly, secondary prevention could be made accessible to those with incipient alcohol problems. Finally, individuals who are actively experiencing problems relating to drinking may receive tertiary prevention, the category in which we consider RP to have a role. The term "tertiary prevention" may be preferable to "treatment," in order to underscore a nondisease approach to alcohol problems, as well as to emphasize the continuity between the various levels of prevention. This broad-based approach is consistent with a public health model. At all phases of the intervention process, the goal remains to minimize the degree of harm associated with alcohol consumption. Cost effectiveness, both personal and societal, is increased to the extent that we can prevent problems from occurring. Thus, for many individuals, relapse

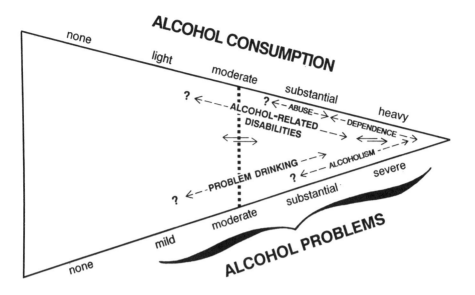

FIGURE 2.1. Alcohol problems. From *Broadening the Base of Treatment for Alcohol Problems* (p. 212) by the Institute of Medicine, 1990, Washington, DC: Institute of Medicine Press. Copyright 1990 by the Institute of Medicine Press. Reprinted by permission.

may best be prevented not at the end of their drinking career but at the beginning.

The concept of "harm reduction" encourages us to broadly reconsider our current approach to dealing with alcohol problems (see Marlatt & Tapert, in press). For example, at all levels of prevention, social and economic factors are of undeniable importance and must be taken into account in our efforts to prevent problematic drinking. To date, the promise of the biopsychosocial model has been fulfilled largely within the biological and psychological domains, to the possible neglect of equally relevant social issues. Just as we should not expect any single form of treatment to be effective for all individuals, we should consider the hypothesis that for some individuals, clinic-based treatment is simply not the appropriate method of intervention (Alexander, 1990).

Just as we may be neglecting some opportunities in the realm of primary prevention, it is important not to overemphasize tertiary interventions. Many programs offer a standard battery of interventions to all individuals seeking treatment. As an alternative to this "shotgun" approach, a minimal intervention stepped-care approach might be implemented.

The distinction between these approaches may be framed within the context of the familiar "journey" metaphor (see Marlatt, 1985a). The goal of treatment may be likened to the summit of a coveted peak. It is important, before embarking on this voyage, to determine the height of the chosen mountain and how far one is currently from the summit. Many treatment programs proceed as though the goal of all patients is to ascend a standard peak, and as though each individual climber is presently standing at its base. Within RP, we presume that no two ascents are alike, that although individuals are embarking on journeys that seem similar, their course and destination will inevitably differ. Individuals will also differ in their level of fitness to embark on the proposed voyage. They will have entered the consulting room already having made differing degrees of progress toward their summit. Moreover, they will reach their goals in differing periods of time. While some clients may in fact be standing far in the shadow of their looming objective, others may have made substantial progress toward this imaginary peak and may need a clinician's assistance to overcome a particular crux along the way. In recognition of these discrepancies in a client's needs, a stepped-care approach is utilized (Marlatt, 1988). Rather than treating all clients as though they need to be airlifted to the summit from a distant clearing, RP begins by considering whether a particular client may benefit from some relatively simple advice or feedback (e.g., joining a self-help group) in navigating his/her course around a particular obstacle. If a minimal intervention is not effective, then more intensive interventions may be tried. The final step in a hierarchical approach to treatment might be in-patient care or community-based interventions (e.g., Azrin, Sisson, Meyers, & Godley, 1982), which would be implemented as a last resort.

In keeping with the goal of harm reduction, the stepped-care approach is sensitive to the potentially disruptive effects of treatment on a client's life. The costs associated with many treatment programs, both in time and money, may exceed the needs and resources of many potential clients. In our experiences working with at-risk youth, it has become clear that few youths will consent to participate in extended treatment programs lasting 14 or 28 days. Fortunately, less invasive procedures have been shown to lead to sustained reductions in alcohol consumption within this population. The results of recent comparative research indicate that a single session of professional advice can lead to reductions in drinking among at-risk youth (Baer, Kivlahan, Fromme, & Marlatt, 1988). The impact of this single-session intervention was comparable to the results of more extensive interventions such as classroom and correspondence conditions lasting several weeks. It therefore appears that the professional advice session is the most cost-effective intervention among those tested. A possible explanation of these findings is that individuals will utilize alcohol-related information in accordance with their motivation for change. Although additional information may be taught to individuals, it does not necessarily follow that they will utilize this information to alter their drinking behavior. For many youths, a single session may appropriately match a level of information to their own interest and willingness to change.

In our current work with young, high-risk drinkers, we have implemented a stepped-care approach that further matches levels of intervention to each individual's needs and motivation for change. At all stages of our intervention we incorporate the "motivational interviewing" technique (Miller, 1983). A basic goal of this technique is to assess, in an ongoing manner, the clients' perception of their drinking, as well as their preparedness to change their behavior. Based on this assessment, the clinician works with the client to increase his/her awareness of alcohol-related consequences and to enhance the motivation for changing problematic behavior. Prior to any clinical intervention, clients are asked to complete a series of self-report measures as well as to monitor their drinking for a period of 2 weeks. The results of these assessments serve the dual function of providing information to the clinician as well as sensitizing clients to a number of alcohol-related matters. This sets the stage for the first step in our intervention strategy, which consists of a single session of detailed feedback. The general outline of these sessions includes discussion of the client's previous and current drinking levels; a review of the client's alcohol-related risk factors, including family history information and alcohol-dependence symptoms; discussion of physiological effects of alcohol, including blood alcohol concentration and the biphasic response; and elaboration of the role of expectancy and setting factors in drinking experiences. In addition, moderation and limit-setting strategies are introduced. As suggested by the previous research cited, this single session may be an appropriate and effective intervention for many individuals. However, others may require additional measures to reduce their harmful drinking. Such individuals are then referred to the next step in the sequence of interventions, which consists of one or more follow-up appointments at our clinic. Subsequent steps in the progression of interventions include attendance in an alcohol information and skills-training class; ongoing counseling; and, finally, referral to more intensive treatment. Clients are matched to services on the basis of clinical concern, as well as the client's preparedness for change. For example, some individuals may benefit significantly from moving beyond the stage of precontemplation to the point of contemplating that they are experiencing alcohol-related problems. This realization may be a sufficient catalyst leading to self-initiated change on the part of the client. Other clients will require help in making such changes. By making available a graduated series of interventions, we are better able to respond to the needs and wishes of individual clients. Across the spectrum of alcohol problems, we believe that similar client-sensitive approaches to change may be the most promising.

Over the course of the past decade, the RP model has inspired a great deal of clinical interest, research, and debate. As a model of treatment for alcohol problems, RP has demonstrated effectiveness. However, RP cannot afford to become associated with any fixed repertoire of techniques. Instead, RP should be a goal toward which we focus all of our available resources. In addition to the research directions suggested by the stepped-care model and treatment-matching hypotheses, environmentally based interventions might be further assessed. Alcohol problems exact an immense toll in many countries, while health care professionals are able to directly intervene with only a fraction of those affected. As a self-management strategy, RP encourages clients to change themselves largely by learning to change their environment. Future research could focus on identifying the environmental factors that lead to sustained changes in drinking, as well as those factors that undermine the change process. In clinical settings, the relationship between efficacy-enhancing experiences and the maintenance of change is well supported. The challenge remains to export these experiences beyond the walls of the clinic and into the daily lives of those people whom they may benefit.

REFERENCES

Alexander, B. K. (1990). *Peaceful measures: Canada's way out of the "war on drugs."* Toronto: University of Toronto.

Allsop, S., & Saunders, B. (1989). Relapse and alcohol problems. In M. Gossop (Ed.), *Relapse and addictive behaviour* (pp. 11–40). London: Tavistock/Routledge.

Annis, H. M. (1982). *Situational Confidence Questionnaire.* Toronto: Addiction Research Foundation.

Annis, H. M. (1986a). A relapse prevention model for treatment of alcoholics. In W. R. Miller & N. Heather (Eds.), Treating addictive behaviors: Processes of change (pp. 407–433). New York: Plenum.

Annis, H. M. (1986b). Is inpatient rehabilitation of the alcoholic cost effective? Con position. *Advances in Alcohol and Substance Abuse, 5,* 175–190.

Annis, H. M., & Davis, C. S. (1988). Self-efficacy and the prevention of alcoholic relapse: initial findings from a treatment trial. In T. B. Baker & D. S. Cannon (Eds.), *Assessment and treatment of addictive disorders* (pp. 88–112). New York: Praeger.

Armor, D. J., Polich, J. M., & Stambul, H. B. (1978). *Alcoholism and treatment.* New York: Wiley.

Azrin, N. H., Sisson, R. W., Meyers, R., & Godley, M. (1982). Alcoholism treatment by disulfiram and community reinforcement therapy. *Journal of Behavior Therapy and Experimental Psychiatry, 13,* 105–112.

Baer, J. S., Kivlahan, D. R., Fromme, K., & Marlatt, G. A. (1988). Secondary prevention of alcohol abuse with college student populations: A skills training approach. In T. Loberg, W. R. Miller, G. A. Marlatt, & P. E. Miller (Eds.), *Addictive behaviors: Prevention and early intervention* (pp. 157–172). Amsterdam: Swets & Zeitlinger.

Bandura, A. (1977). Self-efficacy: Toward a unifying theory of behavioral change. *Psychological Review, 84*, 191–215.

Bandura, A. (1986). *Social foundations of thought and action.* Englewood Cliffs, NJ: Prentice-Hall.

Bouton, M. E., & Swartzentruber, D. (1991). Sources of relapse after extinction in Pavlovian and instrumental learning. *Clinical Psychology Review, 11*, 123–140.

Brickman, P., Rabinowitz, V. C., Karuza, J., Coates, D., Cohn, E., & Kidder, L. (1982). Models of helping and coping. *American Psychologist, 37*, 368–384.

Chaney, E. F., O'Leary, M. R., & Marlatt, G. A. (1978). Skill training with alcoholics, *Journal of Consulting and Clinical Psychology, 46*, 1,092-1,104.

Cooney, N. L., Baker, L., & Pomerleau, O. F. (1983). Cue exposure for relapse prevention in alcohol treatment. In R. J. McMahon & K. D. Craig (Eds.), *Advances in clinical therapy* (pp. 174–210). New York: Brunner/Mazel.

Cummings, C., Gordon, J. R., & Marlatt, G. A. (1980). Relapse: Prevention and prediction. In W. R. Miller (Ed.), *The addictive behaviors* (pp. 291–321). New York: Pergamon.

Daley, D. C. (1991). *Kicking addictive habits once and for all: A relapse-prevention guide.* Lexington, MA: Lexington Books.

Donovan, D. M., & Chaney, E. F. (1985). Alcoholic relapse prevention and intervention: models and methods. In G. A. Marlatt & J. R. Gordon (Eds.), *Relapse prevention: Maintenance strategies in the treatment of addictive behaviors* (pp. 351–416). New York: Guilford Press.

Drummond, D. C., Cooper, T., & Glautier, S. P. (1990). Conditioned learning in alcohol dependence: Implications for cue exposure treatment. *British Journal of Addiction, 85*, 725–743.

Fawcett, S., Clark, D. C., Aagesen, C. A., Pisani, V. D., Tilkin, J. M., Sellers, D., McGuire, M., & Gibbons, R. D. (1987). A double-blind, placebo-controlled trial of lithium carbonate therapy for alcoholism. *Archives of General Psychiatry, 44*, 248–256.

Finney, J. R., Moos, R. H., & Chan, D. A. (1981). Length of stay and program component effects in the treatment of alcoholism: A comparison of two techniques for process analysis. *Journal of Consulting and Clinical Psychology, 49*, 120–131.

Fitzgerald, J. L., & Mulford, H. A. (1985). An experimental test of telephone aftercare contacts with alcoholics. *Journal of Studies on Alcohol, 46*, 418–414.

Grabowski, J. (1986). Acquisition, maintenance, cessation and reacquisition: An overview and behavioral perspective of relapse to tobacco use. In F. M. Tims & C. G. Leukefeld (Eds.), *Relapse and recovery in drug abuse* (National Institute on Drug Abuse Research Monograph 72) (pp. 36–48). Rockville, MD: Department of Health and Human Services.

Gorski, T. T., & Miller, M. (1982). *Counseling for relapse prevention.* Independence, MO: House-Independence Press.

Hall, S. M., & Havassy, B. E. (1986). Commitment to abstinence and relapse to tobacco, alcohol and opiates. In F. M. Tims & C. G. Leukefeld (Eds.), *Relapse and recovery in drug abuse* (National Institute on Drug Abuse Research Monograph 72) (pp. 118–135). Rockville, MD: Department of Health and Human Services.

Heather, N., & Stallard, A. (1989). Does the Marlatt model underestimate the importance of conditioned craving in the relapse process? In M. Gossop (Ed.), *Relapse and addictive behaviour* (pp. 180–208). London: Tavistock/ Routledge.

Institute of Medicine. (1990). *Broadening the base of treatment for alcohol problems*. Washington, DC: National Academy Press.

Ito, J. R., & Donovan, D. M. (1986). Aftercare in alcoholism treatment: A review. In W. R. Miller & N. Heather (Eds.), *Treating addictive behaviors: Process of change* (pp. 435–456). New York: Plenum.

Ito, J. R., Donovan, D. M., & Hall, J. J. (1988). Relapse prevention and alcohol aftercare: Effects on drinking outcome change process, and aftercare attendance. *British Journal of Addiction, 83*, 171–181.

Janis, I. L. (1983). The role of social support in adherence to stressful decisions. *American Psychologist, 38*, 143–160.

Janis, I. L., & Mann, L. (1977). *Decision making*. New York: The Free Press.

Jones, S. L., Kanfer, R., & Lanyon, R. I. (1982). Skill training with alcoholics: A clinical extension. *Addictive Behaviors, 7*, 285–290.

Litman, G. (1980). Relapse in alcoholism: Traditional and current approaches. In G. Edwards & M. Grant (Eds.), *Alcoholism: treatment in transition*. London: Croon Helm.

Litman, G. (1986). Alcoholism survival: The prevention of relapse. In W. Miller & N. Heather (Eds.), *Training addictive behaviors* (pp. 391–405). New York: Plenum.

Litman, G., Eiser, J., Rawson, N., & Oppenheim, A. (1977). Towards a typology of relapse: A preliminary report. *Drug and Alcohol Dependency, 2*, 157–162.

Ludwig, A. M. (1972). On and off the wagon: Reasons for drinking and abstaining by alcoholics. *Quarterly Journal of Studies on Alcohol, 33*, 91–96.

Marlatt, G. A. (1978). Craving for alcohol, loss of control and relapse: A cognitive behavioral analysis. In P. E. Nathan, G. A. Marlatt, & T. Loberg (Eds.), *Alcoholism: New directions in behavioural research and treatment* (pp. 271–314). New York: Plenum.

Marlatt, G. A. (1985a). Cognitive assessment and intervention procedures for relapse prevention. In G. A. Marlatt, & J. R. Gordon (Eds.), *Relapse prevention: Maintenance strategies in the treatment of addictive behaviors* (pp. 201–279). New York: Guilford Press.

Marlatt, G. A. (1985b). Relapse prevention: Theoretical rationale and overview of the model. In G. A. Marlatt & J. R. Gordon (Eds.), *Relapse prevention: Maintenance strategies in the treatment of addictive behaviors* (pp. 3–70). New York: Guilford Press.

Marlatt, G. A. (1988). Matching clients to treatment: treatment models and stages of change. In D. M. Donovan & G. A. Marlatt (Eds.), *Assessment of addictive behaviors*. New York: Guilford Press.

Marlatt, G. A. (1990). Cue exposure and relapse prevention in the treatment of addictive behaviors. *Addictive Behaviors, 15*, 395–399.

Marlatt, G. A. (in press). Harm reduction: Reducing the risks of addictive behavior. Newbury Park, CA: Sage.

Marlatt, G. A., & Gordon, J. R. (1980). Determinants of relapse: Implications for the maintenance of behavior change. In P. Davidson & S. Davidson (Eds.), *Behavioral medicine: Changing health lifestyles* (pp. 410–457). New York: Plenum.

Marlatt, G. A., & Gordon, J. R. (Eds.). (1985). *Relapse prevention: Maintenance strategies in the treatment of addictive behaviors*. New York: Guilford Press.

Marlatt, G. A., & Tapert, S. (in press). Harm reduction: Reducing the risks of addictive behavior. In J. S. Baer, G. A. Marlett, & R. J. McMahon (Eds.), *Addictive behaviors across the lifespan: Prevention, treatment and policy issues*. Newbury Park, CA: Sage.

Meacham, A. (1991). Understanding relapse: Do we need a new definition? *U.S. Journal of Drug and Alcohol Dependence, 5*, 1–10.

Miller, W. R. (1983). Motivational interviewing with problem drinkers. *Behavioural Psychotherapy, 11*, 147–172.

Miller, W. R. (1985). Motivation for treatment: A review with special emphasis on alcoholism. *Psychological Bulletin, 98*, 84–107.

Miller, W. R., & Hester, R. K. (1986). The effectiveness of alcoholism treatment: What research reveals. In W. R. Miller & N. Heather (Eds.), *Treating addictive behaviors: Process of change* (pp. 121–174). New York: Plenum.

Miller, W. R., Leckman, A. L., Delaney, H. D., & Tinkcom, M. (in press). Long-term follow-up of behavioral self-control training. *Journal of Studies on Alcohol*.

Miller, W. R., & Sovereign, R. G. (1988). *A comparison of two styles of therapeutic confrontation*. Unpublished manuscript, University of New Mexico, Albuquerque.

Office of Technology Assessment. (1983). *The effectiveness and costs of alcoholism treatment*. Washington, DC: Author.

Persons, J. B. (1990). Psychotherapy outcome studies do not accurately represent current models of psychotherapy. *American Psychologist, 46*, 99–106.

Prochaska, D. O., & DiClemente, C. C. (1982). Transtheoretical therapy: Toward a more integrative model of change. *Psychotherapy: Theory, Research and Practice, 19*, 276–288.

Prochaska, D. O., & DiClemente, C. C. (1983). Stages and processes of self-change in smoking: Towards an integrative model of change. *Journal of Consulting and Clinical Psychology, 51*, 390–395.

Rosenberg, H., & Brian, T. (1986). Cognitive–behavioral group therapy for multiple-DUI offenders. *Alcohol Treatment Quarterly, 3*, 47–65.

Sandahl, C., & Ronnberg, S. (1990). Brief group psychotherapy in relapse prevention for alcohol dependent patients. *International Journal of Group Psychotherapy, 40*, 453–476.

Saunders, B., & Allsop, S. J. (1987). Relapse: A psychological perspective. *British Journal of Addiction, 83*, 417–429.

Saunders, B., & Allsop, S. (1989). Relapse: A critique. In M. Gossop (Ed.), *Relapse and addictive behaviour*. London: Tavistock/Routledge.

Siegal, S. (1983). Classical conditioning, drug tolerance and drug dependence. In Y. Israel, F. B. Glaser, R. E. Popham, W. Schmidt, & R. G. Smart (Eds.), *Research advances in alcohol and drug problems* (Vol. 7, pp. 207–246). New York: Plenum.

Shiffman, S., & Wills, T. A. (Eds.). (1985). *Coping and substance use*. New York: Academic Press.

Sobell, L. C. (in press). Natural recoveries from alcohol problems: A lifespan perspective. In J. S. Baer, G. A. Marlatt, & R. J. McMahon (Eds.), *Addictive behaviors across the lifespan: Prevention, treatment, and policy issues*. Newbury Park, CA: Sage.

Sobell, L. C., Sobell, M. B., & Nirenberg, T. D. (1988). Behavioral assessment and treatment planning with alcohol and drug abusers: A review with an emphasis on clinical application. *Clinical Psychology Review, 8*, 19–54.

Solomon, K. E., & Annis, H. M. (1990). Outcome efficacy expectancy in the prediction of post-treatment drinking behaviour. *British Journal of Addiction, 85*, 659–665.

Wanigaratne, S., Wallace, W., Pullin, J., Keaney, F., & Farmer, R. (1990). *Relapse prevention for addictive behaviours*. London: Blackwell Scientific Publications.

Westermeyer, J., & Neider, J. (1984). Predicting treatment outcome after ten years among American Indian alcoholics. *Alcoholism, Clinical and Experimental Research, 8*, 179–184.

CHAPTER 3

SMOKING

Robin J. Mermelstein
Tracy Karnatz
Simona Reichmann
THE UNIVERSITY OF ILLINOIS AT CHICAGO

Smoking is the leading preventable cause of morbidity and mortality in the United States today, accounting for more than one of every six deaths (U.S. Department of Health & Human Services [USDHHS], 1989). Considerable progress has been made over the past three decades in reducing the prevalence of cigarette smoking; more than 40% of the adult population smoked in the early 1960s, while by the late 1980s, overall smoking prevalence was less than 29% (USDHHS, 1989). However, for continued progress to be made in reducing smoking, several areas need to be addressed, including lowering initiation rates, targeting and tailoring interventions to hard-to-reach groups, and preventing what still appears to be the most likely outcome of a cessation attempt—relapse.

Much of the research on smoking cessation during the past 10 years has focused on the widespread problem of relapse. Researchers have done a good job of describing the situational determinants of relapse (e.g., Shiffman, 1982; 1986; Marlatt & Gordon, 1980; Baer & Lichtenstein, 1988; O'Connell & Martin, 1987), moderately well at finding a wide range of predictors of relapse (e.g., Condiotte & Lichtenstein, 1981; Baer, Kamarck, Lichtenstein, & Ransom, 1989; Harackiewicz, Sansone, Blair, Epstein, & Manderlink, 1987; Mermelstein, Cohen, Lichtenstein, Baer & Kamarck, 1986; Niaura et al., 1988), but unfortunately, not at all well at relapse prevention (RP) (Glasgow & Lichtenstein, 1987; Carmody, 1990). Rather, two facts have been confirmed: (1) relapse remains common; and (2) relapse is best seen as one stage in a dynamic process in which smokers

frequently cycle back and forth between smoking and abstinence (Prochaska & DiClemente, 1983).

Most current smokers are relapsers. Only about one third of current
smokers have never tried to quit before (USDHHS, 1989), and most
smokers make several serious attempts at quitting before they ultimately
are successful at maintaining abstinence (USDHHS, 1989). This chapter
reviews findings about the patterns and processes of relapse and the
effectiveness of treatments that have been designed to prevent relapse
following cessation and makes recommendations for future RP interventions.

DEFINING "RELAPSE"

Definitions of relapse first require clear definitions of abstinence. Ossip-
Klein et al. (1986) outlined criteria for distinguishing among abstinence,
slips, and relapse. These authors suggest a minimum criterion of 24 hours
of complete abstinence for a "quit episode." However, for investigations
of relapse, we recommend distinguishing between "quit episodes" and
"abstinence periods," defined by a longer criterion, such as 48 hours or 7
days. Quit episodes lasting only 24 hours may not be long enough to
establish a clear pattern of abstinence from which one is eligible to
relapse. Ossip-Klein et al. (1986) recommend that relapse be defined as 7
consecutive days of smoking at least one puff per day. They also recommend an additional definition of relapse that encompasses more unusual
smoking patterns: Relapse may also be defined as seven consecutive slips
within a specified interval. Slips, or lapses, are defined as not more than 6
consecutive days of smoking following at least 24 hours of abstinence.
Thus, both relapses and slips are defined by a pattern of behavior and not
by the amount smoked.

Once criteria for abstinence and relapse are established, relapse
rates can be calculated by comparing rates of abstinence over time.
However, because of the considerable variation in ways of reporting
abstinence throughout follow-ups, it is not always possible to calculate
accurate relapse rates. For example, the most commonly reported abstinence rate, a point-prevalence measure, actually hinders drawing conclusions about rates of relapse. We briefly review the different ways of
reporting abstinence rates and their implications for discussions of relapse.

Point-prevalence measures of abstinence reflect the percentage of
individuals who are abstinent at a given point in time, regardless of their
status at previous measurement waves. At follow-ups, point-prevalence
measures of abstinence comprise individuals who have a variety of be-

havioral patterns, including those who have remained abstinent through-out the time period from end of treatment through follow-up point; individuals who were smoking at a previous measurement wave but who now are abstinent; and individuals who were abstinent previously, had relapsed, and now are abstinent again. Thus it is possible for point-prevalence rates to increase over time or to remain stable as people move in and out of smoking and abstinence. In general, because of the heterogeneity of smoking and abstinence patterns that comprise point-prevalence rates, relapse rates cannot be computed accurately from these figures.

Multiple-point-prevalence rates are often assumed (incorrectly) to be synonymous with measures of continuous abstinence. Multiple-point-prevalence rates are sequential cross-sectional measurements of absti-nence that do not take into account behavior between the measurement waves, thus allowing for the possibility of slips, or even relapse followed by recovery. Continuous abstinence, defined as no smoking at all, not even a puff, between measurement waves, is the most stringent criterion to meet. Cohen et al. (1989) compared abstinence rates across ten studies of self-quitters using two definitions of continuous abstinence—one a multiple-point-prevalence measure and the other a continuous, "not a puff," measure. Six of the ten studies had data reported for the two types of measures at 6 months follow-up. The abstinence rates, when measured by a multiple-point-prevalence definition, ranged from 4.6% to 16.3%. These rates dropped when the stricter "not a puff" definition was used and ranged from 2.5% to 10.1%. When differences between the rates are compared for each of the six individual studies, it becomes apparent that between 13.6% and 45.6% (median approximately 33.5%) of those in-dividuals who reported abstinence at all measurement waves up to the 6-month follow-up had smoked at least one cigarette. By the 12-month follow-up, the percentage of individuals who reported abstinence by the multiple-point criterion but who had smoked in between measurement waves ranged from 0% to 48.8% (median of 20.4%). These data illustrate that multiple-point-prevalence measures may mask important patterns of slipping or relapsing that continue to occur at least through 12 months after cessation. Thus, if one's interest is in the patterns of change and the process of relapse, single- or multiple-point-prevalence measures should be avoided in favor of continuous (no-smoking-at-all) measures.

The primary problem in assessing continuous abstinence, though, is that it is not easily verifiable. Point-prevalence rates, whether single or multiple, are more readily verified through biochemical measures such as cotinine, thiocyanate, or carbon monoxide, which will detect smoking over short periods of time (less than 24 hours to several days). A second problem with continuous abstinence rates is that they rely more heavily on retrospective self-report, which becomes more questionable the longer the interval between follow-up assessments and the more detailed the information required.

Interpretations of abstinence and relapse rates also depend on how attrition is handled. Most studies report some subject loss during follow-up. If one conservatively assumes that all missing subjects are smoking, then relapse rates might be artificially high. Alternatively, one could report rates only for those subjects who provided data at all measurement waves, in which case relapse rates might be spuriously low. The choice of how to handle missing data may depend in part, on the analytical question and the demand characteristics of the study. It may be fruitful for researchers to investigate a variety of models of attrition, using different assumptions about the probability of smoking among missing subjects based on their prior patterns of behavior and individual differences in factors related to relapse.

THE NATURAL HISTORY OF RELAPSE

The previous discussion should serve as a caution to drawing conclusions about the rate and timing of relapse, given that much of the literature is based on point-prevalence rates or unclear definitions of relapse. Nevertheless, several important questions can be asked: When does relapse occur? Are relapse rates constant over time or do they rapidly decrease? Is there a safe point beyond which relapse is unlikely to occur? Do all slips lead to relapses? What are the rates of recovery following a relapse?

When Does Relapse Occur?

Hunt, Barnett, and Branch (1971) provided the first and still very influential examination of relapse rates. They plotted survival rates (proportion of participants not relapsing) over time from the end of treatment through 12 months posttreatment. Their curve was derived by combining cross-sectional abstinence rates from a large number of treatment studies. There were two striking aspects to their curve. First, the vast majority of treatment successes relapse, and most of these relapses occur within 3 months. Second, the rates stabilize over time and appear to plateau. Although this first finding has been well confirmed, the second is open to debate and will be discussed later.

Brandon, Tiffany, Obremski, and Baker (1990) provided one of the few detailed examinations of the process of relapse. These researchers followed 129 abstinent subjects for 2 years after treatment; 92 of the subjects smoked during the 2-year follow-up. Brandon et al.'s study is important in that it distinguished between lapses (defined as any smoking) and relapses (defined as 3 consecutive days of smoking). Nearly all subjects who smoked had their first lapse during the first 3 months posttreatment. The mean number of days to first lapse was 58. Over the 2 years, 88% of the subjects who smoked a single cigarette relapsed. However, relapses did not immediately follow lapses; on average, 41 days separated a lapse from a relapse. The majority of relapses occurred within 7 months of treatment, and one third of all relapses occurred during the first month after treatment. Brandon et al. do not report any lapses or relapses after 15 months. Cummings, Jaen, and Giovino (1985) report similar findings. In a sample of 69 relapsers followed for a year after treatment, 19% relapsed during the first week after treatment, and 68% relapsed within the first 3 months. Cummings et al. (1985) defined relapse as "having smoked a cigarette," which may be more similar to Brandon et al.'s (1990) definition of lapse, rather than relapse. The median number of days to relapse was 57.

Swan and Denk (1987) examined relapse from a more dynamic perspective, modeling transitions between abstinence to relapse and relapse to abstinence. Their subjects were 381 smokers who had been abstinent for 3 months, and who they followed for 1 year. Relapse rates remained constant from 3 to 15 months after initial abstinence, averaging 3.9% per month for males and 3.6% per month for females. These researchers also recalculated relapse rates from Hunt et al.'s (1971) data to arrive at relapse rates of 22% per month before 3 months, and 4% per month after 3 months. Based on their finding of a constant relapse rate after 3 months, Swan and Denk (1987) conclude that there is no safe point beyond which relapse does not occur.

Is There a Safe Point?

The question of a safe point for maintaining abstinence is difficult to answer without follow-ups beyond 1 year. The Multiple Risk Factor Intervention Trial (MRFIT) is one of the few studies to provide long-term follow-ups. Subjects in this trial were all middle-aged men at risk for heart disease who were randomly assigned to either special intervention or usual care groups. At the 48-month follow-up, 56.2% of the subjects who had quit at the end of the intensive intervention were still abstinent (Hughes, Hymowitz, Ockene, Simon, & Vogt, 1981). Most of the relapses occurred within 3 months after the intervention. However, approximately one third of the remaining relapsers relapsed more than 1 year after the intervention.

Two studies of smokers who quit with no or minimal assistance provide more detailed data on relapse rates beyond 1 year. In a sample of

118 New Year's Day quitters, Marlatt, Curry, and Gordon (1988) found that at a 4-month follow-up, almost two thirds of the subjects could be classified as relapsers, approximately 15% were slippers, and about 20% were abstainers. Twelve percent of the subjects who were abstinent at 1 year relapsed by the 2-year follow-up. Mermelstein et al. (1990) examined rates of relapse and recovery from relapse in a sample of 344 abstinent subjects who had quit smoking in conjunction with a televised smoking-cessation program. By 6 months after the intervention, 47.4% of those who were abstinent at the end of the program had relapsed; 29.8% of subjects who were abstinent at both the end-of-program and 6-month measurements relapsed between 6 and 12 months; and, importantly, 13.4% of subjects who were abstinent at all measurement points through the 12-month interview relapsed between 12 and 24 months, a number very similar to that of Marlatt et al. (1988). Thus, although the rate of relapse declines with increasing time abstinent, a significant proportion of individuals who are abstinent 12 months after an intervention will relapse later. As Swan and Denk (1987) note, a safe point for maintenance has not yet been identified.

Do All Slips Lead to Relapse?

Without a doubt, slips increase the probability of relapse. As noted above, Brandon et al. (1990) reported that 88% of their subjects who slipped later relapsed. Baer et al. (1989) found that 79% of their subjects who slipped relapsed by a 1-year follow-up. Marlatt et al. (1988) found that slippers were more likely to become subsequent relapsers than were abstainers. Overall, 59% of the subjects they classified as abstainers and 91% of the slippers at the 1-month follow-up were classified as relapsers at the 2-year follow-up. Mermelstein et al. (1990) found that subjects who slipped had approximately three times the odds of relapsing than subjects who did not slip.

A given slip, however, may not lead directly to a relapse. As noted previously, Brandon et al. (1990) found that, on average, 41 days separated a slip from a relapse. We also know that a significant proportion of abstainers at any given point in time have had prior slips. For example, Baer et al. (1989) reported that 24% of those subjects who were abstinent at a 1-year follow-up had at least one documented slip. Recall, too, the data reported previously from the Cohen et al. (1989) study, indicating that a good number of subjects who were abstinent at 12 months had at least one slip during the follow-up period. It is clear that slips are common and that they increase the chances of a subsequent relapse, but the mechanism by which this occurs is not clear.

Recovery following Relapse

It is obvious that relapse is not a static end point. The fact that most smokers cycle back and forth between periods of abstinence, no matter how brief, and smoking, speaks to this point. Only a few studies have documented rates of recycling into subsequent quit attempts. Swan and Denk (1987) found that 34% to 38% of relapsers recycled (i.e., had a subsequent period of abstinence) during their 1-year follow-up period. Brandon et al. (1990) found that 25.9% of relapsers reported a subsequent distinct period of abstinence during a 2-year follow-up period, with this second abstinence period occurring on average almost 150 days after the relapse (median of 85 days). Mermelstein et al. (1990) reported that almost 28% of subjects who relapsed recycled into a subsequent period of abstinence at some time during a 2-year follow-up period; and Marlatt et al. (1988) found that 5% of relapsers at the 1-year follow-up became abstainers at the 2-year follow-up.

Documenting the rate and speed of recycling following a relapse is a first step in understanding the process of relapse from a more dynamic, longitudinal perspective. Some basic questions will need to be answered, though, such as whether to encourage rapid recycling following a relapse or, instead, to allow for a longer latency in order for the smoker to rebuild high levels of motivation, confidence, and commitment. Encouraging rapid recycling stems from an assumption that it is better to "strike while the iron is hot" and not allow smoking to become reestablished. Allowing for a longer latency assumes that the smoker may need to recover from feelings of discouragement, failure, and lowered efficacy. More data on the sequelae of relapse would help to answer these questions.

THEORIES OF SMOKING RELAPSE

Marlatt's model of the relapse process (Marlatt & George, 1984; Marlatt & Gordon, 1980, 1985) has provided the cornerstone for much of the research on RP over the past decade. This is a rich model, so only a brief overview will be presented here. The model starts with the assumption that the newly abstinent individual experiences a sense of perceived control until he/she encounters a high-risk situation. The most common high-risk situations are ones associated with negative emotional states, interpersonal conflict, social pressure, and the presence of other smokers or alcohol (Cummings, Gordon, & Marlatt, 1980; Marlatt & Gordon, 1980; Shiffman, 1982). If an individual can cope effectively in the high-risk situation, perceived control and self-efficacy will increase and the

probability of a relapse will decrease. The longer an individual is abstinent, and the more high-risk situations he/she is able to master, then the
more sense of control and self-efficacy increase, thus continuing to decrease the probability of relapse.

Obviously, many newly abstinent individuals do not cope successfully with high-risk situations. The hypothesized consequence of the
failure to cope is decreased self-efficacy not only for that particular high-
risk situation, but also for subsequent difficult situations. The probability
of a relapse is further enhanced if the individual holds positive expectations about the effects of smoking. For example, believing that
smoking will make one more relaxed and better able to cope with stress is
likely to lead to smoking when this belief is coupled with an inability to
cope effectively in a high-risk situation.

What if the individual does slip and smoke a cigarette? Whether the
slip turns into a full-blown relapse depends on the individual's reactions
to the slip and on his/her perceptions of the cause of the slip. A common
reaction to a slip is summarized by the abstinence violation effect (AVE)
(Curry, Marlatt, & Gordon, 1987; Marlatt & Gordon, 1985). The intensity
of the AVE varies as a function of a number of factors, including how long
the individual has been abstinent and how much the individual is committed to abstinence. The AVE has two components: (1) a cognitive–
dissonance effect; and (2) a personal attribution effect. Cognitive–
dissonance and guilt are aroused to the extent that the slip is perceived to
be inconsistent with one's self-image as an ex-smoker. The dissonance can
be resolved by altering one's self-image to fit the new behavior; thus,
smoking more will redefine one as a smoker. If the individual also
attributes the slip to stable personal or internal factors, then the probability of the slip's turning into a relapse increases further. Data from Curry
et al. (1987) and from O'Connell and Martin (1987) lend support to
components of the AVE. Both of these research groups found that relapsers, as compared to lapsers, made more internal and stable attributions
for their smoking.

Shiffman et al.'s (1986) conceptualization of relapse proneness com-
plements Marlatt's model. Relapse proneness refers to the risk of relapse
at any particular time. Changes in relapse proneness may occur as the
result of three mechanisms: (1) continuously and relatively slowly over
time as a result of the cumulative effect of a variety of background
variables (to be described later); (2) more suddenly, brought about by
discrete, precipitous events that trigger relapse, and (3) the two previous
mechanisms operating together such that discrete events may raise relapse proneness above a threshold level, but these events occur within
the context of background changes in relapse proneness.

Shiffman (1989) has elaborated further on these concepts and suggested that variables that influence relapse may be divided into three groups: (1) enduring personal characteristics, (2) background variables, and (3) precipitants. Each of these groups of variables forms the basis for a model of relapse risk. The first, a personal characteristics or constant risk model, emphasizes stable individual differences such as demographic or dependence variables. The personal characteristics model focuses on the question of individual vulnerability and predicting who will relapse based on factors that tend not to change over time. This model's strength is that it identifies a high-risk group of individuals, but its limitation is that it does not lead to treatment suggestions. A second model of relapse risk, the background factors or cumulative risk model, focuses on changes in background factors during the maintenance period. Examples of background factors include stress, mood, withdrawal symptoms, and motivation level. Background factors serve to "set the stage" for relapse and may reach a threshold level above which relapse is likely. The treatment implications of this model are relatively clear; once appropriate background factors have been identified, they can be monitored and modified in order to keep relapse proneness below a threshold level. The third model, the precipitating factors or episodic risk model, as noted previously, suggests that relapse crises follow sudden, intense events. One potential treatment implication of this model is to provide individuals with the necessary coping resources to handle these unexpected events or alternative resources to buffer against them.

Shiffman (1989) argues that all three models need to be considered simultaneously. However, much of the research on relapse has focused on one model at a time, thus leading to potential inconsistencies in research findings. For example, withdrawal symptoms may serve as a background factor but not as a precipitant. Thus, depending on one's measurement model, conclusions about the role of withdrawal in relapse may vary. Shiffman's conceptualization of models of relapse risk is certainly compatible with Marlatt's theory. Both background and precipitating factors could be viewed as high-risk situations. How an individual reacts to these situations, as determined by a combination of coping skills, self-efficacy, and expectancies, may determine whether the level of relapse proneness crosses a threshold.

Finally, Niaura et al. (1988) have argued that no one theoretical formulation has yet been able to account adequately for the process of relapse. They proposed an integration of social learning formulations, such as Marlatt and Gordon's (1985) and Shiffman's (1989), with conditioning models and arrived at a dynamic regulatory feedback model that integrates both affective and contextual cues. The model hypothesizes that relapse precipitants can include either positive or negative affect states, contextual cues, or some combination. These cues or affect states trigger a series of responses, including urges, positive outcome expectancies, and physiological activation. These responses will further serve as positive feedback to the affective states. Cognitive–behavioral coping efforts, attributions, and self-efficacy expectations all interact with the intensity of these reactions to determine whether initial smoking will occur. This initial lapse also feeds back into the affective state, perhaps further engendering negative affect in some individuals. Efficacy expectations and attributions of controllability may decrease the probability of a lapse's turning into a full-blown relapse. Niaura et al.'s model also has direct treatment implications for RP. Treatments designed to decrease the strength of cue reactivity and to increase the use of coping skills in the presence of cues are both important in preventing relapse.

INTERVENTIONS

Interventions to improve the maintenance of abstinence have come full circle, with numerous enhancements along the way. Early efforts to enhance maintenance simply extended treatment through additional contact or booster sessions. More recently, there has been renewed interest in continued contact as a maintenance strategy. In between, interventions tended to follow one of several approaches: adding cognitive–behavioral skills training and RP techniques based on Marlatt and Gordon's (1980) model to the basic cessation program; adding components that were hypothesized to be related to RP (e.g., social support training, weight control components, cue exposure, and conditioning procedures); or adding pharmacological treatments, either in addition to skills training or alone. We review the findings from each of these intervention approaches.

Maintenance versus No-Maintenance Treatments

The general conclusion from early studies of extended contact and booster sessions has been that boosters alone are ineffective in RP (Schwartz, 1987). One problem with these early interventions was that the booster sessions were often weak, both in the timing of their sessions and in their failure to tailor the content to the individual's stage of change. More recent evaluations of booster or maintenance sessions suggest, though, that they should not be dismissed so readily. Rather, it may be important to evaluate the effects of extended contact by the type of program smokers initially receive. Intensive clinic-based programs may not be enhanced by booster sessions, but more minimal treatment programs might be. For example, a study by Brandon, Zelman, and Baker (1987) evaluated the effects of adding maintenance treatments to a clinic-based cessation program. They compared two maintenance treatments to a nonmaintenance control. Both maintenance treatments comprised coping skills and cue-exposure training, and one also included rapid puffing trials. Maintenance sessions were held 2, 4, 8, and 12 weeks after the end of the cessation treatment. During the maintenance period, the two maintenance conditions had lower relapse rates than did the control; 66% of the maintenance subjects were abstinent compared with only 37% of the controls at 3 months posttreatment. However, once the maintenance sessions ended, the difference between the maintenance and control conditions was no longer statistically significant; at 6-months posttreatment, 47% of the maintenance subjects remained abstinent, compared to 37% of the controls. Brandon et al. (1990) conclude that maintenance sessions prolong abstinence only as long as the sessions last. One could argue, though, that Brandon et al. failed to give their maintenance sessions an adequate test; they simply did not have enough power to detect significant differences with a sample size of only 18 to 20 subjects per condition.

Earlier studies by Lando (1982; Lando & McGovern, 1985) similarly show a lack of superiority of maintenance treatments to no maintenance. Lando's (1982) maintenance treatment included group discussion and behavioral contracts during seven sessions over an 8-week period. If subjects smoked, they contracted to have additional booster sessions of rapid smoking. Lando found marginal effects for the maintenance treatment during the first few months posttreatment, but these effects disappeared by the 12-month follow-up. All treatment conditions showed considerable relapse, however, and relapse rates did not vary by condition. In his later study, Lando (Lando & McGovern, 1985) found no differences between the maintenance and nonmaintenance control at any follow-up point.

More minimal treatment programs, such as self-help guides or physician advice, may benefit from maintenance materials or extended contact (Kottke, Battista, DeFriese, & Brekke, 1988). Davis, Faust, and Ordentlich (1984) conducted a large-scale evaluation of the American Lung Association's self-help cessation manual, *Freedom From Smoking in 20 Days*, and its accompanying maintenance manual, *A Lifetime of Freedom From Smoking*. Smokers ($N = 1,237$) were randomly assigned to one of four conditions: (1) educational leaflets only; (2) leaflets plus the maintenance manual; (3) cessation manual only; or (4) cessation manual plus maintenance manual. The cessation manual contains a number of behavioral strategies and follows a 20-day plan for cessation. The maintenance manual emphasizes techniques for coping with potential high-risk situations. All conditions showed considerable relapse, ranging from 40% to 69% in the first month. By the 12-month follow-up, there was a slight advantage for the maintenance conditions. Continuous abstinence rates for the two maintenance conditions were 4% and 5% compared with 2% and 3% for the nonmaintenance conditions. Thus, the maintenance manual produced higher quit rates than leaflets or the cessation manual alone, but the relapse rate was still very high.

A recent study by Orleans et al. (1991) suggests that extended contact in a minimal assistance program may be of benefit. These investigators found that subjects who received prescheduled phone calls from a counselor at 6, 18, 34, and 60 weeks after receiving self-help materials had higher cessation rates than subjects who did not receive this additional contact. The self-help materials described RP techniques. However, one single reinforcement mailing (a booster that attempted to remotivate and reinforce quitting and use of the self-help guide) sent 1 year after subjects enrolled in the study had no effect on outcome. Thus, serial contacts, close in time to the cessation intervention, may enhance minimal assistance programs.

The above approaches to RP are largely atheoretical and follow a "more is better" philosophy. With minimal assistance programs, this assumption may well be true. However, in clinic-based programs, booster sessions have often been a reiteration of previously presented material and may not have adequately addressed the unique problems associated with the maintenance phase (Brownell, Marlatt, Lichtenstein, & Wilson, 1986).

RP Training

Marlatt and Gordon's model has served as the basis for most of the RP interventions. Typically, interventions based on their model have incorporated several of the following components: identification of high-risk situations, training in coping skills, cognitive reframing, innoculation against the AVE, coping with slips, and life-style balancing. It is rare, though, to find an intervention that contains all the components of their model. Evaluations of RP training have at best been mixed. Early studies (e.g., Brown, Lichtenstein, McIntyre, & Harrington-Kostur, 1984) found no difference between conditions with and without RP, but these studies may have been hampered by insufficient sample sizes for detecting differences.

Davis and Glaros (1986) evaluated RP training within a behavioral analytical framework. In their experimental group, subjects were provided with instruction, modeling, behavioral rehearsal, and feedback and coaching of coping behaviors. Subjects were also trained in the use of general problem-solving skills and had discussion about preventing the AVE and developing rewards. The experimental group was compared with a control group that received only a basic cessation program and with an enhanced control, who, in addition to the cessation program, discussed randomly chosen high-risk situations. At the 12-month follow-up, there was no difference among the groups. Point-prevalence rates were 12% for the control, 21% for the enhanced control, and 13% for the experimental group. Although this study was limited by its small sample size (no more than 16 per condition), low power does not explain why the enhanced control had a trend toward higher (but not significantly so) point-prevalence rates at 12 months. Rather, it may be that the experimental group's intervention was overly complex for too short a time frame. In addition, most of the training occurred before subjects stopped smoking, perhaps further limiting the understanding and utility of RP training.

In contrast to these negative findings, two other studies have found positive results for RP training. Hall, Rugg, Tunstall, and Jones (1984) compared a skills-training RP condition to a discussion control. The skills-training treatment had three components: cue-produced relaxation training, commitment enhancement, and RP skills training (identifying high-risk situations, role-playing alternatives). At the 12-month follow-up, the skills-training condition produced abstinence rates superior to the discussion condition (46% vs. 30%). The skills-training subjects were also more likely to report the use of specific RP strategies.

Stevens and Hollis (1989) also evaluated the effect of individually tailored RP training. Subjects who stopped smoking following an intensive cognitive–behavioral cessation program were randomly assigned to one of three maintenance conditions: (1) a three-session skills-training program in which subjects developed and actively rehearsed, in session, individually tailored coping strategies for high-risk situations; (2) a three-session discussion control; or (3) a no-treatment control. At 1 year, the skills-training condition had significantly higher rates of sustained abstinence (41.3%, defined as no tobacco use in the previous 6 months) than did the other two groups (34.1% for the discussion group and 33.3% for the no-treatment control). Simply adding a discussion group did not enhance success. However, there was a modest, but significant benefit to skills training. Stevens and Hollis (1989) point out the need for both active rehearsal and tailoring for RP training to be successful.

In one of the more rigorous theoretical tests of the RP model, Curry, Marlatt, Gordon, and Baer (1988) compared an RP approach to a "traditional" intervention emphasizing the need for absolute abstinence. The RP intervention, in contrast, emphasizes the gradual acquisition of coping skills and allows for early errors, or slips. These researchers anticipated that the two approaches would produce a different pattern of behavioral change such that the traditional program would have higher initial cessation compared to the RP program, but that there would be more long-term abstainers in the RP approach. Although the two approaches contained some similar program components, such as relaxation training, practicing alternative behaviors, and enlisting social support, they differed in the timing of quit day and hence the amount of postquit support (5 weeks for RP vs. 3 weeks for the absolute-abstinence program) and in other specific strategies as well. The RP treatment included identifying high-risk situations, cognitive restructuring, and role playing, whereas the absolute-abstinence approach included focused smoking, health education, and contingency contracting. Abstinence rates at the 1-year follow-up were not significantly different between the two approaches. However, as expected, the behavioral change patterns did differ. Participants in the RP program were more likely to slip sooner but were also more likely to become abstinent during the follow-up. Curry et al. (1988) suggest that individuals treated with an RP approach will be more likely to be increasingly successful at later cessation attempts. They speculate, though, as have others, that the complexity of the RP intervention may be a problem; it requires participants to learn too much in too short a time. In the absolute-abstinence program, participants concentrate on a smaller number of changes.

One of the more interesting findings to emerge from the Curry et al. (1988) study was the different pattern of treatment effects for men and women. Women were more likely to benefit from the RP program than from the absolute-abstinence program, whereas men were more likely to quit in the absolute-abstinence program than in the RP one. Relatedly, Hall et al. (1984) had found that the benefits of their RP skills training was limited to lighter smokers; there were no treatment differences for participants smoking more than 20 cigarettes a day at baseline. It may well be that RP training is most efficacious among certain subgroups and that one of the goals of future interventions should be to identify characteristics of individuals most likely to benefit from this type of intervention.

RP and Additional Components

Hoping to improve on the disappointing effects of RP treatments alone, researchers have attempted to supplement interventions with components found to be related to relapse. We review three areas that have had great appeal either theoretically or clinically: social support, weight control, and affect regulation.

High levels of social support for quitting have consistently been associated with better cessation outcomes (Cohen & Lichtenstein, 1990; Coppotelli & Orleans, 1985; Mermelstein, Lichtenstein, & McIntyre, 1983; Mermelstein et al., 1986). The notion behind adding social support components was to extend the support of the clinic into the participant's natural environment and through the maintenance phase. However, clinic-based interventions aimed at increasing social support have, for the most part, been unsuccessful at improving long-term success rates above those of RP treatments alone (Lichtenstein, Glasgow, & Abrams, 1986). Lichtenstein et al. (1986) and Cohen et al. (1988) reviewed the early social support interventions and identified problems that may have precluded their finding positive results, including a failure in some cases to influence the level of support received (McIntyre-Kingsolver, Lichtenstein, & Mermelstein, 1986; Malott, Glasgow, O'Neill, & Klesges, 1984); confounding by dual-role subjects (i.e., both helper and recipient) (McIntyre-Kingsolver et al., 1986); a lack of reinforcement for the partner's or buddy's efforts; and a lack of statistical power. Finally, the social support components may not have had enough salience in the context of already rich, multicomponent programs to show an effect. Cohen et al. (1988) suggested that minimal assistance or community interventions may provide a better context than the clinic-based program in which to test the effects of social support training.

A more recent study has found benefits for social support training in combination with RP in the context of a larger-scale, minimal assistance and community-based intervention. Gruder et al. (1992) evaluated the effectiveness of a brief group intervention that focused on social support and RP as a supplement to a televised self-help cessation program. Smokers ($N = 489$) registering for a televised cessation program who also expressed interest in joining a support group and who had a nonsmoking buddy were randomized to three conditions: (1) no contact control: subjects received a self-help manual and were encouraged to watch the TV program; (2) discussion: in addition to the self-help manual and TV program, subjects were invited to attend three group meetings that provided a review of the cessation program, and were asked to bring a buddy to one meeting; (3) social support and RP training: in addition to the self-help manual and TV program, subjects were invited to attend three group meetings that provided training in social support and RP, and their buddies received social support training in one session as well. Over a 24-month follow-up, abstinence rates were highest in the social support condition (9.3% multiple-point prevalence), followed by the discussion (5.7%), and then the no contact control (2.6%). Importantly, the social support condition successfully influenced the level of support received. Thus, as an adjunct to a minimal intervention, support training along with RP may well provide a means of enhancing long-term success. Unfortunately, the design of the Gruder et al. study did not allow for a separate evaluation of support training compared to the RP training alone.

A second area that has received increased attention recently has been the problem of weight gain following cessation. Weight gain is highly likely following cessation and is often cited as a potential contributor to relapse, especially among women (Klesges, Benowitz, & Meyers, 1991). However, data showing a positive relation between weight gain and relapse are far from compelling, and indeed, there are data showing the opposite (Hall, Ginsberg, & Jones, 1986; Swan & Denk, 1987). Nevertheless, adding a weight-control component to cessation programs has been an appealing idea for trying to prevent relapse. Klesges et al. (1991) reviewed behavioral treatments for postcessation weight gain and concluded that adding weight-control components to multicomponent cessation programs has not been successful thus far. Klesges et al. postulate that there may be several reasons for this lack of success: The resulting programs may be too complex, weight gain may actually protect against relapse, and the subjects most concerned about weight gain may not be the ones who attend clinical programs. What may be more promising is combining pharmacological approaches (e.g., nicotine replacement or d-fenfluramine) to help prevent weight gain with RP (c.f., Spring, Wurtman, Gleason, Wurtman, & Kessler, 1991).

A third area that is starting to receive attention is combining affect regulation approaches with cessation programs as a way to prevent relapse. It is clear that negative affect states play a large role in triggering relapse (Marlatt & Gordon, 1980; Shiffman, 1982). Several researchers have also found that depressed individuals are more likely to relapse following cessation than nondepressed individuals (Anda et al., 1990; Glassman et al., 1990; Hall, 1988). Hall, Munoz, and Reus (1991) recently evaluated the effects of mood-management intervention and found that this approach may be specifically efficacious for smokers who have a history of major depressive disorder. These authors also suggest that the low abstinence rates reported in cessation clinics may be influenced by the large proportion of smokers with a history of major depressive disorder in such settings. Hall et al.'s (1991) data are intriguing and certainly suggest that more work should be done on studying affect regulation approaches as a way to prevent relapse.

In sum, the effects of adding more components to an already complex RP program have been mixed, although the jury is still out on the benefits of affect regulation approaches. In evaluating the past decade of cessation interventions, Lichtenstein and Glasgow (1992) conclude that minor differences in treatments have not led to major differences in outcome, and we are not likely to identify that one "magic bullet" intervention component.

RP and Pharmacological Approaches

Nicotine substitution therapy, using nicotine gum, has been the most successful pharmacological approach to smoking cessation to date. The large set of convincing data documenting the addicting properties of nicotine and the role of withdrawal symptoms in affecting relapse (USDHHS, 1988) has increased interest in combining pharmacological and psychological treatments for cessation. Nicotine gum is most effective when combined with cognitive–behavioral programs (Fagerstrom, 1988; Lam, Sacks, Sze, & Chalmers, 1987; Schwartz, 1987). However, nicotine gum appears to have its greatest benefit on reducing short-term relapse and has less impact on long-term outcomes (Fagerstrom, 1988).

Several studies have evaluated the effects of RP treatments combined with pharmacological manipulations. Goldstein, Niaura, Follick, and Abrams (1989) evaluated the effects of an RP intervention compared to a health education intervention within the context of two different schedules for nicotine gum delivery (fixed or *ad lib*). At 6 months follow-up, Goldstein et al. (1989) found that the RP plus gum treatment was superior to the health education and gum treatment (36.7% abstinent vs. 17.5%). However, their overall success rates were not noticeably better than those obtained in RP programs without a gum component.

It is also important to note, though, two well-designed studies where RP components did not fare as well. Hall, Tunstall, Ginsberg, Benowitz, and Jones (1987) conducted a double-blind trial in which subjects were randomly assigned to one of four conditions. The conditions varied by either active nicotine gum or placebo and by intensity of treatment contact. The low-contact treatment comprised five 1-hour discussion sessions, as compared to the intensive 14-session treatment which included aversive smoking, RP skills training, and commitment enhancement (similar to that used in Hall et al., 1984). Although the active gum produced higher abstinence rates at 1 year than did the placebo (44% vs. 21%), the intensive behavioral treatment was no better than the low contact. In fact, among subjects who received active gum, there was a trend for the low-contact group to have higher abstinence rates at 1 year than did the intensive group (50% vs. 34%). There may be an inherent treatment conflict between external attributions about success fostered by gum treatment and the internal attributions about control fostered by RP (cf. Harckiewicz et al., 1987).

Killen, Fortmann, Newman, and Varady (1990) conducted a large-scale, minimal contact nicotine gum and RP trial. Subjects ($N = 1,218$) who were abstinent for 48 hours were randomized into one of 12 interventions, each of which varied by four levels of a pharmacological factor (nicotine gum *ad lib* or fixed dosage, placebo, or no gum) and by three levels of a psychological treatment factor (self-selected RP modules, randomly assigned modules, or no modules). There were 16 written RP modules providing self-instruction on how to avoid smoking in specific high-risk situations. The modules emphasized performance-based experience by encouraging subjects to practice their plans for avoiding smoking in these situations. Subjects who received active gum had significantly better abstinence rates only through 6 months. The gum did not improve longer-term abstinence rates. Unexpectedly, subjects who received the RP modules did not achieve higher abstinence rates than those who did not receive modules. Killen et al. (1990) hypothesized that the modules may not have provided enough guidance for developing plans for gradual exposure to high-risk situations and that they may have actually discouraged the use of coping skills. Killen et al. (1990) also found that men and women responded differently to the treatments. For men, the nicotine gum produced higher abstinence rates. For women, however, no treatment was superior. Their overall abstinence rates at 12 months (between 18% and 24%) fall short of those found in more intensive clinic-based programs with nicotine gum.

Conclusions about RP Interventions

RP interventions are intuitively appealing; they address factors (e.g., self-efficacy, coping with high-risk situations, slips) that show consistent relations to outcome. However, the empirical evidence supporting them is equivocal. In drawing conclusions about their utility, we need to address two questions. First, have RP interventions been tested adequately, and second, do they produce lower relapse rates than other treatments? Unfortunately, there is no clear answer to either of these questions. Evaluations of RP interventions have fallen short in several ways. Several studies have lacked adequate power to detect significant differences. Many have tried to teach too much information in too little time and may have relied on discussion of coping skills as opposed to training and rehearsing of coping skills. Studies vary, too, in whether RP skills are taught before or after participants stop smoking. In addition, with the exception of the Curry et al. (1988) study, it is difficult to evaluate how close many investigations come to the Marlatt and Gordon (1985) model of RP. For example, important components such as life-style balance, discussion of slips, and avoiding the AVE may not always be addressed.

Are relapse rates lower with RP interventions than with other interventions? Comparing the effectiveness of different intervention strategies is a difficult task. Most problematic are the differences in definitions of abstinence and length of follow-ups across studies. Also frustrating for a discussion of relapse is that most studies report and compare abstinence rates across treatments, rather than comparing relapse rates. Treatments may be superior over the long run because they produce higher initial abstinence rates even if there are no differences in relapse rates. Because most of the studies we critiqued reported only point-prevalence abstinence rates, we were unable to make direct comparisons of relapse rates. In the few cases where relapse rates could be computed, they were often not lower than 50%, even in the most effective treatment condition. For example, the approximate relapse rate at 12 months in Stevens and Hollis's (1989) RP condition was 59%, compared to 66% for their discussion group. Killen et al.'s (1990) relapse rates for all conditions (nicotine gum, placebo, or no gum with or without RP) ranged from 73% to 81%, higher than those found in clinic-based studies. As Curry et al. (1988) propose, one of the advantages of RP interventions may be that they produce more recovery from a relapse than do other treatments. However, because of the way the data are presented in most studies, we are unable to evaluate this hypothesis. We recommend that future intervention studies report both relapse rates and recovery rates more directly.

One of the most important findings to emerge from the above review is that RP programs may be differentially effective for different individuals. Women and lighter smokers, for example, may do better with RP treatments than with other programs (Curry et al., 1988; Hall et al., 1984). Unfortunately, we know the least about how RP works for the subgroups of smokers who increasingly comprise the smoking population—minorities, women, and less educated individuals (Pierce, Fiore, Novotny, Hatziandreu, & Davis, 1989). Clearly, more work needs to be done examining individual differences in treatment responses.

TREATMENT RECOMMENDATIONS

The high relapse rates following cessation emphasize the need to focus on maintenance. Our first treatment recommendation is for clinicians to acknowledge that maintenance is a long-term process. Although the majority of relapses occur within 3 months of cessation, ex-smokers are still vulnerable to relapse throughout the first year, and perhaps beyond. Lengthening treatment to cover at least the first 3 months postcessation may be worthwhile. However, treatment should not be just a reiteration of previously presented material. Rather, assessment of relapse proneness, training new coping skills to criterion, debriefing of slips, and life-style reprogramming should have priority.

Second, maintenance should focus on maintaining skills or behaviors, not just on maintaining the absence of a behavior. However, it is unrealistic for us to expect participants to maintain new coping skills or alternative activities when these behaviors have not been adequately established. As several authors (e.g., Curry et al., 1988) have noted, RP training is often too brief, without adequate checks on whether participants have acquired the necessary skills. It is clear that simple discussions of skills and suggestions for coping, whether presented orally or in written format, do not go far enough. Behavioral rehearsal and competency checks prior to treatment termination are likely to be more effective.

Third, viewing relapse as a process, and not as an all-or-nothing phenomenon, gives us multiple points of intervention before the full-blown relapse crisis occurs. Both slips and changes in background factors, leading to increases in relapse proneness, provide early opportunities to intervene. Marlatt and Gordon's model points to the need to prepare participants for the potential of slipping and experiencing the AVE. This is perhaps one of the more difficult treatment aspects of their model. Therapists must walk a thin line when, on the one hand, they must express confidence in participants' abilities to remain abstinent and to build efficacy while, on the other hand, they must warn about slips and train participants to cope with that possibility. The danger lies in having participants misinterpret the message as giving permission to smoke. Therapists need to watch for new ex-smokers who start to plan slips because they have convinced themselves that slips are not a problem. Therapists need to be clear with their message: Slips are dangerous; they increase the probability of relapse; they should be taken as a warning sign that it is time to increase one's vigilance and attention to maintenance, but slips do not mean that relapse is automatic. The failure is not in having the slip but in ignoring it. In addition, participants need to feel comfortable about reporting slips and debriefing them with therapists. Again, a middle ground must be reached between having participants so comfortable with their slips that they just dismiss them and having them so frightened or embarrassed by their slips that they avoid therapeutic contact.

Fourth, although motivation is usually conceptualized as an important component in the early stages of change, it is equally important during maintenance. Despite its numerous health hazards, smoking (i.e., nicotine) may well provide benefits to the smoker, such as mood management, relaxation, and pleasure (United States Department of Health and Human Services, 1988). As new ex-smokers start to realize the effort involved in maintaining abstinence and as they experience the discomforts of withdrawal, they may start to become discouraged and miss the benefits they derived from smoking. A review of the perceived costs and benefits of quitting is thus useful during maintenance. Of concern are the ex-smokers who, despite being abstinent, have thoughts about wishing they did not have to quit, how difficult quitting is, and how disruptive quitting is to their lives. These cognitions need to be addressed directly rather than hoping that the perceived benefits of quitting will outweigh or mask them. Miller and Rollnick's (1991) motivational interviewing techniques are likely to be of value.

Fifth, smokers need to be prepared for the possibility of withdrawal and offered options for coping. Both pharmacological and cognitive–behavioral strategies are of use. The benefits of nicotine replacement may be better realized with the use of transdermal nicotine patches, as they have the potential for overcoming many of the compliance problems and unpleasant side effects associated with nicotine gum (Transdermal Nicotine Study Group, 1991).

Sixth, RP strategies may also need to be tailored to the changing population of smokers. The population of smokers increasingly comprises lower educated individuals from lower socioeconomic groups (Pierce et al., 1989). Traditional clinic treatment approaches may seem less feasible and less accessible to these smokers who may want more low-cost, time-efficient aids (Glynn, Boyd, & Gruman, 1990). Researchers need to work on incorporating many of the RP components into more accessible and effective modalities.

Finally, RP should not stop at the point of relapse. As we noted earlier, relapse may best be seen as one stage in a dynamic process in which smokers cycle back and forth between smoking and abstinence (Prochaska & DiClemente, 1983). Prochaska and DiClemente's stage model (1983) argues for the need to develop interventions specific to the distinct cognitive and behavioral processes that characterize each stage. In order to do this, we need to learn more about the sequelae of relapse and ways to encourage more successful recycling into subsequent cessation attempts.

Acknowledgments

This chapter was supported in part by Grant No. HL42485 from the National Heart, Lung, and Blood Institute and by Grant No. CA42760 from the National Cancer Institute.

REFERENCES

Anda, R. F., Williamson, D. F., Escobedo, L. G., Mast, E. E., Giovino, G. A., & Remington, P. L. (1990). Depression and the dynamics of smoking. *Journal of the American Medical Association, 264,* 1541–1545.

Baer, J. S., Kamarck, T., Lichtenstein, E., & Ransom, C. C. (1989). Prediction of smoking relapse: Analyses of temptations and transgressions after initial cessation. *Journal of Consulting and Clinical Psychology*, 75, 623–627.

Baer, J. S., & Lichtenstein, E. (1988). Classification and prediction of smoking relapse episodes: An exploration of individual differences. *Journal of Consulting and Clinical Psychology*, 56, 104–110.

Brandon, T. H., Tiffany, S. T., Obremski, K. M., & Baker, T. B. (1990). Postcessation cigarette use: The process of relapse. *Addictive Behaviors*, 15, 105–114.

Brandon, T. H., Zelman, D. C., & Baker, T. B. (1987). Effects of maintenance sessions on smoking relapse: Delaying the inevitable? *Journal of Consulting and Clinical Psychology*, 55, 780–782.

Brown, R. A., Lichtenstein, E., McIntyre, K. O., & Harrington-Kostur, J. (1984). Effects of nicotine fading and relapse prevention on smoking cessation. *Journal of Consulting and Clinical Psychology*, 52, 307–308.

Brownell, K. D., Marlatt, G. A., Lichtenstein, E., & Wilson, G. T. (1986). Understanding and preventing relapse. *American Psychologist*, 41, 765–782.

Carmody, T. P. (1990). Preventing relapse in the treatment of nicotine addiction: Current issues and future directions. *Journal of Psychoactive Drugs*, 22, 211–238.

Cohen, S., & Lichtenstein, E. (1990). Partner behaviors that support quitting smoking. *Journal of Consulting and Clinical Psychology*, 58, 304–309.

Cohen, S., Lichtenstein, E., Mermelstein, R., Kingsolver, K., Baer, J. S., & Kamarck, T. (1988). Social support interventions for smoking cessation. In B. H. Gottlieb, (Ed.), *Creating support groups: Formats, processes, and effects* (pp. 211–240). Beverly Hills: Sage.

Cohen, S., Lichtenstein, E., Prochaska, J. O., Rossi, J. S., Gritz, E. R., Carr, C. R., Orleans, C. T., Schoenbach, V. J., Biener, L., Abrams, D., DiClemente, C. C., Curry, S., Marlatt, G. A., Cummings, K. M., Emont, S. L., Giovino, G., & Ossip-Klein, D. J. (1989). Debunking myths about self-quitting: Evidence from 10 prospective studies of persons quitting smoking by themselves. *American Psychologist*, 44, 1355–1365.

Condiotte, M. M., & Lichtenstein, E. (1981). Self-efficacy and relapse in smoking cessation programs. *Journal of Consulting and Clinical Psychology*, 49, 648–658.

Coppotelli, H., & Orleans, C. T. (1985). Partner support and other determinants of smoking cessation maintenance among women. *Journal of Consulting and Clinical Psychology*, 53, 455–460.

Cummings, C., Gordon, J. R., & Marlatt, G. A. (1980). Relapse: Prevention and prediction. In W. R. Miller (Ed.), *The addictive behaviors: Treatment of alcoholism, drug abuse, smoking, and obesity* (pp. 291–321). New York: Pergamon Press.

Cummings, K. M., Jaen, C. R., & Giovino, G. (1985). Circumstances surrounding relapse in a group of recent exsmokers. *Preventive Medicine*, 14, 195–202.

Curry, S., Marlatt, G. A., & Gordon, J. R. (1987). Abstinence violation effect:

Validation of an attributional construct with smoking cessation. *Journal of Consulting and Clinical Psychology, 55,* 145–149.

Curry, S., Marlatt, G. A., Gordon, J., & Baer, J. S. (1988). A comparison of alternative theoretical approaches to smoking cessation and relapse. *Health Psychology, 7,* 545–556.

Davis, A. L., Faust, R., & Ordentlich, M. (1984). Self-help smoking cessation and maintenance programs: A comparative study with 12-month follow-up by the American Lung Association. *American Journal of Public Health, 74,* 1212–1217.

Davis, J. R., & Glaros, A. G. (1986). Relapse prevention and smoking cessation. *Addictive Behaviors, 11,* 105–114.

Fagerstrom, K. O. (1988). Efficacy of nicotine chewing gum: A review. In O. F. Pomerleau & C. S. Pomerleau (Eds.), *Nicotine replacement: A critical evaluation* (pp. 109–128). New York: Alan R. Liss.

Glasgow, R. E., & Lichtenstein, E. (1987). Long-term effects of behavioral smoking cessation interventions. *Behavior Therapy, 18,* 297–324.

Glassman, A. H., Helzer, J. E., Covey, L. S., Cottler, L. B., Stetner, F., Jayson, E. T., & Johnson, J. (1990). Smoking, smoking cessation, and major depression. *Journal of the American Medical Association, 264,* 1546–1549.

Glynn, T. J., Boyd, G. M., & Gruman, J. C. (1990). Essential elements of self-help/minimal intervention strategies for smoking cessation. *Health Education Quarterly, 17,* 329–345.

Goldstein, M. S., Niaura, R., Follick, M. J., & Abrams, D. B. (1989). Effects of behavioral skills training and schedule of nicotine gum administration on smoking cessation. *American Journal of Psychiatry, 146,* 56–60.

Gruder, C. L., Mermelstein, R., Kirkendol, S., Hedeker, D., Wong, S. C., Schreckengost, J., Warnecke, R. B., Burzette, R., & Miller, T. Q. (1992). Effects of social support and relapse prevention training on the long-term effectiveness of a televised smoking cessation intervention. *Journal of Consulting and Clinical Psychology.*

Hall, S. M. (1988, August). *Smoking, sweets, and sadness: Dependence, treatment failure, and regularity systems.* Paper presented at the annual meeting of the American Psychological Association, Atlanta, GA.

Hall, S. M., Ginsberg, D., & Jones, R. T. (1986). Smoking cessation and weight gain. *Journal of Consulting and Clinical Psychology, 54,* 342–346.

Hall, S. M., Munoz, R., & Reus, V. (1991, June). *Depression and smoking treatment: A clinical trial of an affect regulation treatment.* Paper presented at the Fifty-Third Annual Scientific Meeting of the Committee on Problems of Drug Dependence, Palm Beach, FL.

Hall, S., Rugg, D., Tunstall, C., & Jones, R. (1984). Preventing relapse to cigarette smoking by behavioral skill training. *Journal of Consulting and Clinical Psychology, 52,* 372–382.

Hall, S. M., Tunstall, C. D., Ginsberg, D., Benowitz, N. L., & Jones, R. T. (1987). Nicotine gum and behavioral treatment: A placebo controlled trial. *Journal of Consulting and Clinical Psychology, 55,* 603–605.

Harackiewicz, J. M., Sansone, C., Blair, L. W., Epstein, J. A., & Manderlink, G.

(1987). Attributional processes in behavior change and maintenance: Smoking cessation and continued abstinence. *Journal of Consulting and Clinical Psychology, 55,* 372–378.

Hughes, G. H., Hymowitz, N., Ockene, J. K., Simon, N., & Vogt, T. M. (1981). The Multiple Risk Factor Intervention Trial (MRFIT) V: Intervention on smoking. *Preventive Medicine, 10,* 289–294.

Hunt, W. A., Barnett, L. W., & Branch, L. G. (1971). Relapse rates in addiction programs. *Journal of Clinical Psychology, 27,* 455–456.

Killen, J. D., Fortmann, S. P., Newman, B., & Varady, A. (1990). Evaluations of a treatment approach combining nicotine gum with self-guided behavioral treatments for smoking relapse prevention. *Journal of Consulting and Clinical Psychology, 58,* 85–92.

Klesges, R. C., Benowitz, N. L., & Meyers, A. W. (1991). Behavioral and biobehavioral aspects of smoking and smoking cessation: The problem of postcessation weight gain. *Behavior Therapy, 22,* 179–199.

Kottke, T. E., Battista, R. N., DeFriese, G. H., & Brekke, M. L. (1988). Attributes of successful smoking cessation interventions in medical practice. *Journal of the American Medical Association, 259,* 2883–2889.

Lam, W., Sacks, H. S., Sze, P. C., & Chalmers, T. C. (1987). Meta-analysis of randomized controlled trials of nicotine chewing gum. *Lancet, 2,* 27–30.

Lando, H. A. (1982). A factorial analysis of preparation, aversion, and maintenance in the elimination of smoking. *Addictive Behaviors, 7,* 143–154.

Lando, H. A., & McGovern, P. G. (1985). Nicotine fading as a nonaversive alternative in a broad-spectrum treatment for eliminating smoking. *Addictive Behaviors, 10,* 153–161.

Lichtenstein, E., & Glasgow, R. E. (1992). Smoking cessation: What have we learned over the past decade? *Journal of Consulting and Clinical Psychology.*

Lichtenstein, E., Glasgow, R. E., & Abrams, D. B. (1986). Social support in smoking cessation: In search of effective interventions. *Behavior Therapy, 17,* 607–619.

Malott, J. M., Glasgow, R. E., O'Neill, H. K., & Klesges, R. C. (1984). Co-worker social support in a worksite smoking control program. *Journal of Applied Behavior Analysis, 17,* 485–495.

Marlatt, G. A., Curry, S., & Gordon, J. R. (1988). A longitudinal analysis of unaided smoking cessation. *Journal of Consulting and Clinical Psychology, 56,* 715–720.

Marlatt, G. A., & George, W. H. (1984). Relapse prevention: Introduction and overview of the model. *British Journal of Addiction, 79,* 261–273.

Marlatt, G. A., & Gordon, J. R. (1980). Determinants of relapse: Implications for the maintenance of behavior change. In P. O. Davidson & S. M. Davidson (Eds.), *Behavioral medicine: Changing health lifestyles* (pp. 410–452). New York: Brunner/Mazel.

Marlatt, G. A., & Gordon, J. R. (Eds.). (1985). *Relapse prevention: Maintenance strategies in the treatment of addictive behaviors.* New York: Guilford Press.

McIntyre-Kingsolver, K. O., Lichtenstein, E., & Mermelstein, R. (1986). Spouse training in a multicomponent smoking cessation program. *Behavior Therapy, 17,* 67–74.

Mermelstein, R., Cohen, S., Lichtenstein, E., Baer, J. S., & Kamarck, T. (1986). Social support and smoking cessation and maintenance. *Journal of Consulting and Clinical Psychology, 54,* 447–453.

Mermelstein, R., Gruder, C. L., Koepke, D., Kirkendol, S., & Warnecke, R. B. (1990, April). *Patterns and predictors of relapse and recycling in a minimal smoking cessation intervention.* Paper presented at the annual meeting of the Society of Behavioral Medicine, Chicago, IL.

Mermelstein, R., Lichtenstein, E., & McIntyre, K. O. (1983). Partner support and relapse in smoking cessation programs. *Journal of Consulting and Clinical Psychology, 51,* 465–466.

Miller, W. R., & Rollnick, S. (1991). *Motivational interviewing: Preparing people to change addictive behavior.* New York: Guilford Press.

Niaura, R. S., Rohsenow, D. J., Binkoff, J. A., Monti, P. M., Pedraza, M., & Abrams, D. B. (1988). Relevance of cue reactivity to understanding alcohol and smoking relapse. *Journal of Abnormal Psychology, 97,* 133–152.

O'Connell, K. A., & Martin, E. J. (1987). Highly tempting situations associated with abstinence, temporary lapse, and relapse among participants in smoking cessation programs. *Journal of Consulting and Clinical Psychology, 55,* 367–371.

Orleans, C. T., Schoenbach, V. J., Wagner, E. H., Quade, D., Salmon, J. A., Pearson, D. C., Fiedler, J., Porter, C. Q., & Kaplan, B. H. (1991). Self-help quit smoking interventions: Effects of self-help materials, social support instructions, and telephone counseling. *Journal of Consulting and Clinical Psychology, 59,* 439–448.

Ossip-Klein, D. J., Bigelow, G., Parker, S. R., Curry, S., Hall, S. M., & Kirkland, S. (1986). Classification and assessment of smoking behavior. *Health Psychology, 5,* 3–11.

Pierce, J. P., Fiore, M. C., Novotny, T. E., Hatziandreu, E. J., & Davis, R. M. (1989). Trends in cigarette smoking in the United States: Projections to the year 2000. *Journal of the American Medical Association, 261,* 61–65.

Prochaska, J. O., & DiClemente, C. C. (1983). Stages and processes of self-change of smoking: Toward an integrative model of change. *Journal of Consulting and Clinical Psychology, 51,* 390–395.

Schwartz, J. L. (1987). *Review and evaluation of smoking cessation methods: The United States and Canada, 1978–1985* (NIH Publication No. 87-2940). Bethesda, MD: U.S. Department of Health and Human Services, Public Health Service, National Institute of Health, National Cancer Institute, Division of Cancer Prevention and Control.

Shiffman, S. (1982). Relapse following smoking cessation: A situational analysis. *Journal of Consulting and Clinical Psychology, 50,* 71–86.

Shiffman, S. (1989). Conceptual issues in the study of relapse. In M. Gossop (Ed.), *Relapse and addictive behavior* (pp. 149–179). New York: Tavistock/ Routledge.

Shiffman, S., Shumaker, S. A., Abrams, D. B., Cohen, S., Garvey, A., Grunberg, N. E., & Swan, G. E. (1986). Models of smoking relapse. *Health Psychology, 5,* 13–27.

Spring, B., Wurtman, J., Gleason, R., Wurtman, R., & Kessler, K. (1991).

Weight gain and withdrawal symptoms after smoking cessation: A preventive intervention using d-fenfluramine. *Health Psychology, 10,* 216–223.

Stevens, V. J., & Hollis, J. F. (1989). Preventing smoking relapse using an individually tailored skills-training technique. *Journal of Consulting and Clinical Psychology, 57,* 420–424.

Swan, G. E., & Denk, C. E. (1987). Dynamic models for the maintenance of smoking cessation: Event history analysis of late relapse. *Journal of Behavioral Medicine, 10,* 527–554.

Transdermal Nicotine Study Group. (1991). Transdermal nicotine for smoking cessation: Six-month results from two multicenter controlled clinical trials. *Journal of the American Medical Association, 266,* 3133–3138.

U.S. Department of Health and Human Services. (1988). *The health consequences of smoking: Nicotine addiction—A report of the Surgeon General* (DHHS Publication No. 88-8406). Washington, DC: U.S. Government Printing Office.

U.S. Department of Health and Human Services. (1989). *Reducing the health consequences of smoking. A report of the Surgeon General* (DHHS Publication No. CDC 89-8411). Washington, DC: U.S. Government Printing Office.

OBESITY

William Fremouw
Diana Damer
WEST VIRGINIA UNIVERSITY

O besity is the biological condition of excessive body fat. Depending on the criteria used, 10%–50% of the United States population is obese (Bray, 1987). The prevalence of obesity is even greater among some ethnic groups and tends to increase as age increases and social class decreases (Stunkard, 1975). Approximately 90% of the obese population is mildly obese (20%–40% overweight), while 9% are moderately obese (41%–100% overweight) and severely obese (greater than 100% overweight), respectively (Stunkard, 1984).

Obesity is recognized as one of the most serious and prominent health problems in the United States. Obesity has been associated with impairments of pulmonary function, gallbladder disease, trauma to weight-carrying joints, and cancer (Bray, 1987). In addition, an excess accumulation of fat in the abdominal region rather than total fat mass increases the risk of cardiovascular disease (Bjorntorp, 1985). Overall, obesity is associated with an increase in mortality in both males and females. In a prospective study by the American Cancer Society, the mortality ratio for major diseases was computed in relation to degree of overweight. The mortality rates were five times greater for men and almost eight times greater for women who were 40% or more overweight. Overall, obesity is a very serious medical and psychological problem in the United States.

DEFINITION OF "OBESITY"

Unlike many of the other problems reviewed in this book, obesity is not a behavioral disorder. Rather, it is a biological condition that is the product of a complex interaction between heredity, metabolism, and eating-exercise behaviors. The most common way to define "obesity" has been by the measurement of weight at given heights. The 1960 and 1983 Metropolitan Company Weight Tables are the most widely used for this purpose. These tables define "obesity" as a minimum of 20% above the ideal weight for a particular height. However, height–weight tables can often be misleading if they are used as the sole indicator of a weight problem. A person may exceed the ideal weight for his/her height but not be obese. Muscular athletes may be overweight for their height, but their bodies contain little fat. A typical adult male's body is composed of 14% fat, while the average adult female has 24% body fat (Stuart & Davis, 1972). To directly assess percentage of body fat, more specialized techniques are needed, such as measures of skin-fold thickness. This requires an experienced evaluator and skin-fold calipers measuring skin thickness at three to four body sites. An even more accurate means for measuring obesity is hydrostatic weighing. A person is submerged in a body of water and the amount of water displaced is determined. This procedure, while accurate, is expensive and seldom available. Overall, obesity is typically first defined by weight at least 20% greater than the height–weight norms accompanied by a self-definition of the client that he/she is obese.

TREATMENTS

While most obese Americans are in the mild range and have few medical complications, as the degree of obesity increases the risk of medical and health-related problems dramatically increases. Each year, millions of dollars are spent on weight loss programs, books, and products.

The history of behavioral programs for weight loss can be divided into three generations of research (Brownell & Jeffery, 1987). The first generation of studies were initial demonstrations of specific behavioral techniques for weight loss. Based on 15 studies in 1974, the average program lasted 8 weeks and only produced an 8-pound weight loss. Follow-ups were done an average of 8 weeks after the program (Brownell & Jeffery, 1987). These initial programs with such modest weight losses clearly did not produce major improvements for anyone who is moderately or severely obese. After these initial demonstration studies of specific components, combinations of treatment components were used for weight loss. The combinations usually included self-monitoring, teaching of stimulus control techniques, and financial and social reinforcement strategies. Several treatment manuals were published and major community programs, such as Weight Watchers, adopted many of these procedures (Stuart, 1978; Mahoney & Mahoney, 1976). In spite of their widespread popularity and acceptance, the programs did not produce dramatic weight losses and maintenance successes. These programs conducted in 1978 averaged a length of treatment of 10½ weeks and produced a 1-pound loss per week. Follow-ups were extended to 30 weeks and showed that on the average, participants had lost 9 pounds from the beginning of the program. Thus, these programs with longer follow-ups did not demonstrate continued weight loss or major improvement from the initial generation of behavioral studies. Stunkard and Penick (1979) reviewed the results of these follow-up studies and concluded that clinically important weight losses obtained by behavioral treatments were rare and that those losses that did occur were not well maintained.

These discouraging results after the initial enthusiasm for behavioral treatments led to more intensive efforts to improve weight loss and maintenance. For example, Fremouw, Callahan, Zitter, and Kattell (1981) treated four moderately obese women in a single-subject design format for 25 weeks while monitoring and changing specific behaviors such as location of eating, snacking, and meal duration. Three of the four subjects lost between 18 and 22 pounds and maintained total weight losses of 14 to 20 pounds for 3 months after treatment. In Kattal, Callahan, Fremouw, and Zitter (1979), another case study was reported of a behavioral treatment that included fasting and a liquid protein diet. This individualized program led to specific behavioral changes and included a 54-pound weight loss that was maintained for 1 year. Other researchers such as Perri, Shapiro, Ludwig, Twentyman, and McAdoo (1984) demonstrated group mean weight loss of 18.9 pounds, while Brownell and Stunkard (1981) achieved 18.2-pound weight losses.

As summarized by Brownell and Jeffery (1987), six large-scale studies conducted in 1986 with subjects' initial weights averaging 210 pounds reported a mean of 22-pound weight loss after 16 weeks. The follow-up period for these six studies was 44 weeks and showed that the final weight losses were 14 pounds from the original weight, still well above the ideal target weight. These more intensive programs included refined reinforcement procedures, incorporated cognitive components, and used long-term maintenance strategies such as regular exercise and techniques to increase social support. Another major difference in these latter and more successful programs was the length of treatment, 22 weeks. Brownell and Jeffery (1987) concluded that programs less than 16 weeks are not long enough to produce any meaningful weight loss or maintenance. They suggest that if programs are at least 4 months in duration and include additonal components such as exercise, social support, and the standard behavioral techniques, then a 20–30-pound weight loss can be achieved. These studies lead to the larger question of the appropriate goal for treatment. Since few behavioral treatments lead to the moderate to severely obese person's reaching the ideal weight, the goal to maintain weight loss may be premature. Maintaining a 20-pound weight loss while a person is still 40 to 60 pounds overweight is statistically significant but may not clinically alter the medical or psychological problems associated with that degree of obesity. A newer goal of treatment programs may be to create long-term weight loss based on previously learned techniques as opposed to just maintaining a partial reduction of obesity. New generations of studies may require continued involvement in permanent long-term programs such as Weight Watchers to provide overall success for the obesity treatment program, since initial treatment efforts seldom reach the ultimate goal weight. This would be comparable to recovering alcoholics who continue their involvement in Alcoholics Anonymous even years after they last consumed alcohol.

Because of the great difficulty in achieving meaningful weight loss and maintaining it, some reviewers have challenged the assumption that mild obesity, without medical complications, should be treated at all. For example, Wooley and Wooley (1984) and Smith and Fremouw (1987), after reviews of the treatment literature, questioned both the effectiveness and the wisdom of the continued effort to treat mild or moderate obesity unless a medical problem exists. Research with laboratory rats dramatically demonstrated the lasting negative effect of unsuccessful attempts at weight loss on subsequent body weight (Brownell, Greenwood, Stellar, & Shrager, 1986). Rats were given free access to high-fat foods until they became obese. They were then put on diets and later refed for two cycles of weight loss and gain. The rats lost weight during the second cycle at only half the rate of the first, and they regained their weight at three times the rate of the first cycle. After these cycles of weight loss or weight gain, rats had a significantly elevated number of fat cells and a higher percentage of body fat than controls who did not diet. These results show that weight cycling increased the amount of fat and metabolic efficiency among laboratory animals. These data suggest that this may occur with humans in that repeated unsuccessful dieting significantly improves metabolic efficiency, which makes further weight loss difficult (Brownell, 1988). Based on these concerns (e.g., Wooley & Wooley, 1984), some argue for a change of treatment goals from just weight loss with a high risk of relapse to altering the self-image and attitudes that create the motivation to lose relatively small amounts of weight.

GOALS AND RP

Relapse prevention (RP) for obesity is often discussed in the context of RP for alcohol abuse, smoking, and drug use (Brownell, Marlatt, Lichtenstein, & Wilson, 1986). However, there is one fundamental difference between obesity and these other problem areas. As discussed by Corcoran (1987), obesity is a biological state that is a combination of both physiological and behavioral components. It is not directly parallel to problem behaviors such as alcohol abuse or smoking. Many obese people do not eat more than those who are not obese (Jeffery, Wing, & Stunkard, 1978). Therefore, excessive eating behaviors are not always the problem in the treatment of obesity. Instead the combination of eating behavior, exercise, genetics, and metabolic rate must be considered.

Furthermore, with eating, in contrast to smoking or drinking, the goal of abstinence is not appropriate. Obviously, everyone must eat. The goal for obesity treatment is the development of healthy or controlled eating and exercise habits, not the elimination of certain problems or behaviors. Therefore, the definition of "relapse" is more difficult. Rosenthal and Marx (1981) suggested that a lapse or slip for obesity be operationally defined as any 24-hour period during which a person did not use a method of weight control. They further defined "relapse" as having gained 5 pounds during a 60-day period of the treatment program.

This definition combines and confuses process behaviors (slips) with biological outcomes (e.g., weight gains) (Corcoran, 1987). Other researchers have just defined maintainers or relapsers according to varying weight gains at different points of follow-up. For example, Wing and Jeffery (1978) defined "maintenance" as a regain of less than 20%, while Gormally, Rardin, and Black (1980) used a definition of regaining no more than 30% as successful maintenance. Overall, there is no clear definition of "relapse" in the obesity area. Furthermore, an experimenter-defined definition of "relapse" does not consider the person's own definition of successful maintenance or failure. A 5-pound regain of weight may be acceptable to one client while viewed as utter failure by another. Overall, this whole area is cloudy. Within the cognitive–behavioral RP model (Marlatt & Gordon, 1985), a slip or lapse is the first consumption of a target substance after a period of abstinence. Since, in obesity, abstinence is not the appropriate goal, a slip would constitute the uncontrolled use of food after a period of controlled use. A problem becomes defining the difference between the controlled and uncontrolled consumption of food. Obviously, it is much easier in other areas such as alcohol and smoking, since any consumption of alcohol or cigarettes is a clear violation of treatment goals. In the weight loss area, daily calories consumed can be a general treatment goal on which to base slips or lapses. Over time, the comsumption of an excessive number of calories will lead to an unwanted weight gain.

Because of the difficulty in defining specific behavioral targets for changing the biological state of obesity, Fremouw, Seime, and Wiener (1987) conceptualized the goal for treatment of eating disorders as increasing the number of healthy days a person has each week. A healthy day is defined as eating at a prescribed moderate level of calorie consumption, accompanied by moderate levels of exercise and absence of unhealthy eating-related behavior such as fasting, vomiting, or using laxatives. By the use of this multidimensional behavioral goal, a "lapse" or "slip" could be defined as the absence of a healthy day and "relapse" could be defined as the accumulation of more than three lapses in a given week. Unfortunately, these suggested definitions have not yet been widely adopted as obesity treatment goals.

FACTORS PRODUCING LAPSES AND RELAPSES

In a study of factors influencing obesity treatment relapse, Sternberg (1985) reported that 67% of 28 subjects had regained 5 pounds or more during a 60-day posttreatment period. Of the people who did not relapse, 89% reported that they had continued to self-monitor calorie intake as a major strategy for weight maintenance compared to only 53% of those who regained during this period. Sternberg (1985) also found that interpersonal factors were associated with 52% of slips for dieters. These interpersonal factors included positive emotional states such as celebrations or parties, social pressure, and/or interpersonal conflict. Negative emotional states preceded 32% of the dieting slips and positive emotional states preceded another 11% of noninterpersonal situations. Overall, 75% of the relapses for dieters were preceded by either positive or negative emotional states.

In another examination of lapses and relapses, Grilo, Shiffman, and Wing (1989) allowed their subjects to define "lapses" according to their own criteria and not depend on a weekly calorie goal. The subjects also self-defined temptations to overeat. Interestingly, what constituted a lapse differed widely. Two thirds of lapses were eating binges of 2,000 to 3,400 calories at one episode while one third of lapses involved only the consumption of forbidden foods without excessive caloric intake. This approach to self-definition of lapses begins to address the subjective problem of subject-defined violations while still providing some objective data on the significance of the lapse. Using cluster analyses, the data from the lapses showed that approximately half of the diet lapses occurred in social mealtime situations. Approximately 10% of the lapses occurred during an emotional upset such as anger, and the third group showed that the remaining 40% of the lapses occurred during periods of solitude, low arousal, or "downtimes." From this study, two major factors emerged as antecedents for eating lapses: (1) food-specific cues and (2) affective states. The presence of strong affective states such as anger reduced controlled eating. The authors also reported that the difference between a temptation that is successfully controlled and a lapse is not the situation itself but the person's ability to engage in coping responses when the temptation occurs. The study identifies two general high-risk situations: foods and social situations and affective emotional situations and a major psychological coping skill. Based on their findings, specific coping strategies in these situations should be included in obesity RP programs.

RP STRATEGIES

In a recent integrative review of RP in smoking, alcoholism, and obesity, Brownell et al. (1986b) organized long-term maintenance strategies into three categories: (1) extend treatment by adding booster sessions, (2) add more components to the treatment package, and (3) adopt a model of lifelong treatment. The authors recommend prevention of both lapses and relapses at three stages of change (motivation and commitment, initial change, and maintenance).

At the first stage, Brownell et al. (1986b) propose methods to enhance motivation and commitment, primarily contingency management (e.g., financial contracts) and screening procedures. With screening, clients who are not appropriate for behavioral treatment (i.e., do not meet established criteria) can be referred to other programs or cautioned to wait until their motivation is higher. At the second stage, initial behavioral change, the authors suggest that decision making, cognitive restructuring, coping skills, and cue extinction be employed, The final stage is maintenance, which entails continued monitoring, social support, general life-style change, programmed relapse, and a special role for exercise. The remainder of this chapter deals with maintenance, although RP may be appropriate at any of the three stages. Several maintenance strategies will now be reviewed.

Long-term monitoring appears to be very effective in the maintenance phase of treatment. Evidence suggests that as therapeutic contacts increase during follow-up, maintenance improves (Perri et al., 1984). Early empirical evaluations of booster sessions were disappointing; however, as the programs have become more complex, their efficacy has increased (Dubbert, Terre, Holm, & Brown, 1987). Unfortunately, the issue of where treatment ends and where maintenance begins may become blurred, and continued contact with a therapist may simply postpone rather than prevent relapse (Brownell et al., 1986b). Brownell and Jeffery (1987) recommend that obesity should be conceptualized as a chronic problem analogous to hypertension or diabetes. The implication is that treatment should be maintained on a relatively permanent basis.

Increasing social support has often been offered as a strategy to enhance long-term weight loss; studies designed to evaluate the effects of social support have generated inconsistent results. Brownell et al. (1986) note that variability among social relationships may be largely responsible for the lack of consistent findings across studies. Some social interactions may facilitate weight loss, while others may sabotage it. Craighead and Agras (1991) suggest that combining pharmacological treatment (anorexiant and antidepressant medication) with behavioral therapy over the long term may enhance weight loss. Pharmacological treatment has not been shown to be effective alone; however, it may prove useful in combination with behavioral therapy for persons not responding well to behavioral therapy alone. Life-style change (Marlatt & Gordon, 1985), the idea that eating can be replaced by other rewarding and incompatible behaviors, is often offered as a strategy for long-term weight loss. Exercise is a major predictor of long-term weight loss success (Cohen, Gelfand, Dodd, Jensen, & Turner, 1980) and may play an integral role in life-style change. Numerous possible explanations for why exercise may help prevent relapse have been offered. Exercise (e.g., running) has been described as a positive addiction (Glasser, 1976), which may replace negative addictions (e.g., bingeing) or function to enhance self-esteem and increase self-efficacy. Alternatively, exercise may provide a peer group that encourages healthy habits or may decrease the appetite through direct physiological processes (Brownell et al., 1986b) (although anecdotally many people report increased appetite following exercise). A final possible explanation is that adherence is a relatively dichotomous phenomenon—a person who is dedicated enough to follow an exercise regimen is more likely to also comply with dietary recommendations.

A more direct approach is to address the relapse phenomenon specifically. Assuming relapse involves a specific chain of events, developing the skills to identify high-risk situations and learning strategies to counteract the detrimental psychological consequences of relapse should prove helpful (Brownell & Jeffery, 1987). Programmed relapse has received attention but has not gained wide acceptance or been proven to be effective. In programmed relapse, the individual purposefully binges in a safe environment (i.e., in the presence of the therapist) after being instructed in coping strategies. This, it is hoped, allows the client to experience the lapse, cope successfully, and prevent the lapse from developing into a relapse (Brownell et al., 1986).

OUTCOME OF MAINTENANCE AND RP STUDIES

Several studies have evaluated the efficacy of maintenance treatments with different components. Kramer, Jeffery, Snell, and Forster (1986) assigned successful weight losers to one of three maintenance treatments: (1) monthly financial contingencies for weight maintenance, (2) monthly financial contingencies for participation in skills-training sessions to solidify behavioral changes, and (3) nontreatment. All clients had been initially 130%–150% above ideal and had lost at least 10% of their body weight during a 15-week behavioral weight loss program. The subjects had initially deposited $195, $75 of which was used during the weight loss program. The remaining $120 was used to provide incentives for maintenance.

Controls received a refund of $100 immediately and the final $20 was returned at the 1-year follow-up. Subjects in the other two conditions met in groups once a month for 1 year. In the skills focus group, clients were taught to practice selecting appropriate foods and engaging in healthy exercise. Ten dollars was returned for attendance at each meeting. Money that was forfeited was later divided among subjects who attended 11 of the 12 groups. In the weight focus group, subjects discussed problems in maintenance. They forfeited $10 for each session if they either did not attend or weighed more than they had posttreatment. Subjects who weighed less than or equal to their posttreatment weight at the end of maintenance received refunds and shared forfeited monies. No significant differences between treatment conditions were found. Substantial regains of 40% of initial losses were reported in all three groups. It should be noted that this program focused strictly on contingency management in maintenance without any specific training in RP.

Other studies have incorporated RP in their maintenance strategies, without labeling the relapse component. Abrams and Follick (1983) evaluated the efficacy of a behavioral weight loss and maintenance program in the workplace. Participants were randomly assigned to three groups matched for percentage overweight. The three groups of subjects received a 10-week behavioral treatment program which included traditional elements such as stimulus control, goal setting, self-monitoring, and cognitive restructuring along with organizational-level social influence procedures (group cooperation and competition techniques such as posting average weight loss for each group). Following the weight loss program, two of the groups received a standard behavioral maintenance program consisting of skills training in generalization and maintenance of weight loss. The other group received a nonspecific maintenance program, involving no new input from therapists. Both maintenance programs involved four biweekly sessions. The structured maintenance program consisted of fading self-monitoring (internalizing the process), structured problem solving, programmed relapse, and enlisting of social support for enhancing maintenance of weight loss. The results indicated that all three groups lost a significant amount of weight, although attrition was high. However, participants in the structured maintenance program successfully maintained their losses while the nonspecific maintenance group did not. The authors concluded that the skills necessary to lose weight are different from those necessary to maintain weight loss.

Similarly, Perri et al. (1988) evaluated the efficacy of four maintenance programs. Twenty men and 97 women were randomly assigned by blocks stratified by percentage over ideal weight to one of five conditions: (1) behavioral therapy only; (2) behavioral therapy plus a posttreatment therapist-contact maintenance program; (3) behavioral therapy plus posttreatment contact plus a social influence maintenance program; (4) behavioral therapy plus posttreatment therapist contact plus aerobic exercise maintenance program; or (5) behavioral therapy plus posttreatment therapist contact plus both the aerobic exercise and social influence maintenance programs.

Behavioral therapy alone consisted of 20 weekly group sessions in which clients were instructed in self-control procedures such as self-monitoring, stimulus control, and self-reinforcement. In the first maintenance treatment, subjects received the behavioral therapy program plus a posttreatment maintenance program involving 26 biweekly therapist contacts, which included weigh-ins, reviewing self-monitoring, and problem solving. In the second maintenance treatment, clients received the behavioral treatment, the posttreatment therapist-contact programs, and a program of social influence strategies designed to maximize motivation. This involved monetary group contingencies for program adherence and continued weight loss, active participation in preparing program content, and instruction on providing support for peers via periodic telephone contacts. In the third maintenance treatment, the clients received the initial behavioral treatment, the posttreatment therapist contact, and an aerobic exercise maintenance program that involved a new set of exercise goals for the posttreatment period and exercise during the biweekly posttreatment sessions. During the initial 6 months of the maintenance program, the intensity of the exercise was gradually increased. In the final maintenance treatment, clients were given the initial behavioral program, the posttreatment contact programs, and the aerobic exercise and social influence maintenance programs.

At the end of treatment, all five programs resulted in significant amounts of weight loss (27.39 pounds) and did not differ significantly from one another. At the 6-month follow-up however, the four maintenance conditions exhibited significantly better weight loss than the behavioral-therapy-only condition. The final most inclusive program (behavioral therapy, posttreatment contact, and both the aerobic exercise and social influence maintenance programs) demonstrated a significant additional weight loss of 9 pounds. At the 12-month follow-up, all four programs demonstrated significantly better maintenance than the behavioral-therapy-only conditions, which showed relapse. The superiority of the four conditions was maintained at an 18-month follow-up. The posttreatment contact was not labeled RP training, although the problem solving employed was consistent with the RP model. The results of this study were impressive; however, the fact that therapist contact was not controlled renders it difficult to interpret the efficacy of specific components.

In a study that evaluated the efficacy of RP more directly and thoroughly, Sternberg (1985) assigned 43 subjects to a standard behavioral or RP condition. The standard program consisted of components such as record keeping, stimulus control procedures, and assertiveness training. The treatment program consisted of nine weekly 2-hour sessions. The first hour was devoted to weigh-ins and training in large groups. The second hour involved small groups discussions. Participants in the RP program attended the same standard behavioral program for the first hour. During the second hour they also met in small groups. Although the total therapist contact time was equal for the two programs, the RP program involved new information during the small group format. The major emphasis of their small group component was changing thoughts and self-statements regarding high-risk eating situations. Subjects were first taught to identify high-risk situations and classify them into general problem categories. Then they engaged in discussion during which alternative ways of coping with these difficult situations were generated.

Next, participants were instructed to keep a record of "wants" and "shoulds" and attempt to achieve a good balance of these types of activities. They were then taught Marlatt and Gordon's (1980) notion of apparently irrelevant decisions, the idea that a person makes small decisions over time that bring him/her closer to a relapse. Participants learned to identify these decisions early in the chain of events. For example, they might use the strategy of examining their thoughts when they felt tempted to buy food that might eventually lead to a relapse. The next component involved a discussion of lapses, relapse, and self-efficacy. Participants discussed lapses and relapses and how they handled them. They were instructed to evaluate their thoughts and feelings before, during, and after lapses.

Finally, the abstinence violation effect, a phenomenon in which the entire diet is abandoned after one small slip, was addressed. For example, dieters who reason. "Oh well, I've already eaten one cookie, I might as well go ahead and eat the whole box," were assured that although they may feel guilty if they overeat, it does not mean that they are failures and must totally surrender control of their eating.

Although participants in the two programs lost similar amounts of weight during treatment (average of 10 pounds), more participants in the RP program continued to lose weight posttreatment (41% vs. 22%). Also, more RP subjects maintained their posttreatment weight losses without additional gains than those who received the standard treatment (27% vs. 14%). Overall, this is the first study that directly applied Marlatt and Gordon's (1985) RP model to weight loss; it demonstrated clear superiority over traditional strategies during the maintenance phase.

In a more comprehensive study, Perri et al. (1984) evaluated the effects of both RP training ad posttreatment client–therapist contact (mail and telephone) on maintenance of weight loss. Obese volunteers who were approximately 57% over ideal weight were randomly assigned to one of six experimental conditions: One of three treatment conditions (nonbehavioral therapy, behavioral therapy, or behavioral therapy plus RP training) coupled with one of two posttreatment contact conditions (no posttreatment contact or therapist contact by phone and mail). In the nonbehavioral therapy group, subjects were told that restriction of calories combined with increased exercise would yield weight losses. They were provided with the American Diabetes Association exchange plan along with an exercise program. Identifying the "underlying reasons" for eating was also emphasized. The behavioral therapy group was informed that obesity is the result of poor eating habits. The goal of the program was to establish more adaptive eating and exercise patterns. The standard type of behavioral program was employed, including self-monitoring, stimulus control strategies, self-reinforcement, and procedures to control the act of eating.

The behavioral therapy plus the RP training program was designed to enhance the behavioral therapy with techniques aimed specifically at preventing relapse and increasing maintenance of behavioral change and weight loss. Participants first received the standard behavioral therapy program and then received RP training (Marlatt & Gordon, 1985), which consisted of teaching participants to identify high-risk situations and generate coping strategies. Participants then practiced coping with these situations—dinner at an Italian restaurant and a "pitch-in party" with high-risk snack foods. Last, participants were trained in cognitive strategies to cope with the guilt and sense of inefficacy associated with lapses. They were told to view the situation as a learning experience and an opportunity to practice an appropriate coping response.

In the posttreatment contact condition, subjects received 22 postcards and were instructed to return one per week to their therapist during the first 24 weeks subsequent to treatment. Subjects recorded weight-related information (e.g., calories consumed, exercise, weight) the specifics of which depended on the treatment group to which they had initially been assigned. After receipt of the postcard, the therapist called each client to briefly discuss the information the postcard contained. During the first 12 weeks, therapists telephoned once a week. After that, calls were gradually faded. All subjects were successful in losing weight (average = 19 pounds), but the losses were not well maintained during follow-up. The posttreatment contact significantly increased weight loss maintenance for the nonbehavioral treatment and behavioral therapy plus RP training groups but did not improve maintenance in groups that received behavioral therapy only. At 12 months follow-up, subjects in the behavioral therapy plus RP training with posttreatment contact were the only ones who maintained their posttreatment weight loss. This ambitious study begins to show that successful maintenance of moderate weight loss may require RP training plus continued contact to maintain motivation.

CLINICAL AND RESEARCH RECOMMENDATIONS

Overall, the study of RP for obesity suffers from several major problems. First, the definition of "relapse" in the obesity treatment field needs to be clarified. Researchers have used both weight gain and failure to maintain behavioral change strategies as definitions of relapse. There is no generally accepted amount of weight gain or appropriate time period for loss of behavioral control. These definitions also fail to consider the individual's perception of success or failure. A 3-pound weight gain may be considered failure to one subject and an acceptable amount of fluctuation to another. Second, the appropriate definition of a lapse or slip needs clarification. Without clear behavioral definitions for controlled eating and/or exercise, it is difficult to define a violation of the behavioral change program. Without clear definitions of lapses and relapses this research will not easily progress.

The foregoing review suggests that maintenance strategies that do not specifically incorporate RP strategies are not as effective. Most of the studies employing RP (e.g., Sternberg, 1984; Perri et al., 1984) have met with positive results. However, there is also evidence that RP needs to be supplemented by additional posttreatment contact (Perri et al., 1984). Furthermore, Grilo et al.'s (1989) findings suggest that future RP training should specifically address the two most common high-risk situations: (1) food-social settings and (2) emotional-affective states. Additional training in resisting temptations is also needed to prevent the initial lapses.

Overall, it appears that Brownell and Jeffery's (1987) recommendation that obesity be conceptualized as a chronic disease similar to diabetes in need of constant monitoring may be quite necessary for long-term success. Most time-limited efforts at weight loss are doomed to failure; permanent and continuing changes in eating, exercise, thinking, and life-style are probably needed for successful obesity treatment.

Significant challenges exist at each stage of the weight loss process: getting people to lose weight, getting people who lose weight to maintain those losses, and one recently coming to the fore, preventing people who lose weight and maintain those losses from becoming too obsessed with weight. In our clinical experience, many recent referrals for treatment of anorexia have been formerly obese (often morbidly) individuals. Therefore, an additional challenge is to motivate people to lose weight for the proper reasons and in a healthy manner. Finally, as discussed earlier in the chapter, weight loss treatment may not be indicated in all obesity cases. Before accepting these challenges, it should be determined that obesity treatment is appropriate for the individual.

REFERENCES

Abrams, D. B., & Follick, M. M. (1983). Behavioral weight-loss intervention at the worksite: Feasibility and maintenance. *Journal of Consulting and Clinical Psychology, 51,* 226–233.

Bjorntorp, P. (1985). Obesity and the risk of cardiovascular disease. *Annals of Clinical Research, 17,* 3–9.

Bray, G. A. (1987). Overweight is risking fate: Definition, classification, prevalence, and risks. *Annals of the New York Academy of Sciences, 499,* 14–28.

Brownell, K. (1988, January). Yo-yo dieting: Repeated attempts to lose weight can give you a hefty problem. *Psychology Today,* pp. 20, 22–23.

Brownell, K. D., Greenwood, M. R. C., Stellar, E., & Shrager, E. E. (1986a). The effects of repeated cycles of weight loss and regain in rats. *Physiology Behavior, 38,* 459–464.

Brownell, K. D., & Jeffery, R. W. (1987). Improving long-term weight loss: Pushing the limits of treatment. *Behavior Therapy, 18,* 353–374.

Brownell, K. D., Marlatt, G. A., Lichtenstein, E., & Wilson, G. T. (1986b). Understanding and preventing relapse. *American Psychologist, 41,* 765–782.

Brownell, K. D., & Stunkard, A. J. (1981). Couples training, pharmacotherapy, and behavior therapy in the treatment of obesity. *Archives of General Psychiatry, 38,* 224–1,229.

Cohen, E. A., Gelfand, D. M., Dodd, D. K., Jensen, J., & Turner, C. (1980). Self-control practices associated with weight loss maintenance in children and adolescents. *Behavior Therapy 11,* 26–37.

Corcoran, K. J. (1987). Relapse and obesity: A comment. *American Psychologist, 42,* 825–826.

Craighead, L. W., & Agras, W. S. (1991). Mechanisms of action in cognitive–behavioral and pharmacological interventions for obesity and bulimia nervosa. *Journal of Consulting and Clinical Psychology, 59,* 115–125.

Dubbert, P. M., Terre, L., Holm, F. E., & Brown, M. (1987). Maintenance in behavioral weight reduction programs. *Behavior Therapist, 10,* 225–230.

Fremouw, W. J., Callahan, E. J., Zitter, R. E., & Katell, A. (1981). Stimulus control and contingency contracting for behavior change and weight loss. *Addictive Behavior, 6,* 289–300.

Fremouw, W. J., Seime, R., & Wiener, A. (1987). Self-monitoring forms for bulimia. In P. Keller (Ed.), *Innovations in clinical practice* (Vol. 6, pp. 231–237). Sarasota, FL: Professional Resource Exchange.

Glasser, W. (1976). *Positive addiction.* New York: Harper & Row.

Gormally, J., Rardin, D., & Black, S. (1980). Correlates of successful response to a behavioral weight control clinic. *Journal of Counseling Psychology, 27,* 179–191.

Grilo, C. M., Shiffman, S., & Wing, R. (1989). Relapse crises and coping among dieters. *Journal of Consulting and Clinical Psychology, 57,* 488–495.

Jeffery, R. W., Wing, R. R., & Stunkard, A. J. (1978). Behavioral treatment for obesity: The state of the art in 1976. *Behavior Therapy, 9,* 189–199.

Katall, A., Callahan, E. J., Fremouw, W. J., & Zitter, R. C. (1979). The effects of behavioral treatment and fasting on eating behaviors and weight loss: A case study. *Behavior Therapy, 10,* 579–587.

Kramer, F. M., Jeffery, R. W., Snell, M. K., & Forster, J. L. (1986). Maintenance of successful weight loss over 1 year: Effects of financial contracts for weight maintenance or participation in skills training. *Behavior Therapy, 17,* 295–301.

Mahoney, M. J., & Mahoney, B. K. (1976). *Permanent weight control: A total solution to the dieter's dilemma.* New York: W. W. Norton.

Marlatt, G. A., & Gordon, J. R. (1985). *Relapse prevention: Maintenance strategies in the treatment of addictive behaviors.* New York: Guilford Press.

Perri, M. G., McAllister, D. A., Gange, J. J., Jordan, R. C., McAdoo, W. G., & Nezu, A. M. (1988). Effects of four maintenance programs on the long-term management of obesity. *Journal of Consulting and Clinical Psychology, 56,* 529–534.

Perri, M. G., Shapiro, R. M., Ludwig, W. W., Twentyman, C. T., & McAdoo, W. G. (1984). Maintenance strategies for the treatment of obesity: An evaluation of relapse prevention training and posttreatment contact by mail and telephone. *Journal of Consulting and Clinical Psychology, 52,* 404–413.

Rosenthal, B. S., & Marx, R. D. (1981). Determinants of relapse among dieters. *Obesity and Bariatric Medicine, 10,* 94–97.

Smith, M., & Fremouw, W. J. (1987). A realistic approach to treating obesity. *Clinical Psychology Review, 7,* 449–465.

Sternberg, B. S. (1985). Relapse in weight control: Definitions, processes and prevention strategies. In G. A. Marlatt & J. R. Gordon (Eds.), *Relapse prevention: Maintenance strategies in the treatment of addictive behaviors* (pp. 521–545). New York: Guilford Press.

Stuart, R. B. (1978). *Act thin, stay thin.* New York: W. W. Norton.

Stuart, R. B., & Davis, B. (1972). *Slim change in a fat world: Behavioral control of obesity.* Champaign, IL: Research Press.

Stunkard, A. J. (1975). From explanation to action in psychosomatic medicine: The case of obesity. *Psychosomatic Medicine, 37,* 195–236.

Stunkard, A. J. (1984). The current status of treatment for obesity in adults. In A. J. Stunkard & E. Stellar (Eds.), *Eating and its disorders* (pp. 157–173). New York: Raven Press.

Stunkard, A. J., & Penick, S. B. (1979). Behavior modification in the treatment of obesity: The problem of maintaining weight loss. *Archives of General Psychiatry, 36,* 801–806.

Wing, R. R., & Jeffery, R. (1978). Successful losers: A descriptive analysis of the process of weight reduction. *Obesity and Bariatric Medicine, 7,* 190–91.

Wooley, S. C., & Wooley, O. W. (1984). Should obesity be treated at all? In A. J. Stunkard & E. Stellar (Eds.), *Eating and its disorders* (pp. 185–192). New York: Raven Press.

CHAPTER 5

ANOREXIA NERVOSA AND BULIMIA NERVOSA

Lisa Orimoto
Kelly Bemis Vitousek
UNIVERSITY OF HAWAII

B y clinical reputation, anorexia nervosa and bulimia nervosa are among the most frustrating and recalcitrant forms of psychopathology. Anorexia nervosa is often characterized by open resistance to treatment; in perhaps half of all attempts at intervention, the anorexic determination to remain thin prevails over the therapeutic objective of restoring normal weight. Clients with bulimia nervosa are more likely to share the clinician's agenda for symptom remission, and more likely to fulfill it; however, progress is frequently interrupted by the recurrence of bulimic episodes. In both of these conditions, it would appear that there is an urgent need for clinical strategies designed to prevent relapse—yet to date, no research has been undertaken to examine the contribution of such techniques to treatment outcome. In the absence of data, discussions of relapse prevention (RP) in the eating disorders remain highly speculative.

In the following chapter, we assemble bits and pieces of information about the psychopathology, natural course, and treatment responsiveness of anorexia nervosa and bulimia nervosa in an attempt to identify salient issues that must be addressed by a model of RP in this domain. To the extent that popular analogies between the eating disorders and the affective, anxiety, and addictive disorders are apt, we may be able to extrapolate established principles of RP from these more extensively studied conditions. Yet, we must also attend to the distinctive features of the eating disorders that limit the validity of each of these analogies (Bemis, 1988). If bulimia nervosa shares many of the functional properties of alcoholism, the nature of the "abused substance" imposes major differences in the choice of appropriate treatment goals—clearly, we cannot direct our bulimic clients to abstain from the substance they crave and misuse. If anorexia nervosa in some respects resembles obsessive–compulsive disorder, it is most closely matched with the subtype professing overvalued ideation—the very group for whom conventional exposure-based treatments have restricted application (Foa, 1979). If both of the clinical eating disorders hold elements in common with the affective disorders, they are more likely to show the chronic, unremitting course characteristic of dysthymia rather than the episodic pattern of unipolar depression—again offering, even through analogy, a particular challenge to the treating clinician.

Throughout most of this chapter, we discuss anorexia nervosa and bulimia nervosa separately, with frequent allusions to commonalities across them. Controversy persists regarding the exact nature of the relationship between the two conditions. The central psychopathology of both is the tendency to evaluate the self in terms of body weight and shape (Fairburn & Garner, 1986; Wilson & Walsh, 1991). Bulimic symptoms are present in nearly half of anorexic patients, and many cross diagnostic boundaries from anorexia nervosa to bulimia nervosa after the restoration of normal weight. The disorders are differentiated by distinctive eating patterns (the steady abstemiousness characteristic of restricting anorexia nervosa versus the alternation between restrained eating and bingeing typical of bulimia nervosa and bulimic anorexia nervosa), by the prominence of physical and psychological starvation sequelae, and perhaps by a variety of background characteristics and personality features (e.g., premorbid obesity and problems with impulse control correlate with bulimic symptomatology). Of particular relevance to the present topic, the disorders may also differ in the extent to which symptom resolution is sought, achieved, and maintained by affected individuals.

Another distinction that will quickly become apparent is that the study of these two disorders has followed markedly different developmental sequences. Anorexia nervosa has been the subject of scientific investigation for more than half a century, allowing time for the accumulation of data on the long-term course of the disorder. Astonishingly, however, virtually no controlled studies of psychotherapy have been conducted—perhaps reflecting clinical pessimism about the prospects for obtaining satisfactory results. The state of knowledge on bulimia nervosa has contrasting areas of strength and weakness. As it has been just over a decade since the condition was officially designated a psychiatric disorder, we lack the perspective of extended follow-up research. Yet, as a function of easier access to subjects and/or greater therapeutic optimism, several dozen comparative treatment trials have already been reported, and the field is beginning to embark on second-generation research to identify active treatment components and mechanisms of change.

ANOREXIA NERVOSA

Diagnostic Criteria

Anorexia nervosa is a clinical syndrome that occurs primarily in females (Bemis, 1978). DSM-III-R (American Psychiatric Association, 1987) identifies the cardinal features as (1) refusal to maintain body weight over a minimal normal weight for age and height; (2) intense fear of gaining weight or becoming fat, even though underweight; (3) disturbance in the way in which one's body weight, shape, or size is experienced; and (4) primary or secondary amenorrhea. Issues currently under evaluation for DSM-IV include the specification of "bulimic" and "nonbulimic" subtypes and the addition of the phrase "denial of the seriousness of current low body weight, or undue influence of body shape and weight on self-evaluation" (Wilson & Walsh, 1991).

It should be noted that three of the four existing criteria for anorexia nervosa make reference to a *stance* concerning body weight and shape—a characteristic cluster of attitudes expressing the position that average weight is unacceptable, weight gain intolerable, and current weight liable to distortion. The prominence of beliefs in the definition of anorexia nervosa presages a number of difficulties in our attempts to understand the condition. The essence of its psychopathology is private. Although some of its manifestations will ordinarily be observable, it is possible for an anorexic to retain all of the attitudes consistent with the disorder even when prevented from acting on her beliefs.

Special Issues

The nature of the essential anorexic attitude also hints at one of the most distinctive features of this condition: the egosyntonic quality of its symptoms (Garfinkel & Garner, 1982; Garner & Bemis, 1982; Theander, 1970). The individual with anorexia nervosa does not experience her disorder as intrusive or unwelcome and does not as a rule see herself as afflicted" (Crisp, 1980). Bruch (1973) notes that "the true anorexic is identified with (her) skeleton-like appearance, denies its abnormality, and actively maintains it" (p. 252). Patients are often puzzled by the alarm and disapproval their behavior elicits from others:

Even during their brittle fight about their right to be as skinny as they want to be, they feel that they are not doing anything unusual. On the contrary, since society praises slenderness, they feel they have earned and deserve praise, awe, and respect for the thinness they have accomplished. (Bruch, 1977, p. 6)

Firsthand accounts reiterate the same themes about the sense of pleasure, accomplishment, and moral virtue anorexics derive from their pursuit of thinness:

> When I eventually weighed under 80 pounds and looked at myself in the mirror. . . . I saw someone beautiful: I saw myself. No matter what anyone else thought or said, I was beautiful: I was myself. The clearer the outline of my skeleton became, the more I felt my true self to be emerging. . . . I was, literally and metaphorically, in perfect shape. . . . I was so superior that I considered myself to be virtually beyond criticism. (MacLeod, 1982, pp. 69–70)

> It's like I never knew what self-respect was all about until now. The thinner I get, the better I feel. . . . I'm proud of my stoic, Spartan existence. It reminds me of the lives of the saints and martyrs I used to read about when I was a child. . . . This has become the most important thing I've ever done. (Ciseaux, 1980, p. 1,468)

> I enjoy having this disease and I want it. I cannot convince myself that I am sick or that there is anything from which I have to recover. (Bruch, 1978, p. 2)

In view of the potent positive self-reinforcement anorexics seem to obtain from their symptoms, it is not surprising that they generally have no wish to recover from their condition, or are at best profoundly ambivalent at the prospect (Bemis, 1983). It is also not surprising that they are infamous for their resistance to treatment—indeed, that they are "more determined than all other mental patients to cling on to a symptom they have been protecting tooth and nail against attacks from all sides" (Selvini-Palazzoli, 1978, p. 112). Their lack of interest in change is not limited to the superficial denial of complaints often voiced in the initial stage of therapy; rather it extends to a more basic rejection of average weight and a preference for extreme thinness that persist even after patients have acknowledged that they are underweight and may have some problems for which medical and psychiatric assistance are indicated. Indeed, anorexics often take pride in the fact that their weight is *not* normal, treasuring the sense of "specialness" that this seems to confer; as one former patient explained the distinction, "While I was anorexic, I had

always considered myself to be extraordinary rather than abnormal" (Mac-
Leod, 1982, p. 103).

Whereas many forms of pathological behavior offer some adaptive
advantages to affected individuals, the intensity of the anorexic's attach-
ment to her symptoms may be unique. Vitousek (1991) developed a scale
to assess the range and degree of recognized concerns that psychiatric
patients may harbor about the prospect of recovery from their presenting
problems. Anorexic subjects scored significantly higher than agoraphobic,
simple phobic, alcoholic, and stimulant drug-abusing subjects on virtually
all of the rationally clustered subscales included on this instrument
(Goodyear, 1990; Vitousek, 1991). Discrepancies were especially notable
on those subscales designed to measure the anticipated loss of perceived
benefits associated with the subject's disorder (fear of interpersonal loss,
fear of personal loss, and loss of a sense of identity); anorexics also
received substantially higher scores than comparison groups on an index
of the denial of symptom irrationality. A sample of bulimic subjects
obtained the second highest means on a number of subscales but consistently scored below the anorexic group. The pattern of results supports
the view that, from the perspective of the anorexic individual, the resolution of symptomatology would entail the loss of many valued attributes.
That the continuation of symptomatology will perpetuate the many
adverse consequences of the syndrome occasions less concern; such consequences are subordinated to—or not even attributed to—the pursuit of
thinness.

Long-Term Course

As noted earlier, our knowledge of anorexia nervosa is informed by
numerous studies tracing the status of diagnosed individuals over extended periods of time following diverse and often poorly specified forms
of treatment. (For detailed information about the course of the disorder,
see Schwartz & Thompson, 1981; Garfinkel & Garner, 1982; Steinhausen
& Glanville, 1983; Szmukler & Russell, 1986; Herzog, Keller, & Lavori,
1988; Hsu, 1988; and Remschmidt, Wienand, & Wewetzer, 1990.)

Comparison of outcome across studies is complicated by the usual
problems of nonequivalent samples, inconsistent criteria for recovery,
and unequal duration of follow-up. Some of the most notable sampling
biases include the type of setting in which patients were initially treated
(with medical clinics reliably producing more positive results than psychiatric facilities, to which more severe cases are typically referred) and
the average age of patients at first contact (with pediatric populations
generally carrying a more favorable prognosis). Studies with high failure-
to-trace rates may yield deceptively encouraging figures, since there is

some evidence that subjects lost to follow-up tend to be doing particularly poorly (Vandereycken & Pierloot, 1983).

Across all investigations reporting subject status from study means of 4 to 33 years after assessment, it is evident that no "typical" outcome of anorexia nervosa can be forecast within or between samples. A substantial proportion of cases qualify for the "good" outcome designation at follow-up; the reported range varies from 27% to 69%, with most studies classifying approximately 40% in this category. An "intermediate" status is attained by 11%–37% of cases, while from 14%–42% are judged to be doing poorly. Death rates from starvation or suicide vary from 1% to 18%, with the longest follow-up studies consistently producing the most troublesome figures. This superficially obvious finding is in fact quite informative: It tells us that anorexia nervosa does not simply pose an acute crisis that will be resolved favorably or unfavorably soon after the initiation of treatment but can take a chronic deteriorating course over the span of decades. For this reason, a 10 to 20 year follow-up period is recommended (Szmukler & Russell, 1986).

Only a few investigators have examined the pattern of recovery, chronicity, and relapse through the duration of follow-up. Two of the longest studies in the literature report remarkably consistent findings (Ratnasuriya, Eisler, Szmukler, & Russell, 1989, 1991; Theander, 1985). Tracking the status of cases over a mean of 20 and 33 years, respectively, these investigations determined that entry into the "good" outcome category continued to occur at a fairly stable rate across the first 12 to 15 years following contact and then dropped off sharply. In contrast, the mortality curve did not begin to flatten throughout the period of follow-up.

All reports concur that the immediate response to treatment has no predictive value in anorexia nervosa. Vandereycken and Pierloot (1983) caution that the disorder "is known for its undulating course with periodic remissions and relapses" (p. 241). Russell (1977) warns that although a short-term improvement in clinical state is virtually guaranteed by hospitalization for weight restoration,

> it is rash to accept such a startling improvement as evidence of recovery. In some patients recovery is indeed persistent. In many others, unfortunately, relapse with a progressive loss of weight and return of the previous psychological disturbance occurs within weeks of leaving the hospital. (p. 284)

Others have emphasized that the erosion of apparent progress following inpatient treatment should not be considered relapse, since there is no evidence that such patients were ever sufficiently recovered to qualify for relapse (Dally, 1969; Garfinkel & Garner, 1982; Rankin, 1989).

One study of the hazard rate for first relapses reported an annual rate of 14% during the first year following intervention, dropping to 4% by the second year and an average of 3% for the remainder of the 12-year study period (Isager, Brinch, Kreiner, & Tolstrup, 1985). In general, experts agree that the anorexic individual has less difficulty preserving a true remission of symptoms than the clinician has in helping her to the point where there is a genuine recovery to sustain. Russell (1977) notes that "the outlook is brighter when it transpires that the patient can maintain a normal weight outside the hospital: the longer this achievement lasts, the more promising the outlook" (p. 277). Theander (1970) estimated the risk of full syndrome recurrence at a relatively modest 12% following a period of sustained recovery.

Criteria for Recovery

It appears from the accumulated data of long-term follow-up studies that a favorable outcome can be attained by perhaps one third to one half of anorexic individuals. Closer examination of the functioning of these subjects, however, suggests that many have failed to achieve a complete resolution of symptomatology. While 48% of the 100 subjects followed by Hsu, Crisp, and Harding (1979) were assigned to the "good" outcome category, only 28% of the total sample were free of excessive concern with weight at reassessment. After an average 8-year follow-up, just 20% of another sample were considered physically and psychologically normal, although 37% qualified for inclusion in the "good" outcome group (Hall, Slim, Hawker, & Salmond, 1984). Ten years after initial treatment, 57% of the 76 subjects described by Eckert (1988) were of normal weight, but only 34% were considered completely or almost completely recovered. In a fourth series, only 27% of subjects were found to be eating normally a full 20 years after initial contact, a figure that matched the percentage of subjects doing well overall (Ratnasuriya et al., 1989, 1991). In general, reviewers conclude that although many anorexic patients can expect a reduction in symptom severity with the passage of time and/or exposure to treatment, complete recovery from anorexia nervosa is rare (Szmukler & Russell, 1986; Theander, 1970).

Since the data clearly suggest that the persistence/cessation of anorexia nervosa is not an all-or-nothing phenomenon, we must contend with the problem of deciding how many residual signs of the disorder we will permit for inclusion in various outcome categories. As the possibility of relapse is predicated upon the achievement of symptom control, these decisions have direct implications for the calculation of relapse rates as well.

At the time of intake, formal criteria force the diagnostician to make a dichotomous decision: The subject being evaluated has "enough" symptomatology to be classified anorexic, or she does not. If we apply the same standard in gauging recovery, we will be forced to designate many slightly subthreshold cases cured (or, at least, no longer anorexic)—and to declare numerous "relapses" when these individuals slip back across the boundary demarcating clinical severity. If, on the other hand, we espouse the conservative position of certifying recovery only with evidence of stable normal weight, exemplary dietary practices, and an absence of concern for weight and shape, we will be imposing standards that are regularly violated by many individuals who have never come close to qualifying for an eating disorder diagnosis.

In addition to setting acceptable levels for the focal symptomatology of anorexia nervosa, we must also decide how much general psychopathology we are willing to tolerate when declaring individuals recovered. Many anorexics whose weight has been normalized continue to struggle with anxiety, depression, and social avoidance (Rosenvinge & Mouland, 1990). Should these cases be considered cured or only partially remitted? Szmukler and Russell (1986) note that the answer to such questions depends on assumptions about the nature of the pathological process in anorexia nervosa; with our present limited knowledge, the most justifiable course in outcome research may be a relatively narrow focus on the specific features used to establish initial diagnoses.

If we turn to DSM-III-R for guidance, it is apparent that only one of the listed criteria is easily applied to the determination of recovery status. The return of menstruation is a relatively verifiable phenomenon that can be used to signal recovery, although even on this index we cannot expect a perfect correspondence between the sign and the syndrome. Amenorrhea sometimes persists well beyond weight restoration, can be masked by the use of exogenous hormones, and is hardly a useful indicator of illness in males or postmenopausal females. Moreover, a few patients continue to menstruate while maintaining extremely low weights—and some lie about the occurrence or nonoccurrence of this private event.

The remaining criteria are considerably more difficult to interpret. The criterion "refusal to maintain a minimal normal weight" implies both a quantifiably subminimal weight and an attitude about that weight. One can be at normal weight involuntarily or reluctantly in conjunction with tube feeding, hyperalimentation, or the manipulation of powerful environmental contingencies, while still refusing to *accept* that normal weight—and such is the position of many treated anorexics. In practice, most investigators attend only to actual weight status in the assessment of outcome, specifying an acceptable range of ± 15% around matched population mean weight, sometimes qualified by reference to the individual's premorbid weight status (Szmukler & Russell, 1986). It should be noted that DSM-III-R makes no mention of the abnormal eating behaviors typically associated with anorexia nervosa. Follow-up studies differ in the extent to which restrictive or ritualistic dietary habits are considered in gauging outcome, but most recent studies specify that bulimic symptomatology is incompatible with a rating of "recovered."

The most challenging problems are posed by the "intense fear" and "body image disturbance" items. These criteria are important aspects of the central psychopathology of anorexia nervosa, of which low weight status and amenorrhea are in some senses mere markers—yet the former are much more subjective and elusive phenomena. Even at the time of initial assessment, the presence of these attitudes must often be inferred from subjects' behavior, since they may be denied by these notoriously defensive individuals in an effort to protect their symptomatology from outside interference. The standardized questionnaires that are widely used to quantify concerns about weight, shape, and food do not resolve the problem of distortion in self-report, and may not demonstrate discriminant validity (Vitousek, Daly, & Heiser, 1991; Wilson & Smith, 1989). A variety of creative strategies have been devised in an attempt to measure body image distortion; however, method variance has produced highly inconsistent findings, and it remains unclear what it is that size estimation techniques are actually assessing (see Ben-Tovim, Walker, Murray, & Chin, 1990; Bowden, Touyz, Rodriguez, Hensley, & Beumont, 1989; Cash & Brown, 1987; Garner, Garfinkel, & Bonato, 1987; Hsu & Sobkiewicz, 1991; Meerman, Napierski, & Vandereycken, 1988; Slade, 1985).

In the past few years, there have been several promising developments in the assessment of attitudes toward weight and shape. Semistructured interviews such as the Eating Disorder Examination appear to be more sensitive than questionnaires to the subtleties of anorexic and bulimic psychopathology, and better differentiate these groups from comparison samples (Cooper & Fairburn, 1987; Cooper, Cooper, & Fairburn, 1989; Wilson & Smith, 1989). Another useful approach may be the adaptation of nonobvious assessment strategies derived from cognitive science. Such techniques may reduce dependence on self-report concerning the salience of food and weight preoccupation by examining variables such as response latency, attentional biases, and memory for schematic information (for an extended discussion, see Vitousek & Hollon, 1990). Alternative methods of minimizing distortion and denial in self-report include indirect questioning strategies, the use of collateral informants, and the separation of clinical and research contexts (Vitousek et al., 1991).

Relapse Rates following Treatment

As we noted at the beginning of the chapter, there are virtually no controlled psychotherapy studies of anorexia nervosa; the few distinguished exceptions report follow-up periods of 1 year or less. The persistent lack of comparative therapy trials with this disorder is somewhat puzzling. All commentators agree that the early weight-restoration phase of treatment, which usually occurs in the hospital, is vital but in some senses trivial; all concur that the real therapeutic challenge comes during the prolonged second phase, usually involving individual and/or family therapy on an outpatient basis. Yet, while the former has been extensively studied, the latter remains almost unexamined.

Several reasons can be advanced to explain this curious gap in the literature, which contrasts sharply with the state of research on bulimia nervosa (Vitousek & Ewald, in press). Anorexia nervosa is a rarer condition, and the common expedient of assembling bulimic samples through solicitation is not available to the anorexia specialist, since most anorexics shun treatment. The recommended course of psychotherapy is longer for anorexia nervosa (often 1–2 years) than for bulimia nervosa (as little as 3–4 months). This extended period of treatment increases the likelihood of subject attrition, which will further reduce sample size and undo randomization, and places investigators reinforced for publication frequency on a schedule of dysfunctionally deferred gratification. The "crisis" phase of short-term weight restoration also seems to distract research attention from the long course of therapy that must follow. Moreover, the first stage is appealingly direct and specific; the issues that must be addressed subsequently are heterogeneous, and clinician–researchers seem to have more difficulty formulating the therapeutic task for the middle and late phases of intervention.

Perhaps one more reason should be added from the perspective of a recovered anorexic well versed in the state of research concerning her disorder:

> It is difficult not to gain the impression from the literature on anorexia nervosa that individual therapy has been devalued because (among other reasons) psychotherapists do not like anorexics, and anorexics do not like psychotherapists. (MacLeod, 1982, p. 122)

Whatever the validity of these explanations, we are left with a very limited data base to scan for clues about relapse and RP in the treatment of anorexia nervosa. A number of comparative studies have been conducted to examine different methods (operant conditioning, milieu therapy, pharmacotherapy, and hyperalimentation) for producing weight gain on an inpatient basis (e.g., Eckert, Goldberg, Halmi, Casper, & Davis,

1979; Kreipe & Kidder, 1986; Pertschuk, Forster, Buzby, & Mullen, 1981; Weizman, Tyano, Wijsenbeek, & Ben David, 1985). Few of these reported follow-up figures on the differential relapse rates associated with various regimens; if they were available, it is not clear that such figures would be particularly informative. It may not be possible to assess the long-term outcome of such brief treatment modalities in any meaningful way because a great variety of confounding variables are likely to intervene between a 1- or 2-month hospitalization and a follow-up assessment conducted years later (Halmi, 1985).

In general, reviews of early-phase treatment research concluded that no specific method seems to confer an increased or reduced risk of subsequent relapse (Bemis, 1987a; Garfinkel, Moldofsky, & Garner, 1977). With reference to the effects of short-term programs designed to promote weight gain, most experts would still endorse a judgment pronounced more than 20 years ago: "Relapses and final outcome are similar, whatever initial treatment is given" (Dally, 1969).

If initial treatment directed exclusively toward weight gain bears no discernible relationship to the course of anorexia nervosa, it seems plausible that subsequent psychotherapy might exert more influence—and perhaps that different forms of therapy might yield differential rates of relapse. Several controlled trials have been reported to date.

Hall and Crisp (1987) compared two brief (12 sessions) outpatient interventions with a sample of 30 anorexic patients. The psychotherapy condition delivered an unspecified blend of psychodynamic and family therapy; the dietary advice program involved the provision of nutritional counseling and an examination of relationships between mood and eating behavior. Subjects in both conditions showed modest improvements in physical and psychological symptomatology. The dietary advice group recorded more consistent gains in weight, while the psychotherapy group improved more on indices of social and sexual adjustment. At 1 year follow-up, most patients maintained improvements over their intake status, but a majority in both groups remained underweight and amenorrheic. Three patients in the psychotherapy condition experienced serious "relapses" during the interval before follow-up. Continuing therapy was indicated for all of the dietary advice subjects and 73% of the psychotherapy subjects.

Russell and his colleagues reported a study in which subjects were randomly assigned to family therapy or individual therapy upon discharge from a hospital program for weight restoration (Russell, Szmukler, Dare, & Eisler, 1987). The family therapy modality was based on the prescriptions of Minuchin and Selvini-Palazzoli; parents were encouraged to gain control over their daughter's disturbed eating and to examine its role in preserving family stability. The individual therapy was described as

supportive, educational, and problem-oriented, and included elements of
cognitive, interpretive, and strategic approaches. At the end of a year, the
results suggested an interaction between mode of therapy and the age of
participants. Family therapy appeared more effective than individual
therapy in the treatment of younger patients with a brief duration of
illness, while the reverse was true for patients with an older age of onset.
Bulimic subjects and early-onset patients whose illness had become
chronic benefited equally from either treatment. Across all conditions,
only 23% of subjects were considered recovered following the 1-year
treatment course.

A third study compared behavioral and cognitive–behavioral therapy
conditions with an unspecified treatment-as-usual cell (Channon, de Silva, Hemsley, & Perkins, 1989). Both the behavioral and cognitive–
behavioral interventions included self-monitoring of intake and dietary
planning. In addition, subjects in the behavioral condition were taught
relaxation and distraction techniques and were exposed to graded
hierarchies of feared foods and situations. Subjects in the cognitive–
behavioral treatment were taught to identify and challenge dysfunctional
thoughts about food and weight, using the combined didactic and collaborative approach described by Garner and Bemis (1982, 1985). After 6
months of active treatment and a 6- and 12-month follow-ups, all groups
were significantly improved; few differences were obtained between conditions. No group could be considered clinically recovered by the end of
the trial. The cognitive–behavioral modality appeared more acceptable to
 clients and was associated with higher rates of compliance—a finding that
the authors note was of some interest because of the notorious difficulty of
engaging anorexics in treatment. However, while the investigators stated
that the cognitive condition was patterned after the recommendations of
Garner and Bemis, it is not clear how closely it conformed to specified
procedures. It appears that the primary focus of the cognitive–behavioral
treatment was the identification and challenge of irrational beliefs. In
discussing the failure of this condition to demonstrate incremental benefit
over the behavioral treatment, Channon et al. (1989) suggested that in
future it might be "more appropriate to focus on the relative importance
 of thinness as a life goal relative to other goals . . . rather than attempting
to modify individual cognitions" (p. 534). Since the former is precisely
what Garner and Bemis advocate on both practical and theoretical
grounds, it is surprising that this crucial component of cognitive therapy
for anorexia nervosa was apparently omitted from a test of the method's
utility.

One clear conclusion seems warranted from the few controlled studies published: Most anorexic patients cannot be said to be in remission 1
year after treatment. In most cases, any deterioration occurring at this

point could not be designated a relapse since recovery had yet to take place. On the basis of the long-term studies discussed earlier, one would predict that nearly half of these subjects will eventually attain a normal weight and resume menstruation—and can anticipate that a subgroup of these will experience true relapses in the future.

Issues Related to Relapse following Treatment

Clinical observation and anecdotal accounts are the only available sources of information about factors contributing to relapse in anorexia nervosa, since data on the process of relapse have never been collected systematically. Both sources tend to attribute symptom recurrence to the distinctive feature of anorexia nervosa highlighted earlier: the egosyntonic nature of its symptoms.

Even after stabilizing weight at acceptable levels, many anorexics continue to cherish the symptoms they are holding in abeyance. Hall (1982) observes that the recovered patient may go through a "mourning process for her (anorexic) self, for an identity and a way of life which has been hers for so long" (p. 642). Branch and Eurman (1980) comment that former anorexics "sometimes regret losing their slender selves and the sense of control inherent in the illness" (p. 632).

Certainly, individuals who have given up other valued but maladaptive behaviors such as smoking and substance abuse may also experience nostalgia for the habits they have foresworn, but there is a depth and fierceness to this longing in the aftermath of anorexia nervosa that is most eloquently conveyed by anorexics themselves:

> For the past 17 years, I've passed for "normal." And yet not a single day in all those years has elapsed that I didn't feel scourged. . . . The moment I surrendered myself to my parents' wishes that I eat—in other words, when I refused to be responsible any more for what I was to become, a fat powerless person—I felt my self-esteem evaporate. . . . As the inevitable flesh coated my bones anew, people commented that they were glad to see I was "getting better." How DARE anyone get satisfaction out of seeing me fail at something I had sought so desperately! (Ciseaux, 1980, p. 1469)

Perhaps the most chilling account is provided by a weight-recovered young woman in the form of a letter written to her previous anorexic self:

> I know you're still there . . . and I can feel your hate at what I've done to your work of art. I can feel it as you shudder and pull back when someone touches me, and I can feel it when tears start welling in my

eyes every time that you see my reflection in the mirror. There are times that I feel terrible about what I've done to you. . . . I can't tell a lot of people this, but I love you, and really do miss you. My college I.D. photograph—smiling, happy, I'm all better now. I can see that smile creeping across your parched lips; we both know better. (Anonymous, 1988, pp. 7–8)

It is clear that the essential anorexic stance concerning weight can survive physical rehabilitation, sometimes for periods of many years. Data on attitudinal measures administered at follow-up confirm the clinical and anecdotal accounts. Clinton and McKinlay (1986) examined a sample of 14 anorexics who were fully weight-recovered after a mean of more than 3 years postdischarge. The investigators stated the major conclusion of their research as follows:

[An] important aspect of anorexia nervosa appears to remain largely unaltered by present treatment methods, namely the distorted attitudes associated with the condition. . . . [There] appears to be a lack of synchrony between the gross physical and behavioral symptoms of anorexia nervosa and the cognitive correlates of the disorder. (Clinton & McKinlay, 1986, p. 66)

While it could not be determined in the Clinton and McKinlay study whether the persistence of the anorexic stance predisposes subjects to relapse, another data set is consistent with this supposition. Channon and de Silva (1985) followed 45 anorexic subjects for 1 year after treatment. They reported that the only psychological predictors of status at follow-up were elevated scores on an inventory of anorexic attitudes and low desired weight at the time of discharge; the same indices administered at the time of admission did not predict follow-up status.

BULIMIA NERVOSA

Diagnostic Criteria

Like anorexia nervosa, bulimia nervosa occurs predominantly in women. Current criteria parallel the essential features proposed by Russell in 1979 and are considerably narrower than those specified in DSM-III. DSM-III-R criteria include (1) repeated episodes of binge eating, occurring at least twice per week for a minimum of 3 months; (2) lack of control over eating during binges; (3) frequent use of practices intended to prevent weight gain, such as self-induced vomiting, laxative abuse, fasting, or excessive exercise; and (4) persistent concern with body shape and weight (DSM-III-R). Proposed modifications for DSM-IV include an attempt to operationalize binges, subclassification into "purging" and "nonpurging" types, and the addition of the statement that "self-evaluation is unduly influenced by body shape and weight" (Wilson & Walsh, 1991).

Special Issues

At least superficially, there is a marked contrast between anorexia nervosa and bulimia nervosa on the dimension that most complicates the treatment of the former: the egosyntonic versus dystonic nature of symptomatology. While anorexics resist intervention, and early-phase treatment is rarely entirely voluntary, bulimics are often eager for symptom remission and are typically self-referred. Yet the desire for recovery in bulimia nervosa often extends only to the symptoms of bingeing and purging. Garner (1986) cautions that their motivation for change may dissipate rapidly with the recognition that treatment must go beyond these symptoms to address the exaggerated concern with weight and shape that is as characteristic of bulimics as of anorexics. When the egosyntonic symptom of pursuing suboptimal weight is challenged, some patients will choose to continue to struggle with bulimia rather than give up their body weight and shape ideals. In this regard, bulimics may be as reluctant as anorexics to relinquish the behaviors that they believe subserve the goal of weight control.

The majority of bulimics also present with a variety of neurotic symptomatology (Fairburn, Cooper, & Cooper, 1986). Depression, anxiety, substance abuse, parasuicidal behavior, and stealing are frequently reported as co-occurring features. Many of these symptoms remit when the bulimic pattern is controlled, but some individuals continue to experience significant and perhaps independent psychiatric problems in diverse areas. The bulimic population appears to be a somewhat more heterogeneous group than anorexics in terms of personality features and psychopathology, so that it may be more hazardous to make generalizations about the etiology and functional significance of symptoms.

Long-Term Course

As discussed earlier, the scientific history of bulimia nervosa is so brief that very little is known about the long-term course of the disorder. The scant data we do possess have been gleaned from studies following subjects for 2 to 6 years after diverse, unspecified, or minimal treatments.

In this section, then, we summarize tentative conclusions about intermediate outcome subsequent to heterogeneous forms of intervention, rather than delineating the extended natural course of the disorder.

At least over short intervals, bulimic behavior does appear to be relatively stable. Research designs incorporating wait-list control conditions have determined that levels of specific and general psychopathology do not abate in the absence of active treatment (Fairburn, 1988). Over longer periods of time, some symptom resolution may occur: In one uncontrolled study, 53% of bulimic subjects who had received no formal therapy were considered improved on the basis of a telephone assessment 12 to 15 months after initial contact (Mitchell, Davis, Goff, & Pyle, 1986).

When interviewed retrospectively about the course of their disorder prior to treatment seeking, bulimics often report fluctuations in their symptomatology. In a series of 275 cases, 67% were found to have experienced at least one episode of symptom remission lasting 2 weeks or more; 19% reported that the suspension of bulimic behavior persisted for at least 3 months (Mitchell, Hatsukami, Pyle, & Eckert, 1986). The investigators concluded that "bulimic behavior is not chronic and ongoing for all patients . . . (rather), symptoms may wax and wane and . . . many patients do gain control for extended periods of time yet relapse back to the behavior" (Mitchell, Davis, Goff, & Pyle, 1986, p. 166).

Although the balance of symptomatic and symptom-free episodes may well shift with intervention, the same investigators observed that the fluctuating course of bulimia nervosa tends to persist after treatment. Noting that only one-third of a combined sample of intensively treated, minimally treated, and untreated subjects remained abstinent from bulimic behavior for more than 1 year following evaluation, Mitchell and his colleagues concluded that "bulimia is not a transient, benign condition which often remits spontaneously" (Mitchell, Hatsukami, Pyle, & Eckert, 1986, p. 449). At the point of follow-up assessment, almost 60% of the subjects acknowledged bulimic episodes in the preceding month, and 44% induced vomiting. A separate study of heterogeneously treated bulimic patients noted that 65% of those who met criteria for recovery during treatment relapsed into a new episode some time during the ensuing year; only 11% of relapsing subjects recovered from this recurrence more than 6 months later (Kelaler et al., 1989).

Several groups of investigators have interviewed bulimic subjects about the occurrence of relapse following periods of symptom control. Winstead (1984) collected the retrospective accounts of 25 bulimics concerning factors that contributed to relapse prior to entry into treatment. In contrast to findings reported in the alcoholism literature, intrapersonal determinants such as irrational beliefs and coping with negative emotional or physical states were much more often associated with relapse incidents than were interpersonal factors. The following precipitants were implicated as contributors to relapse: fear of weight gain (60%), emotional factors (60%), self-control factors (56%), and cognitive factors (28%). Subjects predicted that in the future they would lack the ability to refrain from purging after the consumption of specific kinds and quantities of food, and nominated a variety of situations and time periods as carrying a high risk for bulimic behavior.

Mitchell, Davis, and Goff (1985) conducted telephone interviews with 30 bulimic subjects who relapsed into a regular pattern of binge–purge episodes in the 12 to 15 months following their participation in an intensive outpatient treatment program. One third relapsed within the first month of program completion, and an additional 40% by 3 months. Antecedent conditions included coping with stressful situations (80%), feeling anxious or nervous (23%), and feeling depressed (23%). Few subjects identified problems in interpersonal relationships as precipitants (10%). Contrary to the Winstead (1984) results, only one subject mentioned fear of weight gain as a precipitant; it is unclear whether these differences are a function of the way in which questions were posed in the two investigations.

Root (1990) interviewed a recruited sample of 21 bulimics. A wide majority (81%) experienced at least one relapse after they believed themselves recovered from their bulimic symptomatology. According to this sample, the experiences likely to cause a relapse were weight gain (67%), inability to cope with feelings (62%), attitudes that gave rise to negative affect (48%), and stressful events (48%).

Criteria for Recovery

Currently, there is no accepted set of standards for defining recovery from bulimia nervosa. Bulimia has been described as a multidimensional disorder "whose clinical severity and improvement can be measured in many ways" (Rosen, 1987, p. 465). As in the case of anorexia nervosa, it may be easier to diagnose the disorder than to verify its resolution. If we turn again to DSM criteria to inform us about recovery, we face additional challenges in operationalizing the "absence" of symptomatology.

Binge–purge frequency is probably the most commonly utilized change variable in the treatment outcome literature. Its appeal lies in its status as a seemingly "objective" and quantifiable measure; however, as some have noted (e.g., Rosen, 1987), the binge episode is in fact a subjective phenomenon. On the other hand, purgation by self-induced vomiting or laxative abuse is more readily defined and recognized by both the bulimic informant and the clinician/researcher.

The reliability and validity of binge–purge frequency as an outcome metric may be compromised by the self-report nature of the data. The use of collaterals to verify self-report data is virtually nullified by the secrecy that characterizes bulimic episodes (Wilson, 1987). However, since bingeing and purging are the most distinctive features of bulimia nervosa, they must certainly figure prominently in the assessment of recovery. A liberal definition of symptom resolution would merely require a subclinical frequency of binge–purge episodes (i.e., less than the average of two per week specified for conferral of the bulimic diagnosis). Most clinicians would be reluctant to designate an individual who is still engaging in vomiting on a once-weekly basis "recovered"; therefore, more stringent standards are often applied in the determination of symptom absence than symptom presence. At the same time, the occurrence of occasional slips at widely spaced intervals should not be sufficient to consign an individual to an "intermediate" outcome category. Percentage reductions in binge–purge episodes should be reported alongside abstinence figures; while a decrease from ten to two episodes per week may not appear clinically significant to the outside observer, the partial control of symptoms is quite likely to have clinically significant effects on the daily life of the bulimic herself.

Reassessment of the criterion of "persistent overconcern with weight and shape" poses the same difficulties associated with the measurement of attitudinal variables in anorexia nervosa. Again, it is unclear whether normative standards should be used to gauge meaningful change, since exaggerated concern about weight is extremely prevalent in the general female population.

While measures of the focal symptoms of bingeing, purging, and weight preoccupation are most critical to the determination of outcome, a multidimensional, multimethod approach is essential for studying the process of recovery in bulimia nervosa (Garner, 1987; Wilson, 1987). Additional measures that should be reported routinely include changes in psychological adjustment, interpersonal functioning, comorbid substance abuse, and dietary intake and habits.

Relapse Rates following Treatment

Information regarding the rate of relapse following formal treatment of bulimia is again quite limited. Follow-up intervals tend to be short (typically 3 to 12 months), and outcome data are often reported in a form that makes it impossible to discern rates of relapse. Most studies report the percentage of decrease in episodes and the percentage of abstinent subjects at posttreatment and follow-up; however, it is rarely specified whether the subjects abstinent at follow-up are the same subjects who were abstinent at the end of treatment. Generalizations about treatment efficacy and relapse are also hampered by methodological inadequacies such as high dropout rates, small sample sizes, absence of comparison groups, failure to specify technical operations of treatments, and inadequate measurement of target symptoms (see Garner, 1987; Garner, Fairburn, & Davis, 1987).

Of specific concern to the present chapter, the treatment literature on bulimia nervosa contains no information about the effect of formal RP strategies on the maintenance of treatment gains. In view of the wide currency given to the analogy between bulimia nervosa and the addictive disorders, it is surprising that this element has not been selected for closer examination. Some of the most popular modalities used in the treatment of the disorder do often build in RP components; however, only 8 of the 18 studies summarized in Table 5.1 explicitly mention the use of such strategies. No studies have as yet used a dismantling approach to investigate the specific contribution of RP techniques.

Several excellent reviews of the efficacy of psychological and pharmacological treatments for bulimia nervosa have been published in recent years (e.g., Cox & Merkel, 1989; Craighead & Agras, 1991; Fairburn, 1988; Freeman & Munro, 1988; Garner, 1987; Garner, Fairburn, & Davis, 1987; Laessle, Zoettl, & Pirke, 1987; Mitchell, 1988; Rosen, 1987; Wilson, in press-a). Since it is outside the scope of this chapter to examine the rapidly growing treatment outcome literature, we will simply summarize some of the most consistent findings.

The dominant modality employed in these studies is some form of cognitive–behavioral therapy (CBT), which many commentators currently regard as the treatment of choice for bulimia nervosa (Craighead & Agras, 1991; Wilson, 1989). Although CBT has made an impressive showing in most comparative trials, the originator of the approach cautions against a premature crystallization of theoretical models and treatment techniques, and warned that not every patient benefits from this approach (Fairburn, 1988).

Several variants of behavioral approaches have been tested in controlled treatment outcome research, including exposure and response prevention strategies and a combination of self-monitoring, stimulus control, and dietary planning techniques. Conflicting results have been reported concerning the efficacy of behavioral methods relative to the cognitive–behavioral approach. A few studies examined the use of eclectic approaches that blend psychodynamic, experiential, cognitive, and behavioral elements.

Pharmacotherapy (generally using tricyclic antidepressants) has not proven efficacious in the treatment of bulimia nervosa; while most subjects improve initially, relapse rates are extremely high when medication is discontinued (Craighead & Agras, 1991; Mitchell, 1988). Several

TABLE 5.1 Select Bulimia Nervosa Treatment Studies

Investigators	Orientation	n	Format	R-p[d]	% Reduction pre- to posttreatment		% Abstinent in last week of treatment		% Abstinent/decrease at follow-up		Duration of follow-up
					Bingeing	Vomiting	Bingeing	Vomiting	Bingeing	Vomiting	
Giles et al. (1985)	ERP	34	I	Y	—	—	92%[a]	50%	—	63% abstinent	6½ to 20½ mos.
Kirkley et al. (1985)	CBT	14	G	N	96.5%[b]	95.4%[b]	—	—	—	38%[b] abstinent	3 mos.
	nondirective	14	G	N	63.5%[b]	69.2%[b]	—	—	—	11%[b] abstinent	3 mos.
Schneider & Agras (1985)	CBT	10	G	N	—	90.8%	—	53.8%[b]	—	45.4% abstinent	6 mos.
Luka et al. (1986), follow-up of Schneider & Agras (1985)	CBT	10	G	N	—	90.8%	—	60%	—	75%[a] reduction	30 mos.
Fairburn et al. (1986)	CBT	12	I	Y	87.5%[b]	93.3%[b]	27.3%[b]	36.4%[b]	54.5%[b] abstinent	63.6%[b] abstinent	12 mos.
	focal treatment	12	I	N	82.3%[b]	87.0%[b]	36.4%[b]	27.3%[b]	54.5%[b] abstinent	27.3%[b] abstinent	12 mos.
Wilson et al. (1986)	CR	8	G	Y	50.7%[b]	57.9%[b]	33.3%[b]	33.3%[b]	—	27.3%[b] abstinent	12 mos.
	CR+ERP	9	G	Y	82.7%[b]	88.8%[b]	71.4%[b]	71.4%[b]	83.3%[b] abstinent	100%[b] abstinent	12 mos.

Study	Treatment	N									
Laessle et al. (1987)	BT	8	G	N	—	—	37.5%	62.5%	75% abstinent	75% abstinent	3 mos.
	wait-list	9	G	N	no change	no change	no change	no change	no change	no change	3 mos.
Sohlberg et al. (1987)	psychoanalytic	13	I	N	—	—	—	—	40% reduction	—	2 yrs.
	control	16	?	N	—	—	—	—	58% reduction	—	2 yrs.
Dedman et al. (1988)	CBT	8	G	N	92%[a]	—	37.5%[a]	—	60%[a] abstinent	—	6 mos.
Freeman et al. (1988)	CBT	32	G	N	83.8%[a]	86%[a]	—	—	[e]	[e]	12 mos.
	BT	30	G	N	86.9%[a]	91.6%[a]	—	—	[e]	[e]	12 mos.
	psychoeducational and support	30	G	N	87.3%[a]	93.2%[a]	—	—	[e]	[e]	12 mos.
	wait-list	20	N/A	N/A	35%[a]	-21%[a]	—	—	[e]	[e]	N/A
Leitenberg et al. (1988)	ERP single setting	11	G	N	—	73%	—	36.4%[a]	—	18.2%[a] abstinent	6 mos.
	ERP multiple settings	12	G	N	—	67%	—	33%	—	50%[a] abstinent	6 mos.
	CBT no exposure	12	G	N	—	40%	—	8.3%[a]	—	33.3%[a] abstinent	6 mos.
Agras et al. (1989)	wait-list	19	I	N	—	1.4%[a]	—	5.8%[a]	—	—	6 mos.
	self-monitoring	19	I	N	—	62.6%[a]	—	23.5%[a]	—	18%[a] abstinent	6 mos.

(cont.)

TABLE 5.1 (Cont.)

Investigators	Orientation	n	Format	R-p[d]	% Reduction pre- to posttreatment		% Abstinent in last week of treatment		% Abstinent/ decrease at follow-up		Duration of follow-up
					Bingeing	Vomiting	Bingeing	Vomiting	Bingeing	Vomiting	
	CBT	22	I	Y	—	74.7%[a]	—	56.3%[a]	—	59%[a] abstinent	6 mos.
	CBT + ERP	17	I	Y	—	52.5%[a]	—	31.2%[a]	—	20%[a] abstinent	6 mos.
Cooper et al. (1989)	BT	8	I	Y	97.2%[a]	100%[a]	—	—	100% reduction	100% reduction	12 mos.
Fairburn et al. (1991)	BT	25	I	N	91.3%[a]	95.1%[a]	62%	62%	[c]	[c]	12 mos.
	CBT	25	I	Y	96.7%[a]	94.7%[a]	71%	71%	[c]	[c]	12 mos.
	IPT	25	I	N	89%[a]	66.5%[a]	62%	62%	[c]	[c]	12 mos.
Gray & Hoage (1990)	ERP w/ CR	8	G	Y	—	25% in 7/8 of Ss	—	—	75% abstinent	75% abstinent	12 mos.
Mitchell et al. (1990); follow-up data described in Pyle et al. (1990)	placebo (A)	31	I	N	2.5%[a]	12%[a]	[c]	[c]	*	*	*see Pyle et al. (1990)
	imipramine (B)	54	I	N	49.3%[a]	45.3%[a]	[c]	[c]	[f]	[f]	
	eclectic group + placebo (C)	34	G	Y	89%[a]	84.8%[a]	[c]	[c]	[f]	[f]	
	eclectic group + imipramine (D)	52	G	Y	91.6%[a]	89.6%[a]	[c]	[c]	[f]	[f]	

Study	Treatment group	n									Follow-up
Pyle et al. (1990)	imipramine + support group (originally Mitchell's "D" group)	19	G	N/A	N/A	N/A	N/A	N/A	61% abstinent	61% abstinent	6 mos.
	placebo + support group (originally Mitchell's "D" group)	15	G	N/A	N/A	N/A	N/A	N/A	38% abstinent	38% abstinent	6 mos.
	support group only (originally Mitchell's "C" group)	25	G	N/A	N/A	N/A	N/A	N/A	62% abstinent	62% abstinent	6 mos.
	imipramine only (originally Mitchell's "B" group)	3	med consult only	N/A	N/A	N/A	N/A	N/A	33% abstinent	33% abstinent	6 mos.
	placebo only (originally Mitchell's "B" group)	6	med consult only	N/A	N/A	N/A	N/A	N/A	17% abstinent	17% abstinent	6 mos.
Olmsted et al. (1991)	CBT	30	I	N	82.4%	81%	36%	36%	—	—	3 mos.
	psychoeducational	35	G	N	60.8%	54.9%	20.7%	20.7%	—	—	3 mos.

Note. N/A = not applicable; I = individual therapy; G = group therapy; ERP = exposure and response prevention; CBT = cognitive–behavioral therapy; CR = cognitive restructuring; BT = behavioral therapy; A–D are used to mark the different treatment cells used by Mitchell et al. (1990).

[a] Percent calculated from data presented in the text.

[b] Percent calculated and presented in the text by Garner (1987).

[c] See text for explanation.

[d] Only those studies that explicitly noted an R-P component in their treatment study are noted as "Y."

[e] Results not separated by groups; 21/24 (87.5%) reported as "improved."

[f] See Pyle et al. (1990).

107

reviewers suggest that drugs and cognitive–behavioral therapy may exert their effects on bulimic behavior through directly opposed mechanisms (Craighead & Agras, 1991; Rossiter, Agras, & Losch, 1988; Wilson, 1989). Medication may facilitate dietary restraint through its appetite-suppressant properties, while cognitive techniques seek to decrease restraint by encouraging patients to consume regular, ample meals and reintroduce avoided foods into their diets. If this analysis is correct, it is not surprising that CBT seems to be associated with better maintenance of treatment gains, since restrained eating is often cited as an important etiological variable in the development of bulimic behavior.

Follow-up data from controlled studies provide information relevant to the study of relapse, although as noted earlier, many reports omit the specific figures required for the calculation of relapse rates. Table 5.1 summarizes the results of selected treatment studies that meet the following criteria: (1) sample sizes equal to or greater than 8, (2) clear diagnostic criteria, and (3) specific follow-up data reported after an interval of at least 3 months. For the studies included in Table 5.1, the median abstinence figure for bingeing at follow-up is 61% (range 33%–83%), while the median figure for abstinence from purging is 45.5% (range 11%–100%).

It is apparent that many patients do not derive substantial benefit from treatment; however, the collective results of follow-up studies suggest a somewhat more optimistic picture of the maintenance of treatment gains than would be anticipated on the basis of clinical accounts. Mean reduction in vomiting figures at the time of follow-up are almost the same as those reported at posttreatment assessment (Rosen, 1987). Although a few investigators observed some deterioration in clinical status (Freeman, Beach, Davis, & Solyom, 1985; Kirkley, Schneider, Agras, & Bachman, 1985), long-term follow-ups of other studies report that improvements achieved during treatment can be sustained or enhanced after its completion (Fairburn, 1988; Fairburn, Kirk, O'Connor, & Cooper, 1986).

Since no published research has examined the specific contribution of RP elements to outcome, we will have to search for suggestive information in several groups of studies addressing related issues. The first includes comparative trials in which one of the tested modalities was CBT. The CBT model for the treatment of bulimia nervosa is a complex set of cognitive, behavioral, and educational procedures (Fairburn, 1985). It is based on the theoretical premise that core attitudes about weight and shape represent the essential psychopathology; these must be modified if lasting changes in bulimic behavior are to occur. Many components consistent with an emphasis on RP are built into the CBT approach from the inception of treatment; for example, the identification of high-risk situations, the generation and practice of coping strategies, and the modification of dichotomous thinking about success and failure. Thus, any treatment condition that specifies the use of CBT techniques should be focusing on RP issues to some extent, whether or not such tactics are explicitly identified as comprising an RP unit.

The second set of studies we discuss includes one or more treatment cells with a more explicit emphasis on RP techniques. Many of these are also cognitive–behavioral conditions that specifically note the inclusion of sessions on RP, as recommended by Fairburn (1985).

The third group of studies examined the use of another strategy consistent with a focus on RP: the provision of periodic maintenance sessions following the completion of active-phase treatment.

It should be emphasized strongly that none of these investigations provides direct evidence on the incremental benefit derived from introducing RP components into the treatment of bulimia nervosa. In every instance, the modalities being compared differed on many dimensions other than the inclusion of RP elements, so that it is impossible to determine the specific contribution of the latter to the results obtained.

Studies Using Modalities Consistent with a RP Model

Olmsted and her colleagues conducted a study in which bulimic subjects were nonrandomly assigned to either a psychoeducational group (ED) or individual CBT (Olmsted et al., 1991). The authors indicated that the CBT intervention was fashioned after Fairburn's approach, but did not indicate whether explicit RP training was provided. After the completion of treatment, subjects were assigned to the following categories based on binge–purge frequency: "good" outcome indicated that no more than one binge–purge episode occurred during the 28 days prior to assessment, "moderate" outcome that two to four episodes took place, and "poor" outcome that four or more episodes were reported. Olmsted et al. reported that 18% of the ED group and 22% of the CBT condition qualified for the "good" outcome designation at both posttreatment and 3-month follow-up. They concluded that CBT was more effective than ED for severely symptomatic subjects; however, for those vomiting less than 42 times per month, the treatments proved equally effective. The conclusions that can be drawn from this report are sharply limited by the nonrandom basis for assignment, the confounding of treatment modality with group–individual administration, and the brief duration of follow-up.

Hsu and Sobkiewicz (1989) reported an uncontrolled 4–6-year follow-up investigation of 35 subjects, out of an original group of 45 patients. All subjects originally received at least five sessions of CBT therapy. Among the subjects traced at follow-up (some of whom remained in treatment), 47% were free of bulimic or anorexic symptoms, 16% met criteria for bulimia, and another 16% binged and purged at least occasionally in the previous 6 months. Most of those subjects who relapsed experienced only a brief period of symptom subsidence, although a few appeared recovered for several months before relapsing.

Studies Using an Explicit RP Component

Eight of the studies reviewed in Table 5.1 reported using RP elements in at least one of their treatment cells. Wilson, Rossiter, Kleifield, and Lindholm (1986) described a study comparing 16 weeks of a group cognitive–behavioral intervention (CR) with and without an exposure and response prevention (ERP) (CR or CR+ERP) component. The CR condition employed by Wilson et al. (1986) represented an attenuated form of Fairburn's approach that is best described as cognitive restructuring; the behavioral components Fairburn (1985) considers crucial in the treatment of bulimia were largely omitted. ERP therapy is based on an anxiety-reduction model of bulimia nervosa (Rosen & Leitenberg, 1982, 1985) and consists of two basic ingredients: (1) exposure to the feared stimuli (i.e., the consumption of particular foods or amounts of foods) and (2) prevention of the escape response (vomiting). ERP has proven effective in the treatment of bulimic symptoms in a number of comparative trials (see Craighead & Agras, 1991; Leitenberg & Rosen, 1988; Rosen, 1987).

Wilson et al. introduced RP strategies in the last session of treatment in both modalities. Subjects were asked to anticipate high-risk situations that might trigger a binge and then cognitively rehearse coping strategies for dealing with those situations. They were also asked to plan what they would do if they did slip by consuming something they had not intended to eat. At the end of treatment, both conditions produced a decrease in bingeing and vomiting, with no significant differences between them. Follow-up at 1 year indicated that the majority in the CR+ERP condition had maintained abstinence from bingeing and purging—an unusually positive result that Wilson et al. (1986) speculated might be attributable to the emphasis on RP as a formal component of the treatment package. However, the CR group, which also had the benefit of RP training, did not fare as well. Four of six patients in this group required additional treatment, thereby precluding longer-term follow-up information.

Perhaps the most impressive treatment study of bulimia nervosa was recently reported by Fairburn and colleagues (Fairburn et al., 1991). Subjects were randomly assigned to behavioral therapy (BT), CBT, or interpersonal therapy (IPT). The comparison between BT and CBT represented a dismantling study examining the effectiveness of behavioral techniques in isolation from the combined CBT approach. The IPT condition was included to compare the influence of a nonspecific treatment whose efficacy has been documented with a different psychiatric population (unipolar depression) to an established specific modality (CBT) tailored to the symptoms of bulimia nervosa. IPT is a short-term, directive, psychodynamically oriented therapy focusing on contemporaneous problems in interpersonal relationships. As implemented in the Fairburn et al. (1991) study, IPT did not include direct focus on attitudes about weight and shape, and did not attempt to change eating behavior. Posttreatment results on purging behavior suggested a superiority of CBT over IPT; however, all three treatments were equally effective in reducing binge episodes. CBT produced a greater reduction in disturbed attitudes to shape and weight relative to BT.

Follow-up data collected 1 year after treatment termination revealed some surprising trends. While subjects in the BT condition were doing quite poorly, IPT subjects had caught up with those in the CBT condition (C. Fairburn, personal communication, February 1991). The finding that CBT had a greater effect than BT on attempts to diet and attitudes to shape and weight is consistent with the postulated mechanisms of change in CBT; however, the unanticipated efficacy of IPT by the time of follow-up raises important questions for dominant theoretical models of bulimia nervosa. Since IPT did not address food or weight directly, through what mechanisms did it exert its beneficial effects on the focal symptoms of this disorder? And how did a modality lacking emphasis on RP prove so successful in maintaining (indeed, enhancing) treatment gains?

Fairburn et al. (1991) speculated that the decrease in bulimic behavior associated with IPT may have been mediated through an effect on negative self-evaluation. They noted that "the patients who respond seem to develop an increased sense of self-worth and competence and, as a result, their tendency to evaluate themselves largely in terms of their shape and weight lessens in intensity" (Fairburn, 1988, p. 641). Improvements in eating behavior are hypothesized to follow from these basic changes in self-concept. If this postulated mechanism is verified, the results of the Fairburn et al. (1991) study may have significant implications for our understanding of symptom maintenance and change in bulimia nervosa.

Studies Using a Maintenance Component

In the study of CR and CR+ERP described previously, Wilson et al. (1986) built a brief "check-in" maintenance strategy into their treatment design. During the follow-up period, patients were telephoned by their therapist on a monthly basis. The investigators noted that this minimal contact seemed to have interrupted incipient relapses for two of the participants.

A more extended examination of the utility of maintenance components was reported by Pyle et al. (Pyle, Mitchell, Eckert, Hatsukami, Pomeroy, & Zimmerman, 1990). This study was an extension of treatment following the completion of a separately reported comparative outcome trial (Mitchell, Pyle, Eckert, Hatsukami, Pomeroy, & Zimmerman, 1990). In the initial study, subjects had been randomly assigned to one of four treatment conditions: imipramine, pill placebo, group therapy plus imipramine, or group therapy plus pill placebo. The group therapy was an intensive program blending elements of behavioral, cognitive, dietary management, and abstinence-based treatment components. It did include one session on RP, in which participants were informed about the pattern and dangers of relapse in bulimia nervosa and instructed to develop written plans of what they would do to avoid relapse and to cope with slips if they did occur. At the end of treatment, the authors concluded that the effects of group therapy were stronger than drug treatment on all measures.

The maintenance program described by Pyle et al. (1990) was provided to all subjects who had responded positively to the active phase of treatment. Patients who had originally received medication were continued on imipramine or pill placebo, while those who had received group therapy were offered participation in a weekly support group. At the 6-month follow-up, the investigators determined that "the most important factor in preventing relapse was initial treatment with group psychotherapy regardless of maintenance treatment" (Pyle et al., 1990, p. 874). Relapse occurred in 21% of the subjects who received group therapy during the active phase (with or without imipramine), versus 78% of those who were in the imipramine-only condition. Attendance at group maintenance sessions did not appear to confer protection from relapses; in fact, there was a trend for higher relapse rates to be associated with increased participation in the maintenance program. The most likely interpretation of this finding is that "attendance at support group sessions reflect the seeking of further treatment and support and that many subjects who were in better control of their eating behavior did not desire further participation in a group" (Pyle et al., 1990, p. 875).

Issues Relevant to Relapse after Treatment

The frequent occurrence of relapse is one of the characteristics of bulimia nervosa that has been cited in support of an addiction model of the disorder. According to this account, binge–vomiting behavior is the manifestation of an underlying progressive disease process. The appropriate model for treatment is the immediate establishment of abstinence; it is considered as futile to attempt psychotherapy with a still-symptomatic as it would be with an intoxicated alcoholic. Even during the course of psychotherapy, intermittent or reduced-frequency binge–vomiting is unacceptable as a basis for treatment because it is an unstable state that generally deteriorates into total relapse. The proper response to a recurrence of symptoms following intervention is a reaffirmation of the validity of the addiction model and an absolute recommitment to the treatment goal of abstinence (Yeary & Heck, 1989).

Many have argued that the extension of abstinence-based treatment to bulimia is inappropriate because it fails to take unique aspects of the disorder into account (Bemis, 1985, 1987b; Wilson, in press-b). The most obvious difference between bulimia and other "addictive" disorders is that abstinence from the abused substance (i.e., food) is impossible. Clearly, abstinence programs for bulimia do not counsel starvation; rather, their objective is a normalized pattern of ingestion of the problem substance. It is interesting to note that this objective is precisely equivalent to the "controlled drinking" model that abstinence programs for alcoholism consider impossible.

Critics of the abstinence approach caution that programs such as Overeaters Anonymous may reinforce dichotomous thinking styles about "good–bad" foods and behaviors, and condone the very restrictiveness in food intake that it should be the business of treatment to modify. Whatever the merits of black-and-white thinking for disorders in which the abused substance *can* be avoided, it is suggested that an understanding of more subtle gradations may be necessary when the only possible treatment goal is moderation. It is also noted that endorsement of an abstinence standard may be unrealistic in view of the high rate of symptom recurrence in bulimia nervosa—and may in fact increase the risk of serious relapse by triggering the abstinence violation effect described by Marlatt and Gordon (1978).

As in the case of anorexia nervosa, desynchrony between the control of symptomatic behavior and the modification of core attitudes about body weight and shape seems common following treatment for bulimia nervosa, and may be a significant contributor to relapse. During the course of CBT, changes in the acceptance of body weight were found to be correlated with reductions in vomiting frequency (Schneider, O'Leary, & Agras, 1987). A separate study reported that body image dissatisfaction at the end of treatment was the most potent predictor of subsequent relapse (Freeman et al., 1985).

CLINICAL RECOMMENDATIONS

Despite our lack of specific knowledge about the relationship between particular therapeutic techniques and the reduction of relapse risk following treatment for anorexia or bulimia nervosa, a variety of clinical strategies for promoting maintenance can be derived from our general knowledge of treatment response in these disorders. Several authors have provided detailed guidelines for incorporating RP training into psychotherapy (e.g., Fairburn, 1985; Johnson & Connors, 1987; Johnson, Connors, & Tobin, 1987); their suggestions and some of our own clinical recommendations are outlined below.

This discussion should be prefaced with a reiteration of one elementary point: The maintenance of symptom control is predicated upon the establishment of symptom control in the first instance. As emphasized earlier, many eating disorder cases entered into the relapse statistics compiled at follow-up are more accurately characterized as examples of symptom persistence. The provision of adequate treatment is the foundation of efforts to prevent relapse.

A corollary point is that many of the same principles and techniques involved in effective treatment will be applicable to the maintenance of changes induced by treatment. To a great extent, successful RP training in the eating disorders will consist of trying to increase the probability that, following treatment termination, individuals will continue to employ the strategies acquired during treatment (e.g., meal planning, weight stabilization, analysis of high-risk situations, examination of dysfunctional beliefs, moderation of dichotomous thinking, development of an expanded repertoire of coping skills, pleasurable activities, and bases for self-evaluation). It is thus somewhat artificial and misleading to discuss prevention tactics separately from a discussion of the therapeutic enterprise as a whole. In the following section, we isolate a few special issues that are particularly relevant to planning for the maintenance of change following treatment; the missing context can be obtained in a number of descriptive articles on therapy for the eating disorders (e.g., Fairburn, 1985; Garner & Bemis, 1982, 1985; Johnson & Connors, 1987; Vandereycken & Meerman, 1984; Wooley & Wooley, 1985).

The Maintenance of Regular Eating Patterns: Settling into a Life without Dieting

Many experts concur with the judgment of Wooley and Wooley (1985) that "*dieting (starvation) itself may be a sufficient condition for the development of anorexia nervosa or bulimia*" (italics in original, p. 393); certainly, continued restrictiveness in food intake is incompatible with a resolution of these conditions.

The first phase of most forms of treatment for the eating disorders involves the replacement of the rigid or chaotic eating habits of these patients with a structured, normalized pattern of intake. In preparing for treatment termination, it is crucial that patients accept the principle that their commitment to adaptive eating behavior may need to be lifelong. Adaptive eating behavior implies the consumption of three adequate meals at spaced intervals, the avoidance of dietary strategies for weight reduction, and the inclusion of a wide variety of foods in the diet— including those the individual considered "dangerous" or "forbidden" when in the throes of her eating disorder.

In the early stages of therapy, the content and scheduling of meals are highly structured; patients are encouraged to eat preplanned menus at designated hours regardless of circumstances or appetite (Fairburn, 1985; Garner & Bemis, 1985). Over time, it is anticipated that patients can become more flexible and responsive to physiological cues and personal preferences; however, clinical experience suggests that premature (often self-initiated) attempts to decrease the structure imposed during treatment may predispose individuals to relapse. An impaired sense of satiety is one of the most persistent effects of semistarvation in normal human beings (Keys, Brozek, Henschel, Mickelson, & Taylor, 1950). In the absence of dependable internal feedback about hunger and fullness, recovering anorexics and bulimics who have abandoned structured meal plans may vacillate between overeating and restrictiveness, often spending inordinate amounts of time trying to figure out just how hungry they "really" feel and how much food will be required to fill the need. A follow-up study of anorexia nervosa confirmed the impression that structured eating is correlated with symptom control (Garfinkel, 1974). All subjects in the "good" and "intermediate" outcome categories were found to be regulating their intake through a variety of artificial systems, rather than attempting to rely on their "stomachs" to determine what they should eat. These improved individuals coped with the lack of recognition of satiety by depending on external cues, while the "poor" outcome group responded to the same deficit by avoiding meals, pursuing food fads, and engaging in purgative practices.

The specific problems encountered by recovering anorexics and bulimics following treatment may differ. Restricting anorexics who have been subsisting on perhaps 500 calories per day and as few as three or four food types are suddenly confronted with the dilemma of choice. Accustomed to controlling their appetites through exclusion, by designating whole categories of foods "off limits," they must now begin to include highly palatable foods in their diet, with all the possibilities for temptation and excess that these introduce. Shortly before treatment termination, a former anorexic client of the second author (KBV) characterized the situation confronting her with this evocative analogy:

> While I was anorexic, being around food was sort of like visiting an art museum. The paintings may be extraordinarily beautiful, but you never start coveting them or feeling sad or envious that they don't belong to you, because it never crosses your mind that you could take them home. Now, being around food is like going to an art gallery rather than a museum. Here, the paintings *can* be purchased and possessed—and you find yourself struggling with the desire to own them.

After starvation has been interrupted, it becomes apparent that the remarkable self-discipline anorexics displayed during the active phases of their illness was in fact quite tenuous, dependent on an all-or-nothing strategy for maintaining control. At this point, some restricting anorexics become vulnerable to the development of bulimic symptomatology, unable to make use of the different set of skills that would support moderation. During the late stages of therapy and after its termination, such individuals may profit from repeated emphasis on the value of continued meal planning, so that they can experiment more safely within the reassuring confines of a structured system. Cognitive reframing is also beneficial; to extend the art gallery analogy, clients can be helped to understand that it is not essential to possess everything that one desires— and it may seem less compelling when one accepts that beautiful objects can be afforded, and will remain available for selection and enjoyment for the remainder of one's life.

For bulimics, the problem of maintaining adaptive eating behavior has somewhat different origins and implications. Unlike their restricting counterparts, who have coped with hunger by declaring most foods "bad" at all times, bulimics have been accustomed to avoiding "bad" foods when they are "being good," while indulging in such foods on occasions when they are "being bad." During recovery, bulimics face the challenge of breaking down not only the distinction between good and bad foods, but also that between good and bad times. They must begin to incorporate previously binge-specific items into their normal daily diet, learning that ingestion of a formerly "bad" food need not be the trigger for initiating a "bad" episode.

In both anorexia and bulimia nervosa, a constant redirection toward moderation is indicated as recovery progresses. Following symptom remission, we rarely worry that anxious individuals will become too mellow or alcoholics too sober, but there is a real risk that anorexics will replace their abstemiousness with bingeing, and bulimics their bingeing with excessive restraint. It should be fully understood by therapists and frequently reiterated to clients that any misuse of food represents symptom persistence rather than recovery.

Accepting Optimal Weight

The most daunting challenge for the eating-disordered individual both during and after treatment involves coming to terms with a body weight and shape that she considers undesirable. In order to recover, anorexics must, by definition, gain substantial amounts of weight and forgo the pursuit of thinness. Bulimics may or may not have to increment their weight in order to stabilize at a level that can be maintained without dieting or purging; in either event, they must give up the idea that a suboptimal ideal weight is compatible with recovery. As we and others have repeatedly emphasized, the tendency to construe the self in terms of weight is the fundamental feature of both anorexia nervosa and bulimia nervosa, and this disposition is exceedingly difficult to modify. As long as it survives intact, the individual will theoretically remain vulnerable to the resumption of symptomatic behavior. Wooley and Wooley (1985) aver that "complete remission of symptoms is possible only when the patient's body image is such that dieting is no longer considered desirable, necessary, or even helpful" (p. 409). They note that an individual can reach this point in several ways: by changing her attitude toward the thin ideal, by accepting her own departure from the thin ideal, or by deemphasizing appearance as a means of regulating her self-esteem.

Few patients seem to be able to abandon the esthetic preference for thinness fostered by contemporary culture; such standards are acquired very early in life and are extremely resistant to modification. Many more are able to acknowledge during the course of treatment that the thin ideal is unattainable for them, and that its pursuit exacts an unacceptable toll in personal suffering and is incompatible with the achievement of other important goals. Following treatment, patients often report that these resolutions are eroded through constant bombardment with messages about the value of thinness from the media, partners, family members, friends, trainers, and physicians. To sustain her recovery, the eating-disordered individual may need to develop attitudes about weight and shape that are markedly discrepant from—and healthier than—those of her peers. Some find it useful to avoid stimuli that exacerbate concerns about weight (e.g., fashion magazines, health spas, and conversations about diet); however, avoidance of exposure to one's own figure (by staying away from the beach or pool) or weight (by throwing out the bathroom scale) is contraindicated. Without exposure to the actual size, shape, and consistency of the body, it is impossible to come to terms with normal proportions. In the absence of objective feedback about weight, more subjective variables such as "feeling fat" will be used to gauge physical status. Recovering individuals should be encouraged to weigh themselves regularly, albeit infrequently, and to establish criteria for detecting trends (e.g., three successive occasions on which increases or decreases are recorded/maintained) to forestall the tendency to react to minor fluctuations in weight. Like reformed smokers and drinkers, some may find that their own recovery is benefited by participation in activities that "carry the message" about the ineffectiveness of dieting and the inappropriateness of the thin ideal.

Identifying and Coping with High-Risk Situations

Anorexic and bulimic clients participating in behavioral, cognitive–behavioral, and most eclectic treatment programs are provided with systematic training in the identification of high-risk situations throughout treatment. In the later stages of therapy, it may be useful to generate a list of the situations the client has already encountered, supplemented with others that she anticipates might be problematic in the future. Strategies that have proven effective in avoiding or responding to these key situations should be reviewed and a formal, detailed plan of action developed for the client's ongoing reference. Fairburn (1985) and Johnson and Connors (1987) have published sample maintenance plans and lists of specific strategies that clients (and clinicians) may find useful; the idiosyncratic techniques generated over the course of each client's own experience in psychotherapy may prove most powerful.

One specific tactic that is often used in high-risk situations involves writing scripts for binge–purge episodes and the avoidance of these episodes. When confronted with an urge to binge, clients are asked to take 10 minutes to compose a detailed account of what would occur if they proceeded with a binge, noting how they would be thinking and feeling during and after a completed episode. They are also instructed to write out an alternative plan for avoiding the binge, describing the thoughts and feelings they would experience in association with that course. The script-writing technique interposes a delay between impulse and the initiation of binge eating and reminds individuals of the predictable adverse effects that occur in the aftermath of a completed cycle.

Responding to Slips

Clients with bulimia nervosa should be prepared for the strong likelihood that episodes of bulimic behavior will recur following successful treatment. Bulimic individuals react to the violation of personally or professionally established abstinence standards in the same manner as the substance abusers described by Marlatt and Gordon (1978), and they respond well to the same sorts of reframing strategies Marlatt and Gordon recommend. The only distinction may be that bulimic subjects seem even more practiced in the art of dichotomous thinking by virtue of many years of experience in its use, and may require frequent repetition of the principles that help to counter it. One disorder-specific requirement is that bulimics who have experienced a binge episode after a period of abstinence should not react to this transgression by suspending their structured eating plan in the hours or days that follow. Bulimics typically believe that they must compensate for the excess calories consumed during a binge by cutting down their subsequent intake; however, this pattern sets up a cycle of deprivation and craving that will increase the risk of subsequent lapses.

Some clinicians strongly advise clients against calculating the duration of abstinent periods in a way that will force them to "restart the clock" following the occurrence of slips. Instead, recovering bulimics are encouraged to credit themselves for the period of time they have coped successfully without resort to binges or purges, recognizing that one episode after a symptom-free week or month represents significant progress for an individual who has been experiencing daily episodes (Bemis, 1985; Johnson & Connors, 1987).

Developing Alternative Bases for Self-Evaluation and Self-Reinforcement

After achieving symptom control, individuals with anorexia or bulimia nervosa must begin to experiment with new sources of enjoyment, new standards for gauging their self-worth, and new strategies for achieving their goals. Anorexics in particular may feel that their lives have lost direction and purpose with the interruption of their quest for thinness. Hall (1982) notes that while "life is barren with anorexia . . . it becomes even more barren and painful without it" (p. 643). Recovering patients may need to develop a whole new repertoire of behaviors to replace the comprehensive, self-contained system that their eating disorder imposed (Slade, 1982). Unfortunately, the satisfactions they will eventually derive from more adaptive self-regulatory and interpersonal skills are seldom apparent in the early phases of recovery. It may be helpful to *predict* this common delay between the suspension of one set of reinforcers and the development of another, and to reassure patients that they will not be abandoned to cope with this difficult period alone.

Many eating-disordered clients seem to believe that they do not deserve to have other complaints; therapists and family members often appear to endorse this view by reducing or withdrawing their attention after the prominent eating and weight symptoms have abated. This regrettable tendency may exacerbate the possibility of relapse by reinforcing any disposition to use the disorder for secondary gain, or simply by leaving significant issues unresolved. While the principal emphasis in treatment is the control of focal symptoms, clinicians should not convey the impression that these constitute the sole concern. The length and frequency of treatment should be determined by the patient's distress rather than tied to her weight and eating behavior.

CONCLUSIONS

At present, we know only a little about the process of relapse in the eating disorders, and nothing whatever about the role of treatment elements designed to reduce its probability. In the case of anorexia nervosa, psychotherapy research is insufficiently advanced to make controlled comparisons of treatment with and without RP components a logical priority. Clearly, we need to establish first that one or another of the therapeutic programs proposed for this disorder is differentially effective in promoting recovery. Moreover, given the extended course of treatment recommended, it may be naive to anticipate that the presence or absence of several sessions of RP work should produce significant group differences at follow-up years later. The study of intervention in bulimia nervosa is developmentally far more advanced, so that dismantling designs varying the prominence of RP would be justified, timely, and potentially informative. It is certainly not premature to initiate research into the relapse process of both disorders through the prospective study of therapeutically and spontaneously remitted individuals.

REFERENCES

Agras, W. S., Schneider, J. A., Arnow, B., Raeburn, S. D., & Telch, C. F. (1989). Cognitive–behavioral and response-prevention treatments for bulimia nervosa. *Journal of Consulting and Clinical Psychology, 57,* 215–221.

American Psychiatric Association. (1987). *Diagnostic and statistical manual of mental disorders* (3rd ed., rev.). Washington, DC: Author.

Anonymous (1988). Letter. *NAAS Newsletter, 11,* 7–8.

Bemis, K. M. (1978). Current approaches to the etiology and treatment of anorexia nervosa. *Psychological Bulletin, 85,* 593–617.

Bemis, K. M. (1983). A comparison of functional relationships in anorexia nervosa and phobia. In P. L. Darby, P. E. Garfinkel, D. M. Garner, & D. V. Coscina (Eds.), *Anorexia nervosa: Recent developments in research* (pp. 403–415). New York: Alan R. Liss.

Bemis, K. M. (1985). "Abstinence" and "nonabstinence" models for the treatment of bulimia. *International Journal of Eating Disorders, 4,* 407–437.

Bemis, K. M. (1987a). The present status of operant conditioning for the treatment of anorexia nervosa. *Behavior Modification, 11*, 432–463.

Bemis, K. M. (1987b). A comparison of abstinence and nonabstinence approaches to the treatment of bulimia nervosa: Must symptoms stop before treatment can begin? Paper presented at the National Conference on the Eating Disorders, Columbus, OH.

Bemis, K. M. (1988). Classifying the eating disorders. *NAAS Newsletter, 11*, 1–3.

Ben-Tovim, D. I., Walker, M. K., Murray, H., & Chin, G. (1990). Body size estimates: Body image or body attitude measures? *International Journal of Eating Disorders, 9*, 283–291.

Bowden, P. K., Touyz, S. W., Rodriguez, P. J., Hensley, R., & Beumont, P. J. V. (1989). Distorting patient or distorting instrument? Body shape disturbance in patients with anorexia nervosa and bulimia. *British Journal of Psychiatry, 155*, 196–201.

Branch, C. H. H., & Eurman, L. J. (1980). Social attitudes toward patients with anorexia nervosa. *America Journal of Psychiatry, 137*, 631–632.

Bruch, H. (1973). *Eating disorders: Obesity, anorexia nervosa, and the person within*. New York: Basic Books.

Bruch, H. (1977). Psychological antecedents of anorexia nervosa. In R. A. Vigersky (Ed.), *Anorexia nervosa* (pp. 1–10). New York: Raven Press.

Bruch, H. (1978). *The golden cage: The enigma of anorexia nervosa*. Cambridge, MA: Harvard University Press.

Cash, T. F., & Brown, T. A. (1987). Body image in anorexia nervosa and bulimia nervosa. *Behavior Modification, 11*, 487–521.

Channon, S., & de Silva, P. (1985). Psychological correlates of weight gain in patients with anorexia nervosa. *Journal of Psychiatric Research, 19*, 267–271.

Channon, S., de Silva, P., Hemsley, D., & Perkins, R. (1989). A controlled trial of cognitive–behavioral and behavioral treatment of anorexia nervosa. *Behaviour Research and Therapy, 27*, 529–535.

Ciseaux, A. (1980). Anorexia nervosa: A view for the mirror. *American Journal of Nursing, 80*, 1468–1470.

Clinton, D. N., & McKinlay, W. W. (1986). Attitudes to food, eating, and weight in acutely ill and recovered anorectics. *British Journal of Clinical Psychology, 25*, 61–67.

Cooper, P. J., Cooper, Z., & Hill, C. (1989). Behavioral treatment of bulimia nervosa. *International Journal of Eating Disorders, 8*, 87–92.

Cooper, Z., & Fairburn, C. G. (1987). The eating disorder examination: A semi-structured interview for the assessment of the specific psychopathology of eating disorders. *International Journal of Eating Disorders, 6*, 1–8.

Cooper, Z., Cooper, P. J., & Fairburn, C. G. (1989). The validity of the eating disorder examination and its subscales. *British Journal of Psychiatry, 154*, 807–812.

Cox, G. L., & Merkel, W. T. (1989). A qualitative review of psychosocial treatments for bulimia. *Journal of Nervous and Mental Disease, 177*, 77–84.

Craighead, L. W., & Agras, W. S. (1991). Mechanisms of action in cognitive–behavioral and pharmacological interventions for obesity and bulimia nervosa. *Journal of Consulting and Clinical Psychology, 59*, 115–125.

Crisp, A. H. (1980). *Anorexia nervosa: Let me be*. London: Academic Press.

Dally, P. J. (1969). *Anorexia nervosa*. New York: Grune & Stratton.

Dedman, P. A., Numa, S. F., & Wakeling, A. (1988). A cognitive–behavioral group approach for the treatment of bulimia nervosa: A preliminary study. *Journal of Psychosomatic Research, 32*, 285–290.

Eckert, E. D. (1988). Ten year outcome in anorexia nervosa. *Journal of Psychiatric Research, 22*, 314.

Eckert, E. D., Goldberg, S. C., Halmi, K. A., Casper, R. C., & Davis, J. M. (1979). Behaviour therapy in anorexia nervosa. *British Journal of Psychiatry, 134*, 55–59.

Fairburn, C. G. (1985). Cognitive–behavioral treatment for bulimia. In D. M. Garner & P. E. Garfinkel (Eds.), *Handbook of psychotherapy for anorexia nervosa and bulimia* (pp. 160–192). New York: Guilford Press.

Fairburn, C. G. (1988). The current status of psychological treatments for bulimia nervosa. *Journal of Psychosomatic Research, 32*, 635–645.

Fairburn, C. G., Cooper, Z., & Cooper, P. J. (1986). The clinical features and maintenance of bulimia nervosa. In K. D. Brownell & J. P. Foreyt (Eds.), *Handbook of eating disorders* (pp. 389–404). New York: Basic Books.

Fairburn, C. G., & Garner, D. M. (1986). The diagnosis of bulimia nervosa. *International Journal of Eating Disorders, 5*, 403–419.

Fairburn, C. G., Jones, R., Peveler, R. C., Carr, S. J., Solomon, R. A., O'Connor, M. E., Burton, J., & Hope, R. A. (1991). Three psychological treatments for bulimia nervosa. *Archives of General Psychiatry, 48*, 463–469.

Fairburn, C. G., Kirk, J., O'Connor, M., & Cooper, P. J. (1986). A comparison of two psychological treatments for bulimia nervosa. *Behaviour Research and Therapy, 24*, 629–643.

Foa, E. B. (1979). Failure in treating obsessive–compulsives. *Behaviour Research and Therapy, 17*, 169–176.

Freeman, C. P. L., Barry, F., Dunkeld-Turnbull, J., & Henderson, A. (1988). Controlled trial of psychotherapy for bulimia nervosa. *British Medical Journal, 296*, 521–525.

Freeman, C. P. L., & Munro, J. K. M. (1988). Drug and group treatments for bulimia/bulimia nervosa. *Journal of Psychosomatic Research, 32*, 647–660.

Freeman, R. J., Beach, B., Davis, R., & Solyom, L. (1985). The prediction of relapse in bulimia nervosa. *Journal of Psychiatric Research, 19*, 349–353.

Garfinkel, P. E. (1974). Perception of hunger and satiety in anorexia nervosa. *Psychological Medicine, 4*, 309–315.

Garfinkel, P. E., & Garner, D. M. (1982). *Anorexia nervosa: A multidimensional perspective*. New York: Brunner/Mazel.

Garfinkel, P. E., Moldofsky, H., & Garner, D. M. (1977). Prognosis in anorexia nervosa as influenced by clinical features, treatment and self-perception. *Canadian Medical Association Journal, 117*, 1041–1045.

Garner, D. M. (1986). Cognitive therapy for bulimia nervosa. In S. C. Feinstein (Ed.), *Adolescent psychiatry: Developmental and clinical studies* (Vol. 13, pp. 358–390). Chicago: University of Chicago Press.

Garner, D. M. (1987). Psychotherapy outcome research with bulimia nervosa. *Psychotherapy and Psychosomatics, 48*, 129–140.

Garner, D. M., & Bemis, K. M. (1982). A cognitive–behavioral approach to anorexia nervosa. *Cognitive Therapy and Research, 6*, 123–150.

Garner, D. M., & Bemis, K. M. (1985). Cognitive therapy for anorexia nervosa. In D. M. Garner & P. E. Garfinkel (Eds.), *Handbook of psychotherapy for anorexia nervosa and bulimia* (pp. 107–146). New York: Guilford Press.

Garner, D. M., Fairburn, C. G., & Davis, R. (1987). Cognitive–behavioral treatment of bulimia nervosa. *Behavior Modification, 11*, 398–431.

Garner, D. M., Garfinkel, P. E., & Bonato, D. P. (1987). Body image measurement in eating disorders. *Advances in Psychosomatic Medicine, 17*, 119–133.

Goodyear, B. (1990). *Resistance to change, expectancies, and dimensions of personality in psychoactive substance use disorders: A construct validity study of the conerns about change scale.* Unpublished doctoral dissertation, University of Hawaii, Honolulu.

Gray, J. J., & Hoage, C. M. (1990). Bulimia nervosa: Group behavior therapy with exposure plus response prevention. *Psychological Reports, 66*, 667–674.

Hall, A. (1982). Deciding to stay an anorectic. *Postgraduate Medical Journal, 58*, 641–647.

Hall, A., & Crisp, A. H. (1987). Brief psychotherapy in the treatment of anorexia nervosa: Outcome at one year. *British Journal of Psychiatry, 151*, 185–191.

Hall, A., Slim, E., Hawker, F., & Salmond, C. (1984). Anorexia nervosa: Long-term outcome in 50 female patients. *British Journal of Psychiatry, 145*, 407–413.

Halmi, K. A. (1985). Behavioral management for anorexia nervosa. In D. M. Garner & P. E. Garfinkel (Eds.), *Handbook of psychotherapy for anorexia nervosa and bulimia* (pp. 147–159). New York: Guilford Press.

Herzog, D. B., Keller, M. B., & Lavori, P. W. (1988). Outcome in anorexia nervosa and bulimia nervosa: A review of the literature. *Journal of Nervous and Mental Disease, 176*, 131–143.

Hsu, L. K. G. (1988). The outcome of anorexia nervosa: A re-appraisal. *Psychological Medicine, 18*, 807–812.

Hsu, L. K. G., Crisp, A. H., & Harding, B. (1979). Outcome of anorexia nervosa. *Lancet, 1*, 61–65.

Hsu, L. K. G., & Sobkiewicz, T. A. (1989). Bulimia nervosa: A four- to six-year follow-up study. *Psychological Medicine, 19*, 1035–1038.

Hsu, L. K. G., & Sobkiewicz, T. A. (1991). Body image disturbance: Time to abandon the concept for eating disorders? *International Journal of Eating Disorders, 10*, 15–30.

Isager, T., Brinch, M., Kreiner, S., & Tolstrup, K. (1985). Death and relapse in anorexia nervosa: Survival analysis of 151 cases. *Journal of Psychiatric Research, 19*, 515–521.

Johnson, C., & Connors, M. E. (1987). *The etiology and treatment of bulimia nervosa.* New York: Basic Books.

Johnson, C., Connors, M. E., & Tobin, D. L. (1987). Symptom management of bulimia. *Journal of Consulting and Clinical Psychology, 55*, 668–676.

Kelaler, M. B., Herzog, D. B., Lavori, P. W., Ott, I. L., Bradburn, I. S., & Mahoney, E. M. (1989). Letter: High rates of chronicity and rapidity of relapse in patients with bulimia nervosa and depression. *Archives of General Psychiatry, 46,* 480–481.

Keys, A., Brozek, J., Henschel, A., Mickelson, O., & Taylor, H. I. (1950). *The biology of human starvation* (Vol. 2). Minneapolis, MN: University of Minnesota Press.

Kirkley, B. G., Schneider, J. A., Agras, W. S., & Bachman, J. A. (1985). Comparison of two group treatments for bulimia. *Journal of Consulting and Clinical Psychology, 53,* 43–48.

Kreipe, R. E., & Kidder, F. (1986). Comparisons of two hospital treatment programs for anorexia nervosa. *International Journal of Eating Disorders, 5,* 649–657.

Laessle, R. G., Waadt, S., & Pirke, K. M. (1987). A structured behaviorally oriented group treatment for bulimia nervosa. *Psychotherapy and Psychosomatics, 48,* 141–145.

Laessle, R. G., Zoettl, C., & Pirke, K. M. (1987). Metaanalysis of treatment studies for bulimia. *International Journal of Eating Disorders, 6,* 647–653.

Leitenberg, H., & Rosen, J. C. (1988). Cognitive–behavioral treatment of bulimia nervosa. In M. Hersen, R. M. Eisler, & P. M. Miller (Eds.), *Progress in Behavior Modification* (Vol. 23, pp. 11–35). Newbury Park, CA: Sage Publications.

Leitenberg, H., Rosen, J. C., Gross, J., Nudelman, S., & Vara, L. S. (1988). Exposure plus response-prevention treatment of bulimia nervosa. *Journal of Consulting and Clinical Psychology, 56,* 535–541.

Luka, L. P., Agras, W. S., & Schneider, J. A. (1986). Letter: Thirty month follow-up of cognitive–behavioral group therapy for bulimia. *British Journal of Psychiatry, 148,* 614–615.

MacLeod, S. (1982). *The art of starvation: A story of anorexia and survival.* New York: Schocken Books.

Marlatt, G. A., & Gordon, J. R. (1978). Determinants of relapse: Implications for the maintenance of behavior change. In P. Davidson (Ed.), *Behavioral medicine: Changing health lifestyles* (pp. 410–452). New York: Brunner/Mazel.

Meerman, R., Napierski, C., & Vandereycken, W. (1988). Experimental body image research in anorexia nervosa patients. In B. J. Blinder, B. F. Chaitin, & R. Goldstein (Eds.), *The eating disorders* (pp. 177–194). New York: PMA Publishing.

Mitchell, J. E., Davis, L., & Goff, G. (1985). The process of relapse in patients with bulimia. *International Journal of Eating Disorders, 4,* 457–463.

Mitchell, J. E., Davis, L., Goff, G., & Pyle, R. L. (1986). A follow-up study of patients with bulimia. *International Journal of Eating Disorders, 5,* 441–450.

Mitchell, J. E., Hatsukami, D., Pyle, R. L., & Eckert, E. D. (1986). The bulimia syndrome: Course of the illness and associated problems. *Comprehensive Psychiatry, 27,* 165–170.

Mitchell, J. E., Pyle, R. L., Eckert, E. D., Hatsukami, D., Pomeroy, C., & Zimmerman, R. (1990). A comparison study of antidepressants and structured intensive group psychotherapy in the treatment of bulimia nervosa. *Archives of General Psychiatry, 47,* 149–157.

Mitchell, P. B. (1988). The pharmacological management of bulimia nervosa: A critical review. *International Journal of Eating Disorders, 7*, 29–41.

Olmsted, M. P., Davis, R., Rockert, W., Irvine, M. J., Eagle, M., & Garner, D. M. (1991). Efficacy of a brief group psychoeducational intervention for bulimia nervosa. *Behaviour Research and Therapy, 29*, 71–83.

Pertschuk, M. J., Forster, J., Buzby, G., & Mullen, J. L. (1981). The treatment of anorexia nervosa with total parental nutrition. *Biological Psychiatry, 16*, 539–550.

Pyle, R. L., Mitchell, J. E., Eckert, E. D., Hatsukami, D., Pomeroy, C., & Zimmerman, R. (1990). Maintenance treatment and 6-month outcome for bulimic patients who respond to initial treatment. *American Journal of Psychiatry, 147*, 871–875.

Rankin, H. (1989). Relapse and eating disorders: The recurring illusion. In M. Gossop (Ed.), *Relapse and addictive behavior* (pp. 86–95). New York: Tavistock/Routledge.

Ratnasuriya, R. H., Eisler, I., Szmukler, G., & Russell, G. F. M. (1989). Outcome and prognostic factors after 20 years of anorexia nervosa. *Annals of the New York Academy of Sciences, 575*, 567–568.

Ratnasuriya, R. H., Eisler, I., Szmukler, G. I., & Russell, G. F. M. (1991). Anorexia nervosa: Outcome and prognostic factors after 20 years. *British Journal of Psychiatry, 158*, 495–502.

Remschmidt, H., Wienand, F., & Wewetzer, C. (1990). The long-term course of anorexia nervosa. In H. Remschmidt & M. H. Schmidt (Eds.), *Anorexia nervosa* (pp. 127–136). Lewiston, NY: Hogrefe & Huber.

Root, M. P. P. (1990). Recovery and relapse in former bulimics. *Psychotherapy, 27*, 397–403.

Rosen, J. C. (1987). A review of behavioral treatments for bulimia nervosa. *Behavior Modification, 11*, 464–486.

Rosen, J. C., & Leitenberg, H. (1982). Bulimia nervosa: Treatment with exposure and response prevention. *Behavior Therapy, 13*, 117–124.

Rosen, J. C., & Leitenberg, H. (1985). Exposure plus response prevention treatment of bulimia. In D. M. Garner & P. E. Garfinkel (Eds.), *Handbook of psychotherapy for anorexia nervosa and bulimia* (pp. 193–209). New York: Guilford Press.

Rosenvinge, J. H., & Mouland, S. O. (1990). Outcome and prognosis of anorexia nervosa: A retrospective study of 41 subjects. *British Journal of Psychiatry, 156*, 92–97.

Rossiter, E. M., Agras, W. S., & Losch, M. (1988). Changes in self-reported food intake in bulimics as a consequence of antidepressant treatment. *International Journal of Eating Disorders, 7*, 779–783.

Russell, G. F. M. (1977). General management of anorexia nervosa and difficulties in assessing the efficacy of treatment. In R. A. Vigersky (Ed.), *Anorexia nervosa* (pp. 277–289). New York: Raven Press.

Russell, G. F. M. (1979). Bulimia nervosa: An ominous variant of anorexia nervosa. *Psychological Medicine, 9*, 429–448.

Russell, G. F. M., Szmukler, G. I., Dare, C., & Eisler, I. (1987). An evaluation of family therapy in anorexia nervosa and bulimia nervosa. *Archives of General Psychiatry, 44*, 1047–1056.

Schneider, J. A., & Agras, W. S. (1985). A cognitive–behavioural group treatment of bulimia. *British Journal of Psychiatry, 146,* 66–69.

Schneider, J. A., O'Leary, A., & Agras, W. S. (1987). The role of perceived self-efficacy in recovery from bulimia: A preliminary examination. *Behaviour Research and Therapy, 25,* 429–432.

Schwartz, D. M., & Thompson, M. G. (1981). Do anorectics get well? Current research and future needs. *American Journal of Psychiatry, 138,* 319–323.

Selvini-Palazzoli, M. (1978). *Self-starvation: From individual to family therapy in the treatment of anorexia nervosa* (rev. ed.). New York: Jason Aronson.

Slade, P. D. (1982). Towards a functional analysis of anorexia nervosa and bulimia nervosa. *British Journal of Clinical Psychology, 21,* 167–179.

Slade, P. D. (1985). A review of body-image studies in anorexia nervosa and bulimia nervosa. *Journal of Psychiatric Research, 19,* 255–265.

Steinhausen, H. C., & Glanville, K. (1983). Follow-up studies of anorexia nervosa: A review of research findings. *Psychological Medicine, 13,* 239–249.

Szmukler, G. I., & Russell, G. F. M. (1986). Outcome and prognosis of anorexia nervosa. In K. Brownell & J. Foreyt (Eds.), *Handbook of eating disorders: Physiology, psychology, and treatment of obesity, anorexia, and bulimia* (pp. 283–300). New York: Basic Books.

Theander, S. (1970). Anorexia nervosa: A psychiatric investigation of 94 female patients. *Acta Psychiatrica Scandinavica, 214* (Suppl.).

Theander, S. (1985). Outcome and prognosis in anorexia nervosa and bulimia: Some results of previous investigations, compared with those of a Swedish long-term study. *Journal of Psychiatric Research, 19,* 493–508.

Vandereycken, W., & Meermann, R. (1984). *Anorexia nervosa: A clinician's guide to treatment.* Berlin: de Gruyter.

Vandereycken, W., & Pierloot, R. (1983). Long-term outcome research in anorexia nervosa: The problem of patient selection and follow-up duration. *International Journal of Eating Disorders, 2,* 237–242.

Vitousek, K. (1991). *Resistance to change in the eating disorders and anxiety disorders.* Unpublished manuscript, University of Hawaii.

Vitousek, K., Daly, J., & Heiser, C. (1991). Reconstructing the internal world of the eating-disordered individual: Overcoming denial and distortion in self-report. *International Journal of Eating Disorders, 10,* 647–666.

Vitousek, K., & Ewald, L. S. (in press). Self-representation in eating disorders: A cognitive perspective. In Z. V. Segal & S. J. Blatt (Eds.), *Self-representation and emotional disorders: Cognitive and psychodynamic perspectives.* New York: Guilford Press.

Vitousek, K., & Hollon, S. (1990). The investigation of schematic content and processing in eating disorders. *Cognitive Therapy and Research, 14,* 191–214.

Weizman, A., Tyano, S., Wijsenbeek, H., & Ben David, M. (1985). Behavior therapy, pimozide treatment and prolactin secretion in anorexia nervosa. *Psychotherapy and Psychosomatics, 43,* 136–140.

Wilson, G. T. (1987). Assessing treatment outcome in bulimia nervosa: A methodological note. *International Journal of Eating Disorders, 6,* 339–348.

Wilson, G. T. (1989). Bulimia nervosa: Models, assessment, and treatment. *Current Opinion in Psychiatry, 2,* 790–794.

Wilson, G. T. (in press-a). Cognitive–behavioral versus pharmacological treatment of bulimia nervosa. *Verhaltenstherapie.*

Wilson, G. T. (in press-b). The addiction model of eating disorders: A critical analysis. *Advances in Behavior Research and Therapy.*

Wilson, G. T., Rossiter, E., Kleifield, E. I., & Lindholm, L. (1986). Cognitive–behavioral treatment of bulimia nervosa: A controlled evaluation. *Behaviour Research and Therapy, 24,* 277–288.

Wilson, G. T., & Smith, D. (1989). Assessment of bulimia nervosa: An evaluation of the eating disorder examination. *International Journal of Eating Disorders, 8,* 173–179.

Wilson, G. T., & Walsh, B. T. (1991). Eating disorders in the DSM-IV. *Journal of Abnormal Psychology, 100,* 362–365.

Winstead, M. L. (1984, August). *Cognitive–behavioral factors of relapse among bulimics.* Paper presented at the American Psychological Association, Toronto, Canada.

Wooley, S. C., & Wooley, O. W. (1985). Intensive outpatient and residential treatment for bulimia. In D. M. Garner & P. E. Garfinkel (Eds.), *Handbook of psychotherapy for anorexia nervosa and bulimia* (pp. 391–430). New York: Guilford Press.

Yeary, J. R., & Heck, C. L. (1989). Dual diagnosis: Eating disorders and psychoactive substance dependence. *Journal of Psychoactive Drugs, 21,* 239–249.

CHAPTER 6

DEPRESSION

Peter H. Wilson
THE FLINDERS UNIVERSITY OF SOUTH AUSTRALIA

T wo features of mood disorders are most striking: their prevalence in the population and their chronic or recurrent course over time. Depression is one of the most common disorders, with a lifetime prevalence of at least 10% (Lehmann, 1971). The recurrent nature of mood disorders is well established as a characteristic of the various problems grouped under this general category (National Institute of Mental Health [NIMH] 1985; Zis & Goodwin, 1979). DSM-III-R (American Psychiatric Association, 1987) makes distinctions between different types of mood disorders. The most relevant to this chapter is major depressive episode (MDE). A diagnosis of MDE (or "unipolar depression") requires the presence of at least five of the following symptoms nearly every day for a period of at least 2 weeks, including one or the other of the first two symptoms: (1) dysphoric mood; (2) loss of interest or pleasure in all (or almost all) usual activities; (3) decreased appetite or weight loss (or increased appetite and weight gain); (4) insomnia or hypersomnia; (5) psychomotor retardation or agitation; (6) loss of energy or feelings of fatigue; (7) feelings of worthlessness or excessive or inappropriate guilt; (8) diminished ability to think, concentrate, and make decisions, and (9) recurrent thoughts of death or suicidal thoughts or actions.

Unipolar depression is distinguished from Bipolar Mood Disorder (also known as manic depressive disorder) in which there is an alternation between depressive and manic periods. Manic episodes generally are characterized by elevated mood, inflated self-esteem or grandiosity, flight of ideas or racing thoughts, increased activity or psychomotor agitation, and psychotic features such as delusions and hallucinations. Of the various other disorders of mood listed in DSM-III-R, dysthymia may be particularly relevant to the discussion of relapse. Dysthymia involves the presence of at least mild depressive symptoms fairly continuously over a period of at least 2 years and may be secondary to another disorder such as substance dependence or anxiety disorder. Although most research in the area of depression focuses on MDE, dysthymia is also worthy of some attention because dysthymic individuals may frequently seek therapy either for their chronic depressive features or for other coexistent problems. Some people appear to experience a MDE superimposed on dysthymia, a condition referred to by Keller, Shapiro, Lavori, and Wolfe (1982) as "double depression." It is difficult to discuss mood disorders without giving some consideration to the major historical debate concerning the classification of depression into two types: depressions that are allegedly caused by alterations in brain biochemistry (endogenous) and those thought to be a result of environmental factors (nonendogenous, neurotic, reactive). These two putative types of depression are thought to be represented by different symptom classes. It is often considered that endogenous depressions are characterized by a number of features such as loss of interest in almost all pleasurable activities, lack of reactivity to pleasurable stimuli, depression worse in the morning, early-morning awakening, marked psychomotor retardation or agitation, and significant weight loss. These depressions often have a clear episodic pattern with almost complete recovery between episodes. Although there is no suggested etiological assumption in DSM-III-R, a person may be diagnosed as having a MDE with features of melancholia if symptoms that are similar to those listed above for "endogenous" depression are present.

Whether all the distinctions between types of affective disorders that are made within DSM-III-R are truly representative of different disorders of separate etiology is an issue beyond the scope of this chapter. However, the foregoing presentation concerning the existence of potentially different subtypes of mood disorders indicates the need for caution in considering virtually any aspect of depression, including relapse and its prevention, since different conclusions might be reached about the different potential subtypes. The main focus here is on unipolar depression and dysthymia, since these are the forms of mood disorder most likely to be successfully treated with cognitive–behavioral interventions. Even within these disorders, however, we may still be dealing with conditions of different etiology that require further differentiation.

One of the difficulties in any discussion of relapse in depression is the definition of the term "relapse" itself. Some researchers (e.g., Klerman, 1978) advocate the need for a distinction between the terms "relapse" and "recurrence." Both terms imply that significant recovery from an index episode has been achieved since one can hardly talk of either relapse or recurrence unless significant initial improvement has occurred. Klerman (1978) defines "relapse" as a return of symptoms within 6 to 9 months of the onset of the index episode. He uses the term "recurrence" to describe the emergence of a new episode, that is, the return of symptoms after a symptom-free period of at least 6 to 12 months from the conclusion of the index episode. The periods recommended by Klerman are based on the general belief that a depressive episode typically lasts for about 6 to 9 months, and that removal from antidepressant medication within that period often results in a reemergence of depressive symptoms. The main problem with the use of this terminology is the conceptual difficulty involved in the distinction between relapse and recurrence. One might well ask: Is there any fundemental difference between a return to symptoms within or outside the time suggested? The assumption in the definition of "relapse" is that the person is experiencing the return of the same episode, but after some period of time, any emergence of symptoms represents a new episode with either a possibly different etiology or a reinstatement of the same causal processes (recurrence). It could be argued that this distinction represents an unnecessary extension of a disease model to the problem of depression and does little to inform us of the critical aspects of the nature of relapse. In the case of dysthymia, which will sometimes worsen in severity to the extent that MDE would be diagnosed, the problem with the temporal criteria suggested by Klerman is exacerbated since it may be difficult to distinguish between symptom-free and symptomatic periods.

The severity of symptoms required for a definition of relapse is also problematic in the area of depression. In some areas, such as exhibitionism, smoking, or obesity, a return of the problem is more clearly distinguished because of the overt nature of the behavior. However, depressive symptoms may occur in varying degrees of severity and over varying periods of time. The result is that the distinction between "relapse," "recurrence," and "normal functioning" is less clearcut. On the other hand, Hollon, Shelton, and Loosen (1991) have argued for a preservation of this relapse–recurrence distinction and have cogently advanced a research design in which the causal concepts and consequences of depression can be more readily disentangled. For the present, the distinction between relapse and recurrence in depression might best be "tentatively" preserved until further empirical evidence results in some greater clarification of its usefulness and validity, although the distinction between short-, medium-, and long-term relapse might be just as useful (see Wilson, Chapter 15, this volume). For the purposes of this chapter, the term "relapse" will be used to denote either relapse or recurrence unless one or another meaning is clearly required.

RELAPSE RATES FOR DEPRESSION

Relapse rates for unipolar depression vary according to the period
covered by the assessment procedure and may be influenced by a number
of methodological features of the research. The National Institute of
Mental Health (NIMH; 1985) considered that "as many as 50% of patients
with recurrent unipolar disorders who recover from a given episode are
reported to have a recurrence within the first 2 years after recovery" (p.
471). It is difficult to know what the natural relapse rate for depression
would be in the absence of any treatment whatsoever. In practice, subjects in most studies have completed a course of treatment for an index
episode. However, studies do vary in the extent to which treatment is
maintained during a follow-up assessment period. The most comprehensive summary of the data on relapse is provided by Lavori, Keller,
and Klerman (1984). They provide a life table, or survival analysis, as
their approach to the problem that reveals an overall decline in the rate of
relapse across time. According to these figures, relapse is highest during
the initial 2 months (about 20%), after which the rate flattens out to about
30% by 6 months, 40% by 1 year, and 50% by the end of 2 years. Thus,
relapse is a considerable risk following successful intervention for depression.

Initial Response and Relapse
following Pharmacotherapy

Pharmacological treatments for mood disorders include antidepressants
(tricyclic antidepressants, monoamine oxidase inhibitors, and several
groups of newer antidepressants) and lithium. The antidepressants are
generally used to treat episodes of depression and have a success rate of
about 60%–70% in the alleviation of initial symptomatology. In their
review of the earlier antidepressant drug studies, Morris and Beck (1974)
report that about two thirds of the studies found superior results for
antidepressants in comparison with placebo medications. Following
symptomatic improvement, antidepressant medication is generally continued at a lower dosage for varying periods, typically for about 9 to 12
months. There is considerable support for the view that this antidepressant maintenance program assists in the reduction of the likelihood
of relapse (e.g., Glen, Johnson, & Shepherd, 1984; Klerman, DiMascio,
Weissman, Prusoff, & Paykel, 1974; Mindham, Howland, & Shepherd,
1973). There is also some evidence for the efficacy of lithium as a prophylactic agent for some patients with recurrent depression (see, e.g.,
Baastrup, Poulsen, Schou, Thomsen, & Amdisen, 1970; Davis, 1976;
Prien & Kupfer, 1986).

Cognitive and Behavioral Therapy

Cognitive therapy (Beck, Rush, Shaw, & Emery, 1979) has emerged as a major approach to the treatment of depression. There is now a large body of research on the efficacy of cognitive (or cognitive–behavioral) interventions for depression (Hollon, Shelton, & Loosen, 1991). Although some distinction might be drawn between purely cognitive treatment and cognitive–behavioral therapies, the term "cognitive" in this chapter implies a combined cognitive–behavioral approach. The studies in this area have been subjected to meta-analyses in at least four different research reports (Dobson, 1989; Nietzel, Russell, Hemmings, & Gretter, 1987; Robinson, Berman, & Neimeyer, 1990; Steinbrueck, Maxwell, & Howard, 1983). Dobson (1989) included 28 studies employing Beck's cognitive therapy (CT) for depression in which the Beck Depression Inventory (BDI) (Beck, Ward, Mendelson, Mock, & Erbaugh, 1961) was used as an outcome measure. The meta-analysis yielded significant effect sizes (ES) in favor of CT in comparison with no treatment (mean ES = –2.15; 10 studies), behavioral therapy (mean ES = –0.46; 9 studies), pharmacotherapy (mean ES = –0.53; 8 studies), and other psychotherapies (mean ES = –0.54; 7 studies). As can be seen, the largest effect is for the comparison with no-treatment controls, suggesting that treatment is superior to no treatment and administration of the assessment devices. The effects for CT versus other treatments, although favorable to CT, are rather smaller than the conventional 1 standard deviation unit, suggesting that CT is similar in effectiveness to other interventions.

Several large-scale studies of cognitive and other treatments for depression have been reported (e.g., Blackburn, Bishop, Glen, Whalley, & Christie, 1981; Elkin et al., 1989; Murphy, Simons, Wetzel, & Lustman, 1984; Hollon et al., 1991; Rush, Beck, Kovacs, & Hollon, 1977). The largest study that has appeared recently is the NIMH Collaborative Depression Project, which involved 239 patients at three research sites (Elkin et al., 1989). In this study, there were four conditions: CT; interpersonal psychotherapy (IPT); pharmacotherapy (imipramine) plus clinical management; and placebo plus clinical management. Overall, there were no significant differences between treatments, although imipramine generally ranked best, placebo worst, and IPT and CT fell in between the other two. For the more severely depressed subjects, imipramine was superior to placebo medication, but CT was not found to be superior to placebo. Overall, the NIMH study and other large treatment outcome investigations generally reveal an equivalence of effects for pharmacotherapy and CT in the short term (at posttreatment), although the NIMH study suggests that severity of depression may be an important predictor of initial treatment response. In the most recent study to appear, Hollon et al. (in press) randomly allocated 107 unipolar nonpsychotic depressed patients to one of four conditions: (1) CT, (2) imipramine without continuation, (3) imipramine with continuation for 1 year, and (4) CT plus imipramine (in which the pharmacotherapy was discontinued at the end of the initial treatment period). As with the other large-scale studies, there were no significant differences between the cognitive and pharmacological treatments at posttreatment. Of the 64 subjects who completed treatment, 44% (14/32) of imipramine subjects, 50% (8/16) of CT subjects, and 69% (11/16) of combined treatment subjects met a strict criterion of clinical success (BDI <=9 and Hamilton Rating Scale for Depression [HRSD] <=6). (Note that the two medication groups are combined here since these groups only differed in relation to continuation of medication during the follow-up period.) Using a more liberal criterion of success, referred to as "partial response" (posttreatment BDI<=15), improvement rates were 75% for the single-treatment modalities and 88% for the combined treatment. The overall "conservative" conclusion that can be reached from the various studies of CT is that it is an effective treatment for patients with mild to moderate depression, with a success rate of about 60%–70%.

LONG-TERM EFFECTS OF CT

It has been suggested that CT is likely to lead to superior maintenance of effects due to the alteration in the depressogenic cognitive style, which is assumed to be either the cause of or an important concurrent feature of depression. Fennell (1983) has also suggested that an important determinant of long-term effects is the learning of cognitive problem-solving skills that can be utilized across a broad range of situations. Regardless of the mechanism, there has certainly been a great deal of interest in the maintenance of long-term effects of cognitive treatments for depression (see Belsher & Costello, 1988; Shaw, 1989; Wilson, 1989). The relapse rates or percentages of patients who were symptomatic at various follow-up assessments for some of these studies are presented in Table 6.1. Only those studies that involved comparisons between CT and pharmacotherapy for which either relapse rates or depression status are reported, and which had a follow-up period of at least 6 months, are presented in Table 6.1. Follow-up results of four of the large-scale studies mentioned previously are provided in separate papers by Kovacs, Rush, Beck, and Hollon (1981), Simons, Murphy, Levine, and Wetzel (1986), Blackburn, Eunson, and Bishop (1986), and Evans et al. (1991). Also included in this table are the results of two other studies. Beck, Hollon, Young, Bedrosian, and Budenz (1985) evaluated the effectiveness of two treatment conditions: CT or a combination of CT and amitriptyline. They report the 6- and 12-month status of these patients, the results of which are displayed in the table. Hersen, Bellack, Himmelhoch, and Thase (1984) conducted a large-scale study of the effectiveness of social-skills training for depression. Subjects were randomly allocated to one of four treatments: (1) social-skills training plus placebo medication, (2) social-skills training plus amitriptyline, (3) amitriptyline, or (4) psychotherapy plus placebo. An unusual feature of this study is that maintenance treatments were conducted in each condition (6–8 sessions for the psychological treatments). No differences were found between the four conditions posttreatment or at the 6-month follow-up assessment. Percentages of patients who failed to meet a fairly strict criterion of recovery (score on the 24-item version of the HRSD < 10 [Hamilton, 1967]) are presented in Table 6.1.

Not displayed in Table 6.1, but still of great interest, are the findings of McLean and Hakstian (1990) who present the results of a 2¼-year follow-up of their earlier investigation (McLean & Hakstian, 1979) with 121 subjects who had received one of four treatments over a 10-week period: (1) behavioral therapy, (2) pharmacotherapy (amitriptyline), (3) relaxation therapy, or (4) nondirective psychotherapy. Assessments took place at 3, 6, 9, 15, 21, and 27 months after the conclusion of treatment. Subjects in the behavioral therapy condition were found to have improved significantly more than the other conditions over the follow-up period on a number of measures including mood, social activity, and personal productivity. McLean and Hakstian (1990) report the percentages of patients who, on a set of mood variables, fell "above a point in the normal, nondepressed distribution . . . that was one standard deviation below the normal group mean" (p. 486) aggregated over the follow-up period. These results are behavioral therapy (63.6%), pharmacotherapy (28.0%), relaxation therapy (25.7%), and nondirective psychotherapy (37.5%), where higher percentages reflect a better outcome. Thus, subjects who received behavioral therapy had a better course than those who received the other treatments on the mood variables in the 2¼ years after treatment.

It should be noted that a number of other studies of CT or behavioral therapy are not included because they did not involve comparisons with pharmacotherapy, they had shorter follow-up periods, or relapse rates (or symptom status) were not calculable from the reports. Of these studies, the one by Beutler et al. (1987) is probably the most important for this chapter. In this study, subjects were assigned (nonrandomly, partly by order of evaluation) to one of four groups: CT plus alprazolam, CT plus placebo, alprazolam plus support, or placebo plus support. Interestingly, from the standpoint of relapse prevention (RP), the final sessions of CT were spent in preparation for termination and reinforcement of changes.

TABLE 6.1. Percentages of Patients Who Relapsed or Were Depressed at Follow-up for Cognitive Therapy (CT) and Tricyclic Antidepressant Medication (TCA)

Study	Rate (%)	Period	Treatment
Kovacs et al. (1981)[a]	44	1 yr.	CT
	65	1 yr.	TCA
Beck et al. (1985)[a]	38	at 6 mos.	CT
	60	at 6 mos.	CT + TCA
	42	at 1 yr.	CT
	18	at 1 yr.	CT + TCA
Blackburn et al. (1986)	6	6 mos.	CT (Maint.)
	30	6 mos.	TCA (Maint.)
	0	6 mos.	CT + TCA (Maint.)
	23	2 yrs.	CT
	78	2 yrs.	TCA
	21	2 yrs.	CT + TCA
Simons et al. (1986)	20	1 yr.	CT
	67	1 yr.	TCA
	43	1 yr.	CT + TCA
	18	1 yr.	CT + Placebo
Evans et al. (1991)[b]	21(30)	2 yrs.	CT
	32(53)	2 yrs.	TCA (Maint.)
	50(70)	2 yrs.	TCA (No Maint.)
	15(46)	2 yrs.	CT + TCA (No Maint.)
Hersen et al. (1984)	33	at 6 mos.	SST + Placebo
	37	at 6 mos.	SST + TCA (Maint.)
	42	at 6 mos.	TCA (Maint.)
	40	at 6 mos.	P/therapy + Placebo

Note. SST = social-skills training; P/therapy = psychotherapy; Maint. = maintenance treatment.
[a]Subjects were not divided into responder/nonresponder categories.
[b]Conservative criterion: Two consecutive fortnightly BDIs of at least 16. Liberal criterion (shown in brackets): BDI score of at least 16 on any one occasion.

The results of a 3-month follow-up are reported on the HRSD (Hamilton, 1960) and the BDI. On the HRSD, only two subjects failed to meet criteria for remission (DSM-III diagnosis and HRSD score > 7), but on the BDI, 29% of the CT subjects and 12% of the non-CT subjects met criteria or improvement (BDI < 7). The inconsistency in the results of these two measures and the lack of totally random assignments lead to some difficulties in the interpretation of the results. Even at best, taking the BDI results, the symptomatic state of these patients is not impressive.

In view of some recent research, IPT also warrants some attention, although it is not the specific subject of this chapter. Weissman, Klerman, Prusoff, Sholomskas, and Padian (1981) found no differences between

IPT, antidepressant medication, and a combination of the two treatments on depressive symptomatology at a 1-year follow-up. It should also be noted that Covi and Lipman (1987) reported a better outcome with CT in comparison with an interpersonally oriented dynamic psychotherapy (IPT). Frank et al. (1990) recently reported the results of a follow-up of five treatment conditions, each of which was delivered during a 3-year maintenance phase that took place after an intensive combined imipramine/IPT had been completed. The five conditions were (1) imipramine, (2) imipramine plus IPT, (3) IPT alone, (4) IPT and placebo medication, and (5) placebo medication. The authors conclude that "survival analysis demonstrated a highly significant prophylactic effect for active Imipramine . . . and a modest effect for monthly interpersonal psychotherapy" (p. 1093). The results obtained with IPT are intriguing, and we await the long-term findings of the large NIMH collaborative trial with a great deal of interest, especially since this study involves a CT comparison group.

As can be seen in Table 6.1, the relapse rate (or depression status percentages) for CT tends to be lower than that obtained with antidepressant medication. However, it should be noted that in several of these investigations, subjects in the antidepressant therapy conditions did not receive maintenance medication as part of the study during the follow-up period. As mentioned previously, the continuance of medication, usually at a lower dosage for at least 4 to 6 months following improvement, generally reduces relapse in comparison with placebo medication (e.g., Mindam et al., 1973) and is widely adopted as the standard therapeutic practice. In the study reported by Blackburn et al. (1986), in which subjects were originally allocated to either CT, antidepressant medication (drug of choice), or a combined treatment condition, subjects continued to receive the relevant treatment in a maintenance format for a further 6 months. Blackburn et al. found that relapse rates were 6% (CT), 30% (pharmacotherapy), and 0% (CT plus pharmacotherapy). While these results are certainly favorable to CT, only tentative conclusions can be reached due to the rather low cell sizes (10–16 per group). The results could be substantially altered by even small sampling variations.

Hollon et al. (in press) report follow-up data on their recently completed study (see description above) in a separate report by Evans et al. (1991). Subjects who responded to the initial treatment, using the liberal criterion for success, were assessed in a clinical interview every 6 months, and completed monthly BDIs for 2 years. Two criteria were used to define a relapse. One, a liberal criterion, required the return of a BDI score of at least 16 on any one occasion. The other, a conservative criterion, required two consecutive BDIs of at least 16, in which the second BDI was administered in the clinic generally at least 1 week after the mail return. Data from a total of 44 subjects were available during the 2-year follow-up period. On the conservative criterion, which is the authors' preferred definition of relapse, relapse rates were 50% (imipramine, no continuation), 32% (imipramine, continuation), 21% (CT alone), and 15% (combined imipramine and CT). On the liberal criterion, relapse rates over a 2-year period were 70% (imipramine, no continuation), 53% (imipramine, continuation), 30% (CT alone), and 46% (combined Imipramine and CT). Overall, it can be seen that imipramine alone, without continuation beyond the initial treatment period, was inferior to the other treatments, a result that was not surprising given the existing literature that supports the prophylactic effect of continuing medication. The important point, however, is that there were no clear differences between the other treatments. Thus, it can be concluded that CT is as effective in preventing relapse as imipramine *when the drug is properly maintained over a 12-month period*. The fact that CT alone, 2 years after termination of the intervention, was at least as effective as maintenance medication is itself worth highlighting, as this finding provides the best support to date for the enduring effects of CT. It is also of interest to note that relapses that occurred in the drug-only condition (without maintenance) were quite early in the follow-up period (mean survival time = 3.3 months) whereas relapses that occurred in the other conditions were considerably later (after approximately 17 months). The one caveat that is worthy of mention is the low cell size for the follow-up analyses, which, as with the Blackburn (1986) study, places some limitation on the strength of the findings.

METHODOLOGICAL PROBLEMS IN STUDIES OF RELAPSE

There are numerous methodological problems in the study of relapse, including the method of reporting outcome, selection of time intervals for assessments, delineation of criteria for relapse, and other difficulties that were discussed in Chapter 1 (Wilson, this volume). One manifestation of these problems in the area of depression has been the mere reporting of means and standard deviations on a specific measure of depression at one point in time. Mean BDI scores at selected points in time can be rather misleading as a guide to the maintenance of treatment effects in depression due to the periodic and cyclical nature of the disorder. Individuals who are symptom free at one point in time may have experienced significant depression in the period between assessments. Thus, average scores on a measure such as the BDI often remain virtually constant for a large sample during a lengthy follow-up period, but this constancy does not necessarily reflect maintenance of improvement for individuals in the sample. The same point can be made about the finding of similar effect sizes for posttreatment and follow-up assessments in meta-analyses (Nietzel et al., 1987; Robinson et al., 1990).

There is also considerable variability in the length and intensity of follow-ups. Many follow-up periods are relatively short, with an assessment at only a single point in time (e.g., at 3 months follow-up). The duration of follow-up has varied from 1 month to 2½ years after the termination of treatment. Clearly, a follow-up of 1 month can only be regarded as providing evidence for the immediate retention of treatment gains, and even 2 years only provides evidence for intermediate maintenance in a highly chronic problem such as depression. The methods of assessment have also varied in intensity. These methods have included telephone contact, physicians' notes, interviews, mail-back testing, administration of self-report scales, and the conduct of clinical ratings. The follow-up period in the study by Blackburn et al. (1986) was 2 years, but psychometric tests were conducted only at 6 months and there was reliance on physicians' notes for the remaining period. In the study reported by Simons et al. (1986), the duration was 1 year with formal assessment at 1, 6, and 12 months. In the follow-up reported by Kovacs et al. (1981), the follow-up duration was 1 year with monthly BDIs. Evans et al. (1991) conducted monthly BDI assessments in a mail-back form, supplemented by interviews if a relapse was indicated. Regular 6 month interviews were also conducted in this study.

The use of different criteria for relapse in each study presents difficulties in making comparisons between studies. For example, Blackburn et al. (1981) set criteria of relapse involving a BDI > 9 and an HRSD score > 8 at 6 months or the indication in the physicians' notes that there was a need for further drug treatment, psychotherapy, or hospitalization, while Simons et al. (1986) used the receipt of more treatment, or a BDI of 16 or more at follow-up interviews held at 6 and 12 months, as their criterion for relapse. Hollon et al. (in press) defined two different criteria for relapse, but their conservative criterion involved the presence of a BDI score of at least 16 on 2 adjacent months (or return to treatment). Finally, in the paper reported by Beck et al. (1985), depression status was assessed using a criterion score of 10 or more on the BDI at the 6- and 12-month follow-ups.

The proportion of subjects who obtain further treatment has been used as a criterion of relapse in some studies but not in others. It is argued that further treatment may reflect a judgment by the subject that their condition has deteriorated. Return to treatment is often included as a criterion in order to eliminate any underestimation of relapse due to the success of further treatment. However, as Simons et al. (1986) have pointed out, return to treatment can be affected by factors other than depression, such as individual differences in help-seeking behaviors. In comparisons between treatments, relapse rates could be affected by the extent to which such behaviors are encouraged or discouraged by the treatments themselves. It is also possible that some depressives may not seek treatment because they are "too demoralized" (Simons et al., 1986, p. 43). Of course, receipt of treatment may also overestimate relapse since some people may be seeking treatment for problems other than depression. Despite these problems, it is certainly better for the return-to-treatment rates to be available, and for relapse rates to be reported both with and without return to treatment as a criterion. An additional but related problem is the possibility that differential retention attrition rates during the treatment itself, or during the follow-up period, may affect the interpretation of comparative treatment trials (Hollon, Shelton, & Loosen, 1991).

A problem that has affected the interpretation of some studies is the failure to separate responders from nonresponders (e.g., Kovacs et al., 1981). Clearly, it is more sensible to examine the course of subjects who have successfully responded to treatment separately from those whose reponse is only moderate or minimal. Baker and Wilson (1985) and Simons et al. (1986) have shown that clear treatment responders have a remarkably good rate of recovery during the first 5 to 6 months after termination, although the relapse rate for responders seems to increase from about the 6-month posttreatment point up to 12 months (Simons et al., 1986). Of course, if responders are separated from nonresponders in the investigation, an additional interpretive problem is posed by the use of different criteria for defining an initial treatment response in the different studies. Overall, it can be seen that there are numerous method-ological problems in the study of relapse in depression. There is clearly a need for a more uniform approach to some of the principal issues involved such as the definition of recovery and relapse, employing a number of replicable criteria.

RP STRATEGIES

There has been relatively little research on the development and evalua-tion of psychological RP strategies in depression. One strategy in attempt-ing to improve long-term effectiveness in other areas has been to provide some form of booster or additional treatment. So far, this strategy has not been successful in treating depression (e.g., Baker & Wilson, 1985; Kavanagh & Wilson, 1989). Baker and Wilson (1985) assigned subjects to one of three conditions: (1) cognitive–behavioral boosters, (2) nonspecific boosters, or (3) no booster control, but found no differences between the three groups in maintenance. However, subjects were not divided into responder and nonresponder categories prior to the maintenance phase and the cognitive–behavioral booster treatment was delivered in a standard format for all subjects in this condition. It could be argued that the additional treatment would have had a greater impact on relapse if the treatment components had been individualized and focused on each person's known skill deficits and anticipated life events. Kavanagh and Wilson (1987) addressed these issues in a separate study by providing a set of additional treatment sessions 3 months after the termination of the initial treatment to half of their subjects who had shown a positive initial treatment response. Allocation to either the booster group or a no-contact control group was random, with control for posttreatment BDI scores. The additional or "booster" treatment was provided in 5 to 7 individual weekly sessions over a median of 11 hours (range 7–13 hours). The sessions focused on further increasing skills regarding mood control and in reducing both the incidence and impact of aversive events. The objectives were to review the material in the original treatment and to provide additional individually tailored interventions as required to (1) decrease the number and intensity of expected critical events, (2) reduce negative reactions to stress, and (3) increase the range and frequency of positive social interactions (especially with the person's spouse or partner). In spite of the effort to preserve an individualized focus, there was no additional beneficial effect found for these booster sessions in comparison with the no-booster control group. Since median relapse time was 9 months, perhaps the commencement of booster sessions at a point about 7 to 8 months after the termination of treatment would be a more useful approach to the provision of maintenance programs. More regular booster sessions spread over a longer period may also provide a more effective strategy.

In the only study designed to evaluate the effects of a RP program, which was administered in an integrative fashion in the initial treatment phase, Berlin (1985) randomly assigned 22 self-critical women to either a standard cognitive–behavioral therapy or to a specially designed RP program. The major interest was in the effects of the RP program on the maintenance of reduced levels of self-criticism rather than on depression per se. The RP program included the identification of high-risk situations and the development of strategies to cope with these situations. Overall, the two programs were equivalent in their effects on maintenance at the 6-month follow-up on measures of depression and self-esteem. It should also be noted that Hersen et al. (1984), in their evaluation of social-skills training, included a set of 6 to 8 maintenance sessions, but they found no differences between this treatment and the other conditions (one of which was continued medication) at the 6-month follow-up. Unfortunately, the design of this study prevents any evaluation of the specific contribution made to the social-skills training by the maintenance sessions. Teasdale, Fennell, Hibbert, and Amies (1984) also scheduled booster sessions at 6 weeks and 3 months after treatment, but their design precludes any evaluation of the specific contribution made by these sessions.

Miller, Norman, and Keitner (1989), in one of the few studies with inpatient depressed subjects, compared cognitive therapy, social-skills training, and a standard hospital treatment involving antidepressant medication (mainly either amitriptyline or desipramine). In the two psychotherapy conditions, subjects received approximately 28 sessions, which began in the hospital setting and continued for 4 months after discharge. There were no differences between groups at discharge, but the two psychotherapy procedures were found to be more effective than the control condition at the end of the 4-month posthospitalization period. There were some differences between the two psychotherapy conditions, but these were inconsistent. The authors conclude, with appropriate caution, that evidence for the superiority of cognitive–behavioral treatment over other treatments for this population is not strong at the present time.

PREDICTORS OF RELAPSE

Several investigators have attempted to isolate predictors of relapse following psychological treatments for depression, including both CT (e.g., Evans et al., 1991; Kavanagh & Wilson, 1987; Simons et al., 1986) and the "Coping with depression" course (Gonzales, Lewinsohn, & Clarke, 1985; Zeiss & Lewinsohn, 1988). Not only may this kind of research may have practical value in the early identification of individuals who are likely to display poor treatment response, but it may also assist in our understanding of the fundamental processes responsible for change during treatment. In a study of long-term response to their psychoeducational approach, Gonzales et al. (1985) found a set of predictors of relapse that were similar to those in the existing psychiatric literature: higher number of previous episodes, higher initial level of depression, greater dissatisfaction with major life areas, other major health problems, and family history of depression. However, these relationships were weak and accounted for only 38% of the variance.

One feature found to be a fairly reliable predictor of poor response is chronicity of depression or number of previous episodes. Keller, Lavori, Lewis, and Klerman (1983) found relapse rates of 8%, 19%, and 35% for those with no history of depression, one to two episodes, and more than three episodes, respectively. In a study of the effectiveness of CT, de-Jong, Treiber, and Heinrich (1986) treated subjects who met criteria for dysthymia and found poorer results than have generally been found with subjects who presented with MDE. This finding is particularly problematic since one would imagine that the dysthymic person is the kind of individual who has a depressogenic schema of the very type that Beck argues to be the basis of depression. Quite apart from the fact that chronic depression represents a problem in its own right, it is also known that chronic, low-level depression is a predisposing factor for MDE. Thus, chronic depression represents an area worthy of considerably more attention from researchers and clinicians, especially those who are interested in RP.

Although the concept of expressed emotion (EE) has been studied most actively in the prediction of relapse in schizophrenia, there is some evidence that high levels of EE are predictive of relapse in depression as well. Indeed, the original schizophrenia study (Vaughn & Leff, 1976) included a depressive comparison group. Vaughn and Leff found that depressed subjects who returned to high EE environments were more likely to relapse in the following 9 months than those who returned to low EE environments. Furthermore, this effect was found when the criterion for high EE was the expression of two or more critical comments by a relative, rather than the critetion of six or seven or more comments used in the schizophrenia studies. More recently, Hooley, Orley, and Teasdale (1986) replicated the effects of the Vaughn and Leff study. They found that the mean number of critical comments made by spouses of patients who relapsed was 10.5, compared with a mean of 6.1 by spouses of patients who did not relapse. The clearest discrimination between relapsers and nonrelapsers was obtained using a criterion of three critical comments made by spouses. Using this criterion, they found that 20 of the 31 (65%) relatives of high EE subjects relapsed compared with none of the relatives of low EE subjects. Unlike the findings in the schizophrenia area, no association was found between the amount of face-to-face contact with a high EE spouse and the likelihood of relapse. One important difference between the studies of schizophrenia and those of depression, as Hooley et al. point out, is that in schizophrenia, the relative is more likely to be a parent, whereas in the depression studies, the relative is more likely to be a spouse (all the subjects were spouses in the Hooley et al. [1986] study and all but two were spouses in the Vaughn and Leff [1976] study). The different nature of this relationship may affect the criterion level of EE at which the relapse effect is obtained, and it may also influence other aspects of the relationship between relapse and EE. Clearly, there is a need for further research on the relationship between EE and relapse in depression.

Several variables are of interest during the postrecovery phase, the most important of which is probably the occurrence of and reaction to life stresses during this period. This variable is important because there is already evidence that depressed patients experience a higher frequency of major life events, especially those involving losses and exits, prior to the onset of a depressive episode (Brown & Harris, 1978; Paykel, 1979; Paykel et al., 1969). Paykel and Tanner (1976) found significantly higher frequency of adverse life events in the 3 months prior to relapse (median number of events = 1.3) than in a comparable period for nonrelapsers (median number of events = 0.73). In comparison with nonrelapsers, about twice as many relapsers reported at least one event in the 3-month period (83% vs. 43% of each group, respectively). Gonzales et al. (1985) investigated the occurrence of life events during the 12 months prior to each of the 1-, 2-, and 3-year follow-up assessments but found no differences between relapsers and nonrelapsers. As pointed out by Belsher and Costello (1990), a possible explanation for this discrepancy is that the measure used by Gonzales et al. (1985) included both desirable and undesirable events and their procedure covered a longer period (12 months cf. 3 months). In contrast, life events during the 12 months prior to the episode itself have been found not to be predictive of relapse in major depression. For example, Zimmerman, Pfohl, Coryell, and Stangl (1987) found that DSM-III Axis IV stress ratings at the initial assessment did not predict relapse in a MDE.

Several researchers have noted that the relapse rate decreases substantially when one considers only those patients who respond extremely well to the initial intervention. For example, Simons et al. (1986) found that the relapse rate for those with a posttreatment BDI < 4 was 0% for CT compared with 67% for nortriptyline and 17% for the combination of CT and nortriptyline. Baker and Wilson (1985) and Kavanagh and Wilson (1987) also found that low posttest BDI was a good predictor of maintenance. In addition, Kavanagh and Wilson (1987) found that low self-efficacy about control over negative cognitions was a significant independent predictor of maintenance independent of severity of depression as measured by the BDI. Presence of dysfunctional cognitions and low self-efficacy about control over negative thoughts has been found to be predictive of relapse in several studies. Hollon, Evans, and DeRubeis (1990) report that higher levels of "residual depression" and a more negative attributional style (*Attributional Style Questionnaire* [ASQ]) (Peterson, Semmel, von Bayer, Abramson, Metalsky, & Seligman, 1982) predicted relapse during a 2-year period. Attributional style was also found to meet a number of stringent tests outlined by Hollon, Evans, and DeRubeis (1990), which suggested that "it emerges as a potential causal mediator of cognitive therapy's prophylactic effect on posttreatment relapse/recurrence" (p. 126). Clearly, these results are encouraging and warrant attempts at replication in future studies. Thus, it seems that long-term success is strongly associated with the short-term outcome of treatment. One recommendation that follows from this finding is that treatment should continue until a clear reduction in scores on the BDI (preferably < 9) and measures of cognitive dysfunction have been achieved.

Of the numerous biological variables that have been studied as a predictor of relapse, probably the dexamethasone suppression test (DST) represents the most important measure. While most research has supported the view that nonsuppressors of cortisol following DST administration have a higher rate of relapse than suppressors, not all results are supportive (see Belsher & Costello, 1988). In addition, there are particular methodological difficulties with this area, such as the fact that the DST is predictive of initial response to antidepressant medication. Overall, there is a need to consider depression from a viewpoint that incorporates both psychological and biological variables (e.g., Free & Oei, 1989). In the end, further progress in understanding the nature of relapse in depression is most likely to come from such integrative approaches to the problem.

In concluding this section, it needs to be said that certain methodological problems exist in the investigation of predictors of initial response or relapse that do not seem to have been given sufficient recognition. In particular, the sample size needs to be considerably larger than has been customary in order to detect potential differences. Another important issue is the range of values for any particular prognostic variable in a given study. Often there appear to be problems of restricted range in variables such as IQ or endogeneity. Such variables may only become significant predictors of response when the potential range of variation in the population is covered adequately in the sample. With few exceptions, predictors that have been selected for examination have not been derived from any theoretical perspective on depression or any clear conceptualization about likely mechanisms of change. Prediction of relapse following intervention poses particular problems that need to be addressed. One problem that fails to be sufficiently recognized is the possible existence of treatment × predictor interactions. Thus, while one variable may predict relapse following a certain type of intervention, the same variable may well predict maintenance of recovery following another intervention.

WHO IS MOST AT RISK FOR RELAPSE?

The previous discussion should be helpful in identifying those clients most at risk for relapse following intervention for depression. Although I offer the following list somewhat cautiously, the most consistent and important variables to date seem to be (1) posttreatment severity (e.g., BDI score); (2) posttreatment cognitive style such as the ASQ or self-efficacy about ability to control negative thoughts (other scales include the *Automatic Thoughts Questionnaire*, Hollon & Kendall, 1980; and the Dysfunctional Attitude Scale, Weissman & Beck, 1979); (3) chronicity of problem (e.g., history of dysthymia, multiple prior episodes); (4) high EE environment; (5) dissatisfaction with major life areas; and (6) coexisting medical problems. Clients who meet any of these criteria might be identified as requiring closer monitoring during a 2 year follow-up period. If the first two criteria are met, further treatment might be considered prior to termination. If criteria (4) through (6) are met, steps might be implemented to deal specifically with these issues before termination. Clients who are at high risk for relapse might receive several pretermination sessions that are aimed at providing RP strategies such as preparation for a predictable adverse life event. The concluding sessions might be gradually spread out over several months.

RP FOR DEPRESSION: PRACTICAL SUGGESTIONS

The lack of positive findings in studies on booster sessions (Baker & Wilson, 1985; Kavanagh & Wilson, 1987) may prompt a reconsideration of RP for depression. As discussed elsewhere in this book, Marlatt and Gordon (1985) proposed a RP program for the addictive disorders that has been highly influential. It is surprising that researchers have not attempted to extend this approach to depression. In its most general form, RP is a self-management approach based on social learning theory in which the goal is "to teach individuals who are trying to change their behavior how to anticipate and cope with the problem of relapse" (Marlatt & Gordon, 1985, p. 3). The conceptual model proposed by Marlatt and Gordon in the addictive disorders may be instructive in our efforts to deal with depression. In Marlatt and Gordon's model, effective initial treatment results in enhanced perception of control (high self-efficacy) over important events. The person learns to recognize and respond to high-risk situations and has positive outcome expectancies about the use of coping responses in such situations. As they come to use such coping strategies in future situations, their sense of mastery increases, facilitating the maintenance of effective coping strategies. This model, developed in the context of addictive disorders, can be extended readily to the problem of depression in which self-efficacy constructs have only been recently applied (e.g., Kavanagh & Wilson, 1987). The purpose of the present section is to explore the application of the RP approach and other cognitive, behavioral, and interpersonal techniques in the treatment of recurrent depression. The study reported by Berlin (1985) represents one such attempt to extend the RP approach to a group of women with high levels of self-criticism. The view presented in the following section is that preparation for relapse should be an integral part of the therapy for depression. Techniques based on Marlatt and Gordon's approach that might be considered in depression are described in the following section.

Identification of High-Risk Situations

What are high-risk situations for relapse in depression? The literature on life events and depression suggests that loss events (personal, financial, status) are particularly prominent in relation to both an initial episode and later episodes of depression. Some of these events may involve lowered availability of reward due to changes in circumstances, illness, moving, etc. Others may be construed more in terms of life stress, especially those stressors that involve a lack of control over important events. Beck's work would suggest that certain cognitions are especially important, such as cognitions related to perfectionism (failure to reach some level of performance) or social acceptance and approval.

The main question one needs to ask is: What type of situation is the specific person most vulnerable to? This question can be addressed by self-monitoring of mood and events during treatment in order to increase awareness of the most common sources of mood change. Interview material and life-events questionnaires can be used to assess the impact of previous major events. Self-efficacy ratings can be utilized in which the therapist lists a range of situations and the person is asked to rate how confident he/she feels that he/she will be able to cope effectively with that situation. An analysis of the history of previous depressive episodes in general could be undertaken during this pretermination phase in order to pinpoint vulnerabilities and other important information (e.g., patterns of time-course). The role of cognitive factors also needs to be examined. These cognitions could include several different types: attributions about events, expectations about the occurrence and outcome of future events, and expectations or attributions about future coping responses.

Preparation for High-Risk Situations

The person needs to view the maintenance period as an opportunity for new learning, that is, for developing new strategies for dealing with high-risk situations. Since it is inevitable that the person who is prone to depression will encounter further high-risk situations, he/she could be assisted to prepare for such events. The client needs to develop (1) recognition skills and (2) response skills in relation to high-risk situations.

Response skills might be discussed by drawing up a list of high-risk situations and having the client provide an account of what he/she actually would do in each situation. Information about how the client has dealt with past events might also be useful. The main aim of this phase is to enhance self-efficacy concerning ability to cope with high-risk situations. One RP strategy that might be useful is the prediction of future negative life events. For example, Kavanagh and Wilson (1987) asked clients to predict the likelihood of the occurrence of each of 30 events and to predict the likelihood of a depressive episode if the event were to occur. This material can then be used as the basis for planning techniques to deal with such events if they occur. The therapist can select the events predicted to occur and subject them to closer scrutiny. It is preferable that such plans be written down so that they can be retrieved easily if the event actually does occur. Of course, some events might occur that were not predicted. Thus, it is important to develop some general strategies for dealing with such events. The precise nature of such strategies will depend on the nature of the problem that has already been the focus of intervention. For example, if the therapist is aware that the client tends to use a particular cognitive distortion such as catastrophization, he/she points out that coping styles used previously tend to be used fairly automatically when there is a new source of stress. General self-statements for dealing with catastrophization can be developed in conjunction with the client, and these can be written down in the termination summary. The general point here is that the therapist should make use of the knowledge gained from working with the client to develop broad strategies for dealing with both predicted and unpredicted stress.

As an illustration of techniques in the case of a predicted event, consider a case in which the client says that he/she may lose his/her job. A number of questions might be asked:

- How can this come about (i.e., under what circumstances)? What is the most likely cause?
- What type of attribution is made of the cause (i.e., locate the cause on the internal–external, global–specific, and stable–unstable dimensions)?
- When is this most likely to occur? Why? How do you know?
- What can you do, if anything, to prevent this from happening? (Draw up a list of possible steps to prevent the occurrence of the event.)
- Has something like this ever happened before? When? What happened? How did you cope with it? What were the negative–positive consequences?
- If this does happen, how will it affect you on this occasion? (If

reaction is likely to be negative, identify specific ways in which such a negative reaction might occur: likely cognitions, behaviors, etc.)

• What do you think you might do to reduce the impact of this event? (Perhaps you can have the client identify similarities between the hypothesized event and any events that have been discussed in the therapy sessions, and draw upon skills used to deal with these events.)

At this point, the therapist can draw up a list of likely cognitions in which the client might be expected to engage if this event were to occur. The therapist can also assist the client to identify appropriate challenging statements in which to enage if he/she experiences such thoughts. These thoughts could be written into the summary sheet. The occurrence of one life event may precipitate other events or changes in levels of engagement in certain activities. In addition to cognitive preparation, some attention can be given to dealing with these likely consequences as well. A questionnaire such as the *Hassles Scale* (Kanner, Coyne, Schaefer, & Lazarus, 1981) can also be used as a means of assessing the likely reaction to everyday events. Some planning for major events, especially when they are predictable, such as retirement of self or spouse, is likely to be fruitful in some cases.

Generalization Training in Cognitive Therapy

If the effects of cognitive therapy are to achieve the maximum generalization, there is a need to develop and build into therapy specific generalization-skills-training elements. During the therapy program, the therapist can maintain a list of automatic thoughts that are the subject of cognitive restructuring. For each situation or event in which an automatic thought is described and analyzed, the therapist can develop a parallel event for later use at the end of therapy. At that point, each parallel event can be presented and discussed in detail with the client, who would be encouraged to produce his/her likely cognitive reactions to each event. For example, if a client reports a situation during therapy such as, "A person who I knew walked past me in the street and failed to acknowledge me," a parallel situation might be, "I was at a party, and I was totally ignored all night by someone I knew," or, "When introduced to this person, they had forgotten that they had already met me once before." The client is then asked how he/she would think in each situation, and if a negative thought is produced, this thought can be subjected to further cognitive restructuring. A list of 20 or so such situations can be developed and used as generalization testing and training prior to termination.

Slip Recovery and Relapse Crisis Debriefing

At some point in the maintenance phase, the person may actually experience a significant depressive mood. Such a period may be viewed by the depressed person as an inevitable setback, only confirming his/her expectations. It may be useful to examine the cognitions about the actual relapse, to identify likely negative self-statements, and to prepare counterstatements in advance of such a relapse. These statements can be written down and retrieved if needed in later sessions. The fact that the person has already been exposed to the issues at a previous time and is now in a position to examine his/her cognitions with the advantage of hindsight would be expected to increase the power of the cognitive modification methods. Some cognitive restructuring of attributions regarding failure associated with relapse may be needed.

Life-Style Modification—
Pleasant and Unpleasant Events

Life-style modification involves the examination of day-to-day activities and general quality of life. In depression, the therapist can consider the following:

1. Assess daily/weekly routines, activities (enjoyment rating; shoulds vs. wants).
2. Assess level of engagement in pleasant activities and sources of relaxation using the pleasant events schedule (MacPhillamy & Lewinsohn, 1982).
3. Assess level of unpleasant activities, looking for sources of stress arising from work, family, friends, external demands, etc. Three questionnaires are especially useful for the purpose of assessing daily stressors. These are the *Hassles Scale* (Kanner et al., 1981), the *Daily Stress Inventory* (Brantley, Waggoner, Jones, & Rappaport, 1987), and the *Unpleasant Events Schedule* (Lewinsohn, Marmelstein, Alexander, & MacPhillamy, 1984).
4. Examine the balance between desirable and undesirable activities. The therapist can ask the person to list things he/she would like to do more often and less often.

The above information can be used to develop strategies to increase the level of engagement in pleasant activities and to decrease the occurrence of unpleasant events (e.g., Lewinsohn, Antonuccio, Steinmetz, & Teri, 1984). The therapist can help the client to select target activities for the day/week ahead, and to plan relaxation into the week. It is useful to identify activities likely to result in continued commitment (e.g., joining a tennis group).

Life-Style Modification— Reducing Areas of Dissatisfaction

In the course of therapy, many clients express dissatisfaction with broad areas of their life, such as work or relationships. Termination represents a good opportunity to review whatever progress has been made in dealing with these problems. Areas of life can be divided into current work; work-related goals and ambitions; relationship with spouse/partner; relationship with children, parents, or other important family members; social relationships outside the family; financial and housing matters; educational pursuits; recreational activities; and general life goals. An assessment can be made of each of these areas, in which the therapist looks for sources of satisfaction and dissatisfaction. The main aim is to increase the person's sources of rewards. If significant sources of dissatisfaction are identified, some sessions can be devoted to establishing a long-term plan to improve the situation. Broad plans can be broken down into specific steps that involve some definable action. The plans and goals can be written into the termination summary. Steps toward the achievement of the long-term plan can be monitored during the follow-up stage.

Interpersonal Aspects

The moderating effect of high-quality social support on the impact of life events has been well documented (Cohen & Wills, 1985). One implication of this research for relapse is the need to assess the quality of social support and, if necessary, to modify the social environment to increase the likelihood of the receipt of social support and social reward. The interpersonal environment has recently become an important focus of attention in the etiology and treatment of depression. The finding of an association between EE and relapse in depression has important implications for relapse prediction and prevention. Cognitive interventions place little emphasis on the role of family factors in the amelioration of depression, and when they do, they focus on the depressed person's misperception of criticism by the spouse. Therapists should be wary to the fact that complaints by depressives about the behavior of their spouse may be, to some extent, realistic. In any case, a routine area of inquiry should include the evaluation of the interpersonal environment. Efforts need to be made to clearly distinguish between correct perception and misperception of the behavior and comments of the spouse. Where there is misperception, CT techniques are appropriate, but where there is correct perception, CT is inappropriate and possibly harmful. In such cases, direct attempts to improve the interpersonal environment are more likely to lead to sustained improvements. Thus, a range of techniques may be used including assertiveness training, marital therapy, and social-skills training. Another interpersonal aspect of depression to which attention may need to be drawn is the role of others in maintaining depression. It is possible that, in some cases, depressive behavior is partly being maintained by the behavior of other people. Finally, it is also possible that the person's depressive behavior is punishing for other people and may be leading to decreased social interaction as a consequence of avoidance.

The above suggestions for a RP program for depression are based primarily on Marlatt and Gordon's RP approach to addictions. The efficacy of such a program in RP in depression awaits evaluation.

CONCLUSIONS AND SUGGESTIONS
FOR FUTURE RESEARCH

CT and continued antidepressant medication have emerged as the principal therapies for the long-term management of depression. Nevertheless, a significant number of recovered depressives experience a relapse or recurrence of symptoms within a 2-year period, and the search for more effective strategies that might be useful for those who still experience further episodes of depression remains a priority. I have suggested an adaptation of the Marlatt and Gordon (1985) approach as one possible avenue. It would also be of considerable interest to evaluate the effects of alternative approaches, such as behavioral marital therapy or other techniques with an interpersonal focus (Weissman et al., 1981) in a group of patients who have failed to enjoy sustained improvement after CT or pharmacotherapy. Patients who fail to maintain their responses to one of these treatments may respond to another intervention, a possibility that has not been sufficiently investigated. The growing body of literature on interpersonal aspects of depression (e.g., Hops et al., 1987), including the work cited earlier on EE, suggests that there may be some benefit from paying increased attention to altering the social environment within a cognitive–behavioral approach. Additionally, samples in most studies have included a high preponderance of subjects with MDE. There are other types of mood disorder in which the use of psychological treatment approaches have been the subject of relatively little study. Dysthymic disorder and bipolar disorder represent two groups that are relatively neglected by cognitive and behavioral researchers. Recent work on life stress (Hammen, Ellicott, Gitlin, & Jamison, 1989) and EE

(Miklowitz, Goldstein, Nuechterlein, Snyder, & Mintz, 1988; Priebe, Wildgrube, & Müller-Oerlinghausen, 1989) in bipolar disorder suggests an important role for social and family factors that might prove to be fruitful for the development of new treatment strategies.

In view of the importance of relapse or recurrence following recovery from depression, the development and evaluation of various maintenance programs are badly needed. Investigations are needed of the psychological, environmental, and biological factors that precipitate relapse in depression. Such studies also offer the possibility for the enhancement of our knowledge of the basic mechanisms involved in the occurrence of depression (Belsher & Costello, 1990), notwithstanding the difficulties involved in making inferences about causality from such investigations (see Wilson, Chapter 1, this volume). It is hoped that the next decade will see more efforts directed toward the prediction, processes, and prevention of relapse in depression.

REFERENCES

American Psychiatric Association. (1987). *Diagnostic and statistical manual of mental disorders* (3rd ed., rev.). Washington, DC: Author.

Baastrup, P., Poulsen, J. C., Schou, M., Thomsen, K., & Amdisen, A. (1970). Prophylactic lithium: Double blind discontinuation in manic–depressive and recurrent-depressive disorders. *Lancet, 2*, 326–330.

Baker, A. L., & Wilson, P. H. (1985). Cognitive–behavior therapy for depression: The effects of booster sessions on relapse. *Behavior. Therapy, 16*, 335–344.

Beck, A. T., Hollon, S. D., Young, J. E., Bedrosian, R. C., & Budenz, D. (1985). Treatment of depression with cognitive therapy and Amitriptyline. *Archives of General Psychiatry, 42*, 142–148.

Beck, A. T., Rush, A. J., Shaw, B. F., & Emery, G. (1979). *Cognitive therapy of depression*. New York: Guilford Press.

Beck, A. T., Ward, C. H., Mendelson, M., Mock, J., & Erbaugh, J. (1961). An inventory for measuring depression. *Archives of General Psychiatry, 4*, 561–571.

Belsher, G., & Costello, C. G. (1988). Relapse after recovery from unipolar depression: A critical review. *Psychological Bulletin, 104*, 84–96.

Berlin, S. (1985). Maintaining reduced levels of self-criticism through relapse-prevention treatment. *Social Work Research and Abstracts, 21*(1), 21–33.

Beutler, L. E., Scogin, F., Kirkish, P., Schretlen, D., Corbihsley, A., Hamblin, D., Meredith, K., Potter, R., Bamford, C. R., & Levenson, A. I. (1987). Group cognitive therapy and alprazolam in the treatment of depression in older adults. *Journal of Consulting and Clinical Psychology, 55*, 550–556.

Blackburn, I. M., Bishop, S., Glen, A. I. M., Whalley, L. J., & Christie, J. E. (1981). The efficacy of cognitive therapy in depression: A treatment trial using cognitive therapy and pharmacotherapy, each alone and in combination. *British Journal of Psychiatry, 139*, 181–189.

Blackburn, I. M., Eunson, K. M., & Bishop, S. (1986). A two-year naturalistic follow-up of depressed patients treated with cognitive therapy, pharmacotherapy and a combination of both. *Journal of Affective Disorders, 10,* 67–75.

Brantley, P. J., Waggoner, C. D., Jones, G. N., & Rappaport, N. B. (1987). A daily stress inventory: Development, reliability, and validity. *Journal of Behavioral Medicine, 10,* 61–74.

Brown, G. W., & Harris, T. O. (1978). *Social origins of depression.* London: Tavistock Press.

Cohen, S., & Wills, T. A. (1985). Stress, social support, and the buffering hypothesis. *Psychological Bulletin, 98,* 310–357.

Covi, L., & Lipman, R. S. (1987). Cognitive–behavioral group psychotherapy combined with imipramine in major depression. *Psychopharmacological Bulletin, 23,* 173–176.

Davis, J. M. (1976). Overview: Maintenance therapy in psychiatry: II. Affective disorders. *American Journal of Psychiatry, 133,* 1–13.

de Jong, R., Treiber, R., & Henrich, G. (1986). Effectiveness of two psychological treatments for inpatients with severe and chronic depression. *Cognitive Therapy and Research, 10,* 645–663.

Dobson, K. S. (1989). A meta-analysis of the efficacy of cognitive therapy for depression. *Journal of Consulting and Clinical Psychology, 57,* 414–419.

Elkin, I., Shea, T., Watkins, J. T., Imber, S. D., Sotsky, S. M., Collins, J. F., Glass, D. R., Pilkonis, P. A., Leber, W. R., Docherty, J. P. Feister, S. J., & Parloff, M. B. (1989). National Institute of Mental Health treatment of depression collaborative research program: General effectiveness of treatments. *Archives of General Psychiatry, 46,* 971–982.

Evans, M. D., Hollon, S. D., DeRubeis, R. J., Piasecki, J. M., Grove, W. M., & Tuason, V. B. (in press). Differential relapse following cognitive therapy, pharmacotherapy, and combined cognitive-pharmacotherapy for depression.

Frank, E., Kupfer, D., J., Perel, J. M., Cornes, C., Jarrett, D. B., Mallinger, A. G., Thase, M. E., McEachran, A. B., & Grochocinski, V. J. (1990). Three-year outcomes for maintenance therapies in recurrent depression. *Archives of General Psychiatry, 47,* 1093–1099.

Free, M. L., & Oei, T. P. S. (1989). Biological and psychological processes in the treatment and maintenance of depression. *Clinical Psychology Review, 9,* 653–688.

Glen, A. I. M., Johnson, A. L., & Shepherd, M. (1984). Continuation therapy with lithium and Amitriptyline in unipolar depressive illness: A randomized, double-blind, controlled trial. *Psychological Medicine, 14,* 37–50.

Gonzales, L. R., Lewinsohn, P. M., & Clarke, G. N. (1985). Longitudinal follow-up of unipolar depressives: An investigation of predictors of relapse. *Journal of Consulting and Clinical Psychology, 53,* 461–469.

Hamilton, M. (1960). A rating scale for depression. *Journal of Neurology, Neurosurgery and Psychiatry, 23,* 56–62.

Hersen, M., Bellack, A. S., Himmelhoch, J. M., & Thase, M. E. (1984). Effects of social skill training, amitriptyline, and psychotherapy in unipolar depressed women. *Behavior Therapy, 15,* 21–40.

Hollon, S. D., DeRubeis, R. J., Evans, M. D., Wiemer, M. J., Garvey, M. J.,

Grove, W. M., & Tuason, V. B. (in press). Cognitive therapy, pharmacotherapy, and combined cognitive-pharmacotherapy in the treatment of depression.

Hollon, S. D., Evans, M. D., & DeRubeis, R. J. (1990). Cognitive mediation of relapse prevention following treatment for depression: Implications for differential risk. In R. E. Ingram (Ed.), *Contemporary approaches to depression* (pp. 117–136). New York: Plenum Press.

Hollon, S. D., & Kendall, P. C. (1980). Cognitive self-statements in depression: Development of an Automatic Thoughts Questionnaire. *Cognitive Therapy and Research, 4,* 383–395.

Hollon, S. D., Shelton, R. C., & Loosen, P. T. (1991). Cognitive therapy and pharmacotherapy for depression. *Journal of Consulting and Clinical Psychology, 59,* 88–89.

Hooley, J. M., Orley, J., & Teasdale, J. D. (1986). Levels of expressed emotion and relapse in depressed patients. *British Journal of Psychiatry, 148,* 642–647.

Hops, H., Biglan, A., Sherman, L., Arthur, J., Friedman, L., & Osteen, V. (1987). Home observations of family interactions of depressed women. *Journal of Consulting and Clinical Psychology, 55,* 341–346.

Kavanagh, D. J., & Wilson, P. H. (1987). Prediction of outcome with group cognitive therapy for depression. *Behavior Research and Therapy, 27,* 333–343.

Kanner, A. D., Coyne, J. C., Schaefer, C. A., & Lazarus, R. S. (1981). Comparison of two modes of stress management: Daily hassles and uplifts versus major life events. *Journal of Behavioral Medicine, 4,* 1–39.

Keller, M. B., Lavori, P. W., Lewis, C. E., & Klerman, G. L. (1983). Predictors of relapse in major depressive disorder. *Journal of the American Medical Association, 250,* 3299–3304.

Keller, M. B., Shapiro, R. W., Lavori, P. W., & Wolfe, N. (1982). Relapse in major depressive disorder: Analysis of the life table. *Archives of General Psychiatry, 39,* 911–915.

Klerman, G. L. (1978). Long-term treatment of affective disorders. In M. A. Lipton, A. DiMascio, & K. F. Killam (Eds.), *Psychopharmacology: A generation of progress* (pp. 1303–1311). New York: Raven Press.

Klerman, G. L., DiMascio, A., Weissman, M., Prusoff, B., & Paykel, E. S. (1974). Treatment of depression by drugs and psychotherapy. *American Journal of Psychiatry, 131,* 186–191.

Kovacs, M., Rush, A. J., Beck, A. T., & Hollon, S. D. (1981). Depressed outpatients treated with cognitive therapy or pharmacotherapy: A one-year follow-up. *Archives of General Psychiatry, 38,* 33–39.

Lavori, P. W., Keller, M. B., & Klerman, G. L. (1984). Relapse in affective disorders: A reanalysis of the literature using life table methods. *Journal of Psychiatric Research, 18,* 13–25.

Lehmann, H. E. (1971). Epidemiology of depressive disorders. In R. R. Fieve (Ed.), *Depression in the 70's: Modern theory and research*. Princeton, NJ: Excerpta Medica.

Lewinsohn, P. M., Antonuccio, D. O., Steinmetz, J. L., & Teri, L. (1984). *The coping with depression course: A psychoeducational intervention for unipolar depression*. Eugene, OR: Castalia.

Lewinsohn, P. M., Marmelstein, R. M., Alexander, C., & MacPhillamy, D. J. (1984). *The unpleasant events schedule: A scale for the measurement of aversive events*. Eugene, OR: University of Oregon.

Marlatt, G. A., & Gordon, J. R. (1985). *Relapse prevention: Maintenance strategies in the treatment of addictive behaviors*. New York: Guilford Press.

MacPhillamy, D., & Lewinsohn, P. M. (1982). The Pleasant Events Schedule: Studies on reliability, validity, and scale intercorrelation. *Journal of Consulting and Clinical Psychology, 50,* 363–380.

McLean, P. D., & Hakstian, A. R. (1979). Clinical depression: Comparative efficacy of outpatient treatments. *Journal of Consulting and Clinical Psychology, 47,* 818–836.

McLean, P. D., & Hakstian, A. R. (1990). Relative endurance of unipolar depression treatment effects: Longitudinal follow-up. *Journal of Consulting and Clinical Psychology, 58,* 482–488.

Miklowitz, D. J., Goldstein, M. J., Nuechterlein, K. H., Snyder, K. S., & Mintz, J. (1988). Family factors and the course of bipolar affective disorder. *Archives of General Psychiatry, 45,* 225–231.

Miller, I. W., Norman, W. H., & Keitner, G. I. (1989). Cognitive–behavioral treatment of depressed inpatients. Six- and twelve-month follow-up. *American Journal of Psychiatry, 146,* 1274–1279.

Mindham, R. H. S., Howland, C., & Shepherd, M. (1973). An evaluation of continuation therapy with tricyclic antidepressants in depressive illness. *Psychological Medicine, 3,* 5–17.

Morris, J. B., & Beck, A. T. (1974). The efficacy of antidepressant drugs: A review of research (1958 to 1972). *Archives of General Psychiatry, 30,* 667–674.

Murphy, G. E., Simons, A. D., Wetzel, R. D., & Lustman, P. J. (1984). Cognitive therapy and pharmacotherapy: Singly and together in the treatment of depression. *Archives of General Psychiatry, 41,* 33–41.

National Institute of Mental Health/National Institutes of Health, Consensus Development Conference Statement. (1985). Mood disorders: Pharmacologic prevention of recurrences. *American Journal of Psychiatry, 142,* 469–476.

Nietzel, M. T., Russell, R. L., Hemmings, K. A., & Gretter, M. (1987). Clinical significance of psychotherapy for unipolar depression: A meta-analytic approach to social comparison. *Journal of Consulting and Clinical Psychology, 55,* 156–161.

Paykel, E. S. (1979). Recent life events in the development of the depressive disorders. In R. A. Depue (Ed.), *The psychobiology of depressive disorders: Implications for the effects of stress* (pp. 245–262). New York: Academic Press.

Paykel, E. S., Myers, J. K., Dienelt, M. N., Klerman, G. L., Lindehtal, J. J., & Pepper, M. P. (1969). Life events and depression: A controlled study. *Archives of General Psychiatry, 21,* 753–760.

Paykel, E. S., & Tanner, J. (1976). Life events, depressive relapse and maintenance treatment. *Psychological Medicine, 6,* 481–485.

Peterson, C., Semmel, A., von Bayer, C., Abramson, L. Y., Metalsky, G. I., & Seligman, M. E. P. (1982). The attributional style questionnaire. *Cognitive Therapy and Research, 6,* 287–300.

Priebe, S., Wildgrube, C., & Müller-Oerlinghausen, B. (1989). Lithium prophylaxis and expressed emotion. *British Journal of Psychiatry, 154*, 396–399.

Prien, R. F., & Kupfer, D. J. (1986). Continuation drug therapy for major depressive episodes: How long should it be maintained? *American Journal of Psychiatry, 143*, 18–23.

Robinson, L. A., Berman, J. S., & Neimeyer, R. A. (1990). Psychotherapy for the treatment of depression: A comparative review of controlled outcome research. *Psychological Bulletin, 108*, 30–49.

Rush, A. J., Beck, A. T., Kovacs, M., & Hollon, S. (1977). Comparative efficacy of cognitive therapy and pharmacotherapy in the treatment of depressed outpatients. *Cognitive Therapy and Research, 1*, 17–37.

Shaw, B. F. (1989). Cognitive–behavior therapies for major depression: Current status with an emphasis on prophylaxis. *Psychiatric Journal of the University of Ottawa, 14*, 403–408.

Simons, A. D., Murphy, G. E., Levine, J. L., & Wetzel, R. D. (1986). Cognitive therapy and pharmacotherapy for depression: Sustained improvement over one year. *Archives of General Psychiatry, 43*, 43–48.

Steinbrueck, S. M., Maxwell, S. E., & Howard, G. S. (1983). A meta-analysis of psychotherapy and drug therapy in the treatment of unipolar depression with adults. *Journal of Consulting and Clinical Psychology, 51*, 856–863.

Teasdale, J. D., Fennell, M. J. V., Hibbert, G. A., & Amies, P. L. (1984). Cognitive therapy for major depressive disorders in primary care. *British Journal of Psychiatry, 144*, 400–406.

Vaughn, C. E., & Leff, J. P. (1976). The influence of family and social factors on the course of psychiatric illness. *British Journal of Psychiatry, 129*, 125–137.

Weissman, A. N., & Beck, A. T. (1979). *The Dysfunctional Attitudes Scale*. Unpublished thesis, University of Pennsylvania, Philadelphia.

Weissman, M. M., Klerman, G. L., Prusoff, B. A., Sholomskas, D., & Padian, N. (1981). Depressed outpatients: Results one year after treatment with drugs and/or interpersonal psychotherapy. *Archives of General Psychiatry, 38*, 51–55.

Wilson, P. H. (1989). Cognitive–behaviour therapy for depression: Empirical findings and methodological issues in the evaluation of outcome. *Behaviour Change, 6*, 85–95.

Zeiss, A. M., & Lewinsohn, P. M. (1988). Enduring deficits after remissions of depression: A test of the scar hypothesis. *Behaviour Research and Therapy, 26*, 151–158.

Zimmerman, M., Pfohl, B., Coryell, W., & Stangl, D. (1987). The prognostic validity of DSM-III Axis IV in depressed patients. *American Journal of Psychiatry, 144*, 102–106.

Zis, A. P., & Goodwin, F. K. (1979). Major affective disorder as a recurrent illness: A critical review. *Archives of General Psychiatry, 36*, 835–839.

CHAPTER 7

SCHIZOPHRENIA

David J. Kavanagh
UNIVERSITY OF SYDNEY

Since Kraepelin's description of dementia praecox in 1896 (Kraepelin, 1896), there has been concern over the outcomes of the disorder that we now know as schizophrenia. As his term for the disorder suggested, Kraepelin saw it as a mental disorder that inevitably involves intellectual deterioration. In his words:

> The course of the illness varies, in that the dementia may proceed at a slow or fast rate, or be halted at different stages. In the most favorable cases the illness ends after a few months or years in a state of severe mental impairment. The condition then remains unaltered for the rest of a patient's life, though at times it would seem that some of the symptoms gradually disappear. The premorbid level of mental ability is never regained. (Kraepelin, 1896, p. 16)

More recently, we have seen the advent of neuroleptic medication, which has greatly improved the control of positive symptoms such as hallucinations, delusions, and formal thought disorder (Cole & Davis, 1969; Dollfus & Petit, 1991). Now we also recognize that understimulation is often a major contributor to apparent deteriorations in intellectual performance (Wing & Brown, 1970). However, concern about the outcome of schizophrenia persists. For example, a 5-year follow-up study by Watt, Katz, and Shepherd (1983) found that only 16% of schizophrenia sufferers had had a single episode with no subsequent symptoms or functional impairment, and another 32% had multiple episodes with little ongoing impairment. A total of 52% had multiple episodes with no return to normality, and in 43% the pattern was of increasing impairment over time. Results of first-episode patients were a little more optimistic, but the proportion who fully recovered was still only 23%, and 33% had multiple episodes with increasing impairments. Results like these are typical of the outcomes in the literature (Breier, Schreiber, Dyer, & Pickar, 1991; Carone, Harrow, & Westermeyer, 1991; Curson et al., 1985; Johnstone, Owens, Gold, Crow, & Macmillan, 1984; Möller, Schmid-Bode, Wittchen, & Zerssen, 1986; Rajkumar & Thara, 1989). In the medium term, between 15% and 20% have good functioning and few if any symptoms; about another third have mild problems, and about half are significantly disabled (Bland & Orn, 1978).

RELAPSE IN SCHIZOPHRENIA

Recurrence of Psychotic Symptoms

As the results of Watt et al. (1983) illustrate, schizophrenia involves a significant risk of further acute episodes. Even when neuroleptic medication is used consistently, about 30% of people with schizophrenia have a major recurrence of symptoms within 2 years (Davis, 1975). Although some of the consequences of hospitalization can be avoided by community treatment during the acute episode (e.g., Hoult, 1986; Stein & Test, 1985), the episode still represents a major disruption in the life of sufferers and their families. Recurrences can also have an indirect and long-term impact on their social and occupational functioning: Friendships and jobs are often lost, and sufferers gain a history of mental disorder that makes readjustment much more difficult. Anything that can be done to prevent or delay relapse is therefore very important.

Unfortunately, the discussion of relapse prevention (RP) continues to be hampered by nonstandard criteria in the literature and by problems in identifying exacerbations in sufferers who have a high level of positive symptoms between episodes (Falloon, Marshall, Boyd, Razani, & Wood-Siverio, 1983). Rehospitalization is not an appropriate criterion because it represents a social reaction to the disorder that is often related to affective symptoms (e.g., Falloon, Watt, & Shepherd, 1978) or to behavioral disturbance rather than to a clear exacerbation of psychotic symptoms. The literature also tends to rely excessively on survival analyses, which are insensitive to changes in the severity, length, or social effects of multiple episodes.

Ongoing Psychotic Symptoms and Functional Deficits

As important as acute relapses are, they do not represent the only risk in schizophrenia. If sufferers are functioning relatively well between these episodes, they may be able to live a relatively normal life. At least as important to their quality of life can be the effects of ongoing symptoms and functional deficits, and as Kraepelin's (1896) observation attested, these features are very common. In Creer and Wing's (1974) study, 74% were socially withdrawn, 54% showed little conversation, and relatives reported that 71% had difficulty mixing socially outside the home. Only 35% of the single patients offered companionship and support to the relatives that was rated as satisfactory, and about 50% were underactive and had few leisure interests (Creer & Wing, 1974). For approximately 30%–40% of sufferers, performance deficits extended to impaired personal care (Creer & Wing, 1974; Johnstone et al., 1984). A significant proportion of sufferers exhibited odd behaviors (34%), odd postures or movements (25%), overactivity (41%), and threats of violence (23%) (Creer & Wing, 1974). Collectively, these problems place significant stress on caregivers (e.g., Gibbons, Horn, Powell, & Gibbons, 1984). In Creer and Wing (1974), 48% of the relatives reported severe effects on their own health and well-being.

Some of these problems may be due to ongoing positive symptoms and attempts by sufferers to cope with them. For example, hostility and violence often appear to be reactions to hallucinations and delusional ideas (Bartels, Drake, Wallach, & Freeman, 1991). Other reactions are attributed to the disorder's so-called negative symptoms (Andreason & Olsen, 1982; Jackson, Minas, Burgess, Joshua, Charisiou, & Campbell, 1989), although there is clearly a risk of circularity in this attribution, and other possible factors should not be neglected. For example, many patients face periods of depressive mood (Siris, 1991), and these are likely to contribute to behavioral problems. Recreational drugs are also used by a significant proportion of people suffering from schizophrenia (Dixon, Haas, Weiden, Sweeney, & Frances, 1991; Mueser et al., 1990), and both the effects of these drugs and the norms of user groups may sometimes contribute to the behavior of suffers (Bartels et al., 1991). Many behavioral deficits can also be due to effects of treatment, such as the side effects of neuroleptic medication (Marder, 1992) or the impact of long-term hospitalization (Wing & Brown, 1970). Since the disorder usually begins in early adulthood (Lewine, 1988), significant gaps in skills training can occur. Some of the functional problems may also reflect reactions to the disorder by employers, friends, landlords, and relatives—reactions that often involve discrimination, rejection, or overprotection.

Depression and Suicide

The combination of schizophrenic symptoms, the disorder's functional deficits, and the effects of medication invoke yet another risk: a high rate of depression and suicide. Johnson (1981b) found that 70% of patients who were maintained on neuroleptics over a 2-year period had episodes of depression, and all of the schizophrenic episodes were accompanied by depression either at the relapse or in the following month. Reports by sufferers suggest that dissatisfaction with their achievements and their circumstances probably contributes to the risk of depression, and some depressive features may also be side effects of the neuroleptic medication (Johnson, 1981a). A disturbing number of suffers end up taking their own life (Caldwell & Gottesman, 1990). In a follow-up over 2–12 years, Breier et al. (1991) found that 38% of patients attempted suicide. Over approximately 13 years, Westermeyer, Harrow, and Marengo (1991) found that 8.8% succeeded in committing suicide. Over 5% of the sample suicided within 6 years of their first hospitalization, and the greatest risks were observed in white males who already showed signs of a more chronic course of disorder.

The prevention of relapse, the maintenance of social functioning, and the prevention of suicide pose difficult and complex challenges for treatment services. Since schizophrenia has a lifetime risk just under 1% (Fremming, 1951), the problem is also a costly one for the community (Andrews, 1991; McGuire, 1991). The development of more effective long-term maintenance strategies must therefore become a high priority for health services.

OUTCOME PREDICTION

Before we can attempt to improve maintenance in schizophrenia, we need to identify some of the predictors of outcome. Since the outcome variables are only moderately correlated with each other (e.g., Gaebel & Pietzcker, 1987), different prediction equations may be required for each one (Strauss & Carpenter, 1978; Fenton & McGlashan, 1987). The general psychological principle applies that past measures of specific behaviors are usually good predictors of future occurrences (Mischel, 1968). So, rehospitalization is predicted by the amount of previous treatment, among other variables (Goldberg, Schooler, Hogarty, & Roper, 1977). Assaultive behavior is predicted by similar instances of violence in the past (Monahan, 1981).

Along the same lines, the best predictors of chronicity are current signs of established chronicity, such as an earlier and insidious onset, a history of previous symptoms, a poor past employment history, and low levels of social functioning in the past (Mantonakis, Jemos, Christodoulou, & Lykouras, 1982; Strauss & Carpenter, 1977; Jonsson & Nyman, 1991). In particular, predictors of "negative symptoms" such as affective flattening and social withdrawal include previous measures of autonomic nonresponsivity, passivity, and social isolation (e.g., Cannon, Mednick, & Parnas, 1990), whereas predictors of "positive symptoms" include past observations of attentional impairment and overactivity (Cannon et al., 1990). Apart from showing evidence of behavioral stability, these data may indicate some variation between sufferers in the type and severity of their biological disorder (Zubin & Spring, 1977). Crow (1980, 1985) proposed a categorization of schizophrenia in which type I was characterized by a predominance of positive symptoms and a dopamine abnormality and type II was related to negative symptoms and structural brain pathology. Type I was seen as having a better response to neuroleptic treatment and a better overall prognosis. While other work has challenged this simple typology (Bentall, 1992), it does seem that neuropsychological tests of frontal lobe dysfunction are associated with outcome levels of negative symptoms and social functioning, rather than with levels of positive symptoms (Breier et al., 1991).

Prognostic scales have been devised using indices of established chronicity and severity (e.g., the Strauss–Carpenter Scale) (Kokes, Strauss, & Klorman, 1977), and such scales have established validity in predicting global outcome (e.g., Gaebel & Pietzcker, 1987). However, much of the predictive research continues to be atheoretical (Avison & Speechley, 1987), and it is not clear what determines many of the observed relationships or what can be done to reduce the risk they pose.

There are some other variables that predict a poorer course and may have implications for management.

Gender

Men have a poorer prognosis for schizophrenia then do women, in terms of both symptoms (e.g., Watt et al., 1983; cf. Opjordsmoen, 1991) and community survival (Angermeyer, Goldstein, & Kuehn, 1989). The reasons for this are unclear. There is some evidence that men have poorer premorbid characteristics and a greater risk of negative symptoms (Salokangas & Stengard, 1990). For example, they have an earlier average age of onset (Gureje, 1991). There is also evidence that men face a less tolerant social reaction to functional impairment (Goldstein & Kreisman, 1988) and may experience greater pressure to assume responsibility. If the social reaction toward men and women is the primary source of their differing prognosis, we may expect the difference to decrease as social roles become more similar.

An Industrialized Context without Extended Families

Several studies have observed a lower risk of psychotic relapse in nonindustrialized countries, especially in rural areas (Verghese et al., 1989;

Warner, 1983; World Health Organization [WHO], 1979; Waxler, 1979). Part of the reason for this may be the availability of a productive social role in non-industrialized cultures (Cooper & Sartorius, 1977) and a greater involvement of extended families in those cultures. El-Islam (1979) observed lower rates of emotional withdrawal in patients who lived in extended families within an Arab culture than in those from nuclear families. Extended families were more tolerant of eccentric behavior and temporary withdrawal, and they encouraged more social activity without taxing the patients' social resources (El-Islam, 1982).

Life Events

There is some evidence of an association between challenging life events and schizophrenic relapse. In Brown and Birley (1968), 60% of schizophrenic patients retrospectively reported a significant life event in the 3 weeks before a schizophrenic relapse, compared with rate of 23% in three preceding periods and a rate of 20% in the general population. Although some subsequent studies have failed to replicate this result (Bebbington & Kuipers, 1992), and the area is subject to a number of methodological problems (Tennant, 1985), it seems likely that environmental stressors increase the short-term risk of a major positive-symptoms exacerbation (Malla, Cartese, Shaw, & Ginsberg, 1990), at least for a subgroup of sufferers (Bebbington & Kuipers, 1992). In particular, patients who are adhering to medication and are rehospitalized are especially likely to report a recent environmental stressor (McEvoy, Howe, & Hogarty, 1984).

Expressed Emotion

Social interactions are an important subgroup of life events experienced by the sufferer. For example, a reanalysis by Harris (1987) of the Brown and Birley (1968) data showed that the effect was particularly strong for "intrusive" interactions by other people. Most of the interest in stressful social events has centered on the concept of expressed emotion (EE) within familes (Kavanagh, 1992a). The evidence for an association between this variable and subsequent relapse in schizophrenia is much stronger than in the rest of the literature on stressful events. In a typical study on EE, individual relatives are administered a standard interview (the "Camberwell Family Interview") at the time of a relapse, and the results are used to predict the subsequent course of the disorder. When an interview with one or more of a patient's relatives displays hostility, high levels of criticism, or "emotional overinvolvement" (i.e., self-sacrifice, overprotection, or overidentification with the patient), the whole family is rated high EE.

Kavanagh (1992a) reviewed the results of 26 outcome studies, with a total sample size of 1,323. The median relapse rate over 9 to 12 months was 21% for low EE as compared with 48% in the high EE group. The difference was in the predicted direction for all but 13% of the studies; it reached statistical significance in 70%. These data provide substantial support for EE as a risk factor for positive symptom relapse. The current evidence discounts the possibility that methodological confounds might be accounting for the prediction (Kavanagh, 1992a; cf. Parker, Johnston, & Hayward, 1988).

Until now, most of the work on EE has focused on the negative influence of family variables. It is possible to score low on EE and be indifferent to the patient's problems. However, the literature on stressful events suggests that social support can act as a buffer against the impact of stressful situations (Katschnig, 1986). This suggests that patients from families that provide nonintrusive social support would have much better outcomes than would those whose families do not (Kavanagh, 1992a). There is some indirect evidence in favor of this view. Among families that show low EE, higher levels of warmth are predictive of lower relapse risks (Brown, Birley, & Wing, 1972). Further research that directly focuses on supportive behaviors is required. Social support may also be needed for other positive outcomes. Most patients also require substantial assistance if they are to survive in the community (Salokangas, Palo-Oja, & Ojanen, 1991). Unfortunately, the social network of the sufferer progressively disintegrates over the course of the disorder (Lipton, Cohen, Fischer, & Katz, 1981), so that the support network focuses on the immediate family, the health providers, and community welfare agencies (Jackson & Edwards, 1992). This places a substantial burden on the supportive resources of the family.

An important thread through the "risk factors" involves the induction of negative affect in the sufferer, or its alleviation through features such as a supportive social environment. So, a shorter duration of community survival by chronic schizophrenia sufferers in Caton, Koh, Fleiss, Barrow, and Goldstein (1985) was predicted by interpersonal conflict in the living environment, absence of social support, and nonadherence to treatment (including medication). The risk factors suggest that interventions that attempt to minimize the risk of positive symptom relapse should help sufferers to avoid situations that provoke emotional distress and develop coping strategies that will enable them to meet higher levels of situational challenge. When designing treatments and rehabilitation strategies for schizophrenia, it is important to note that distress can also be induced by interventions that are very confrontational or provide excessive situational challenge: Just as other sources of distress can increase the risk of relapse, so can the interventions themselves (Drake & Sederer, 1986). This provides a salutary warning to treatment providers.

TOWARD A MODEL OF RISK DETERMINATION

Current thinking on the determination of negative outcomes in schizophrenia is still very heavily influenced by stress/vulnerability models of
the disorder (e.g., Zubin & Spring, 1977; Nuechterlein & Dawson, 1984).
These models propose that episodes of schizophrenia are triggered by the
combined effects of biological vulnerability and reactions to stressful
events and situations, such that the cumulative risk exceeds a critical
level. Despite problems in defining and measuring the factors in the
models, this chapter adopts the general approach that they represent.

    In my recent review of EE (Kavanagh, 1992a), I outlined a variant of
the approach that incorporates reciprocal social influences such as criticism and attempted coercion. This model, which is reproduced in Figure
7.1, is heavily influenced by a social–cognitive perspective on behavior
(after Bandura, 1986; Patterson, 1982) as well as the stress/vulnerability
perspective. It is similar to interactive models that have been advanced in
the past (e.g., Birchwood, Hallett, & Preston, 1988), but it attempts to
describe the process of mutual influence in more detail. The model sees
both the biological vulnerability and the situational challenges as fluctuating through time, and it focuses particularly on the reciprocal behavioral
influences between the patient and other people. Figure 7.1 describes
the determinative influences for a patient's behavior at a particular time,
and the effects that this may have on some later events. It represents a
section of a long chain of reciprocal influences through time.

    For example, some attempts by other people to cope with the
behavior of schizophrenia sufferers may involve critical or intrusive communications. These communications are a variety of social events (in the
middle of the top line in Figure 7.1)—ones that present a high behavioral
challenge and significant potential costs. If the coping challenge to the
sufferer exceeds his/her current skills in resolving the conflict and controlling distress, the resultant negative emotion increases the risk of
positive symptoms and aggressive outbursts (middle of the figure). Risks
are further increased if the current biological vulnerability level is high
(top left of the figure) or if the events occur in the context of other
concurrent events that are difficult and unpleasant (top right)—for example, when the person has been arrested on a driving charge. Unfortunately the sufferer's behaviors (middle of the figure) represent new
coping challenges to other people, and their responses may become new
social events for the sufferer to contend with (bottom of the figure). They
may also induce new external stressors (e.g., when the sufferer gets drunk
and is arrested once again). The events cycle through time until they are
moderated by a change in one of the variables.

The model incorporates two moderator variables: the social perception of the other person's behavior and the coping skills that each can apply to the situation. Interpretations of behavior that attribute a negative intention increase the chance of a negative interaction developing. Similarly, a more confrontational or less skillful coping style will decrease the chance of a more positive outcome to the interaction.

The theoretical approach is not only applicable to negative influences but can also be applied to positive effects. Other people may assist the sufferer in dealing with the challenges imposed by external situations (e.g., by helping them solve problems or offering practical assistance). Similarly, neuroleptic medication appears to moderate the immediate biological vulnerability from the disorder, so that higher levels of other

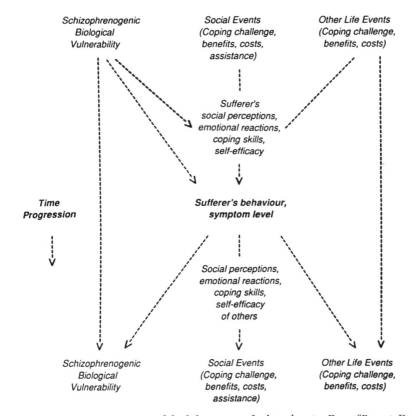

FIGURE 7.1. An interaction model of the course of schizophrenia. From "Recent Developments in Expressed Emotion and Schizophrenia" by D. J. Kavanagh, 1992a, *British Journal of Psychiatry, 160,* p. 611. Copyright 1992a by the *British Journal of Psychiatry.* Reprinted by permission.

stressors may be withstood. An increase in the skills of sufferers or of other people in the social environment may reduce the impact of modifying the extent of the mutual influences.

The implication of the model is that an intervention focusing on any one of the risk factors has the potential to reduce the risk of schizophrenic symptoms and associated behavioral disturbance, as long as other factors have not reached a critical level. However, the interventions that have the greatest potential for maintaining symptomatic control and behavioral functioning through a long period of time will be those that systematically assess the likely risks from each factor and develop effective strategies based on the model as a whole. The evidence for some of the components to such an intervention are discussed here.

INTERVENTIONS

Medication Adherence

Neuroleptic medication provides more than a treatment for acute episodes of schizophrenia: It is a powerful prophylactic. In the first year after a discharge from hospital, 68% of patients on placebo have a relapse (Hogarty, 1984). If they are given neuroleptics, the rate reduces to 41%. The results are even more dramatic when examining patients who have been symptomatically stable for 1 year: When these patients are withdrawn from medication or placebo is substituted, their relapse risk remains at 65%, while those who continue on medication now have a risk of only 15% (Hogarty, 1984). The relapse for unmedicated patients is also likely to be more severe (Johnson, Pasterski, Ludlow, Street, & Taylor, 1983). Neurolepetic medication has such a central role in the treatment of schizophrenia that responsiveness to neuroleptics has emerged as an important predictor of the course of the disorder (Angst, 1988; McGlashan, 1988). A poorer response to medication is associated with problems with information processing (Asarnow, Marder, Mintz, Van Putten, & Zimmerman, 1988), less pretreatment autonomic response (Schneider, 1982), and poorer premorbid functioning (Goldstein, Rodnik, Evans, May, & Steinberg, 1978).

Despite the effectiveness of neuroleptics, 40%–50% of schizophrenia sufferers do not consistently adhere to oral medication (Johnson, 1984), although there is considerable variation across studies (Young, Zonana, & Shepler, 1986). This level of compliance is probably about the same as with those who take medication for chronic physical conditions (Ley, 1979). Perhaps one of the most important targets in schizophrenia is the maintenance of adherence to neuroleptic treatment.

Why do sufferers want to stop taking medication? Among the reasons advanced by sufferers are the side effects of medication, and the level of side effects does seem to be related to adherence (Young et al., 1986; cf. Haynes, 1979). For example, people who experience an early dysphoric response are likely to discontinue medication (Van Putten, May, & Marder, 1984). Many sufferers are also concerned about the long-term risk of tardive dyskinesia, which is a potentially severe movement disorder whose risk probably increases with the dosage of neuroleptic medication and the duration of treatment (Marder, 1992). This is a realistic concern, since 10%–20% of people who are treated with neuroleptics for more than 12 months develop tardive dyskinesia (American Psychiatric Association, 1980), and the disorder can sometimes be irreversible (Marder, 1986).

One recent approach to reducing side effects is to reduce the dosage of the medication. Recent studies suggest that low-maintenance dosages of depot neuroleptics (e.g., 2 ½ to 5 mg of fluphenazine decanoate every 14 days, which is about 10% of the usual dosage) have significantly lower side effects and fewer patients discontinuing treatment. Although there is an increased risk of symptomatic exacerbations, usually these were quickly controlled by increasing the dosage (Marder et al., 1987).

Another aspect of the problem may be limitations to the treatment response. For the 10%–20% of people with schizophrenia who do not show a substantial acute response to standard neuroleptics (Kane, 1989), stopping the drugs may seem to be a rational course of action. Sometimes the acute response to medication can be improved by changing the medication. Recent work on clozapine is especially promising (Safferman, Lieberman, Kane, Szymanski, & Kinon, 1991). Even among treatment responders, effects on positive symptoms are often more marked than the impact on negative symptoms (Carpenter, Heinrichs, & Alphs, 1985) and social functioning (Wallace, Donahoe, & Boone, 1988). In fact, the sedation and akinesia from medication are often confused with negative symptoms from the schizophrenic disorder, and these side effects can also impede the sufferers' progress in reaching rehabilitation goals. The issues of treatment response and side effects become even further intertwined when prescribers react to a poor acute response by increasing the dosage of medication and thereby increasing the severity of the side effects and the perceived aversiveness of the medication.

Two other symptomatic states offer special challenges to adherence. The first occurs when symptoms have been stable for some time. Since the actual risk of relapse may be unabated (Johnson, 1984), maintenance of adherence in this situation is critically important for RP. Another particularly problematic situation occurs when the person becomes suspicious, hostile, grandiose, or anxious (Barofsky & Connelly, 1983; Young et al., 1986). These symptoms can constitute early signs of relapse (Herz & Melville, 1980), and yet they also contribute to the person's discontinuing the very treatment that could prevent the relapse or decrease its severity.

What Can Be Done to Improve Adherence?

A current review of this area is provided by Piatkowska and Farnill (1992). The main strategies appear to be:

1. *Ensure Understanding of Instructions.* In medical disorders, adherence can sometimes be increased by ensuring that instructions are understood by the patient (Ley, 1982). It is not clear whether misunderstanding of instructions is a significant problem in schizophrenia.

2. *Improve Cues and Rewards for Taking Medication.* One way to remind people to take medication is to time the regime to other routines, such as a mealtime or a television program. Other strategies include keeping the medication in a visible location and using a reminder calendar. Reminder strategies like these increase short-term adherence significantly more than either a nonspecific intervention or educational sessions about the disorder and its treatment (Boczkowski, Zeichner, & De Santo, 1985). Adherence may also be boosted by the combination of education and rewards for adherence (Seltzer, Roncari, & Garfinkel, 1980). However, a major challenge for either type of intervention is the maintenance of these gains. For example, gains that rely on extrinsic rewards are unlikely to remain if the contingencies are withdrawn. Unless the behavioral gains can be maintained, the impact on the course of the disorder is likely to be very limited.

3. *Increase Skills in Self-Monitoring and Negotiating Treatment Changes.* When schizophrenia sufferers are given information about medication and its effects and taught to monitor side effects and negotiate treatment changes with their therapists, adherence can be increased significantly (Eckman, Liberman, Phipps, & Blair, 1990).

4. *Provide Supervision.* Adherence is increased when other people help the patient to remember to take the medication (Barofsky & Connelly, 1983). However, close supervision may also trigger conflict or emotional distress and retard progress toward self-management. Excessive protection or interference is one of the factors that is involved in EE, and intrusive supervision of medication may therefore increase the risk of relapse (Kavanagh, 1992). Optimum outcomes are predicted when

the assistance is offered rather than forced on sufferers, when it uses positive rather than negative reinforcement and when prompts are only delivered when self-control strategies are deficient.

5. *Provide Medication in Long-Acting Injections.* Neuroleptic medication can be provided either in an oral form that is taken daily or by depot injections at intervals of 2 to 4 weeks. The oral medication is usually self-administered, whereas the injections are usually given by health staff. Depot injections can increase adherence over a 2-year period to 85% or more (Johnson & Freeman, 1973). While many of the controlled trials of depot injections and oral neuroleptics have found little difference in relapse rates between the two modes of delivery (Glazer, 1984; Kane, 1984), significant improvements from the depot injections may occur when people with poor adherence are allowed to enter the study (Johnson, 1984).

Monitoring and Treating Early Warning Signs

One key behavioral change for RP may be to detect early symptoms and seek rapid treatment. This has been the strategy advocated by Birchwood et al. (1989; Smith & Birchwood, 1990). For this approach to be successful, the relapse has to show a regular and recognizable pattern with enough time to take action before the full-blown episode emerges. In Birchwood et al. (1989), all the relatives thought they could retrospectively identify changes that preceded the full relapse. However, in a 2-year prospective study by Jolley, Hirsch, Morrison, McRink, and Wilson (1990), staff were only able to detect nonpsychotic prodromal signs in 53% of relapses, despite assessments at least once a month.

The most common signs of relapse are anxiety, depression, and irritability or aggression (Herz & Melville, 1980). Half of the patients show hallucinatory behavior. However, the prodromal changes are often very small and there are substantial individual differences in the prodromal pattern (e.g., Subotnik & Nuechterlein, 1988). Variations also occur in subjects' experiences across relapses, although half of the patients in Herz and Melville (1980) believed that the pattern was repeated at each episode. Even if the signs reliably occur before a relapse, it is also necessary to show that they are specific to the relapse before they have clear predictive value. A prospective study by Subotnik and Nuechterlein (1988) confirmed the elevation of depression and anxiety before an episode but suggested that they only attain predictive significance when followed by low-level psychotic symptoms.

The time to take action can also be a problem. Birchwood et al. (1989) found that 75% of relatives recalled that a prodromal period lasted at least 2 weeks. Relapses for patients adhering to medication may have a shorter prodromal phase (with 64% lasting less than 1 week) than relapses for those not on neuroleptics (McEvoy et al., 1984). For some patients, there may be only a very brief window for early intervention. So, although the detection of early signs might help a substantial proportion of subjects avoid a full relapse, it is clearly not a panacea. In order to maximize the beneficial effect: (1) individual patterns of signs need to be established from past episodes, and assessments should focus on these as well as on common features in the literature, (2) assessments must be sufficiently frequent and sensitive to detect early changes for that individual; (3) observations by other people who have frequent contact with the patient may be needed to supplement self-monitoring and clinical assessments; and (4) patients and relatives need to see the consequences of early detection and treatment as beneficial. The last point is important, since patients are often able to hide early symptoms during an assessment interview if they see the consequences as detrimental (e.g., if they anticipate an increase in medication side effects or are concerned about involuntary hospitalization). Some patients and families also attempt to minimize distress by downplaying the significance of possible early signs. Research into the effectiveness of family training that incorporates these features is continuing (Smith & Birchwood, 1990). The challenge, of course, is to maintain vigilance over a long period of time without creating an atmosphere of anxiety over minor changes in behavior or mood.

If the early detection of worsening symptoms is to be useful, there needs to be ready access to 24-hour treatment facilities. Ideally, these facilities should not only offer rapid pharmacological intervention, but also be able to help patients and their families to resolve situational crises that may be contributing to the distress and the psychotic symptoms. Even if the intervention does not completely prevent the psychotic relapse, the community treatment may prevent some of the negative effects of hospitalization (Braun et al., 1981; Hoult, 1986).

Self-Control of Symptoms

Recent surveys of schizophrenia sufferers indicate that they report using a variety of methods to control positive symptoms (Falloon & Talbot, 1981; Tarrier, 1987). The most common strategies included initiating social contact, lying down or going to sleep, and diverting attention from the hallucinations (e.g., by engaging in activity). While individual stratgies are only moderately successful at best, patients who report more control over their symptoms also report using a greater number of strategies. In addition subjects with lower perceived "strain" from the disorder and the medication side-effects are likely to apply behavioral strategies rather than cognitive ones (Wiedl & Schötter, 1991). At this stage, it is not clear whether we can help patients prevent relapse by improving their self-control of symptoms. Promising short-term results have recently been obtained with an intervention that encourages sufferers to monitor their symptoms and systematically apply self-control strategies to them (Tarrier, 1992). It remains to be seen whether this approach decreases the risk of positive-symptom relapse during a follow-up period. Results from uncontrolled studies that apply cognitive strategies to schizophrenic symptoms are also very optimistic (e.g., Kingdon & Turkington, 1991). It is too early to know whether there will be problems for maintenance of symptom control, but it is likely that this will be as much a challenge in this area as it is in other areas of behavioral change.

Control of psychotic symptoms is not the only need in schizophrenia. Other important targets include the prevention of depression (Johnson, 1981b) and violent behavior (Bartels et al., 1991). Cognitive–behavioral strategies after the style of those in Chapter 8 (Brown & Barlow, this volume) have potential to maintain control of depression in this population, but there has been very little research on this topic up to now (West, 1990). Control of violent behavior is another problem that deserves more attention, because of the risks it poses for both sufferers and the people around them and because of the ongoing anxiety it invokes (Creer & Wing, 1974). Unfortunately, the period of increased risk tends to correspond to the times when positive symptoms are high (Yesavage, 1983). This makes it difficult for those patients to apply self-control strategies to their violent behavior (after Novaco, 1985). It also produces acute difficulties for procedures based on contingency management (Paul & Lentz, 1977). Cognitive–behavioral research on problems such as these is still in its infancy.

APPLICATION OF BEHAVIORAL PRINCIPLES
TO FUNCTIONAL IMPROVEMENTS

A major advance in the development of functional skills and performance was the application of token economies to the living and working environments of chronic schizophrenic sufferers (e.g., Ayllon & Azrin, 1968; Paul & Lentz, 1977). In this approach, specific behavioral expectations were established and performances were reinforced by the delivery of tokens that could be used for purchase of goods, activities, or privileges. Token economies have been applied to a range of behaviors including self-care, work tasks, social interaction, symptomatic behaviors, and working on treatment goals. These programs have generally resulted in dramatic behavioral improvements over control interventions as long as the contingencies are maintained. However, the approach has faced problems in ensuring that treatment gains are maintained once the initial program is concluded (Kazdin, 1982).

The most extensive controlled study, by Paul and Lentz (1977), extended over 4½ years with an additional 18-month follow-up and focused on a chronic schizophrenic population. In the follow-up period 93% of the token economy subjects were continuously in the community, as compared with 48% of standard treatment controls. Although only 11% of the token economy subjects attained independent living in the community for a substantial period without a hospital readmission, none of the standard treatment controls reached this level. One of the strengths of this program may have been its focus on the use of tokens to increase skills that were relevant to community tenure and were likely to be maintained by naturally occurring reinforcers. Another seems to have been the use of hostels that continued to apply behavioral principles to the subjects after discharge.

Difficulties with maintenance and generalization have also been faced by other behavioral programs such as social-skills training (Halford & Hayes, 1992). In order to promote the maintenance of generalized behavioral improvements we would expect the following:

1. The trained behaviors need to be relevant to the challenges that clients will face, and the level of skills needs to be enough to meet the challenges successfully.
2. The balance of contingencies needs to continue in favor of the behavior.
3. Either the behavior needs to be strongly associated with the kinds of situations that will be encountered, or the client needs to recall the behavioral concept and perceive its relevance to the situations that do occur.

These criteria represent a significant problem for a behavioral skills-training program—a problem that is often compounded by the range and severity of the behavioral deficits that clients display and by exacerbations in schizophrenic and depressive symptoms that interfere with their performance. Of course, the clients may also have difficulties in attending and interpreting information while the initial training is taking place. For patients with unremitting symptoms and severe behavioral deficits, the maintenance strategy may need to include long-term residential care (Bennett, 1980) with predictable behavioral demands and contingencies and continued prompting by staff. If this care is provided in a community setting, the involvement of patients in community activities can be maximized (Goldberg et al., 1985; Wykes, 1983). For patients who show behavioral gains, the prompts and contingencies can gradually be removed by providing a sequence of progressively less supervised residential environments (Shepherd, 1991).

Another strategy that promotes behavioral maintenance is training other people in the sufferer's living or work environment to acquire skills in modeling, prompting, and rewarding appropriate behavior. One possible source of support that is often underused is the pool of fellow sufferers. The research by Fairweather (1964) and Sanders (1972) showed that supportive groups of chronic sufferers can be established that will live and work as a self-sufficient cooperative. Although the level of schizophrenic symptoms was unchanged, the group intervention resulted in much higher levels of community tenure and social functioning for its members than did an inpatient treatment, and it was much less expensive to deliver. This work shows how clients can support each other in self-care, domestic tasks, and vocational performance. A similar idea is embodied in the "Fountain House" or "clubhouse model," where clients learn skills, take part in enjoyable activities, and provide mutual aid within a club, and the role of professional staff is minimized (Anthony & Liberman, 1986; Beard, Malamud, & Rossman, 1978).

Apart from other patients, the family stands out as the main possible source of support for most schizophrenia sufferers (Jackson & Edwards, 1992). Interventions to assist families to provide appropriate support may therefore be critical to the maintenance of behavioral gains by many schizophrenia sufferers.

Family Intervention

As important as social support may be, most of the recent research on family interventions in schizophrenia has focused on the reduction of stressful family interactions with the sufferer (Kavanagh, 1992b), so that the risk of positive-symptom relapse may be reduced. Table 7.1 displays the published trials of interventions with whole families (including schizophrenic sufferers) in which their effects were compared with those of routine or individual treatments. Each of these studies selected families that exhibited high EE or other signs of distress. As Table 7.1 shows, the outcomes of individual or routine treatment (49% over 9–12 months and 72% over 2 years) were very close to the median results for high EE in the literature (48% and 66%, respectively) (Kavanagh, 1992a). However, subjects who received family intervention had cumulative relapse rates of only 8% at 9 to 12 months and 33% at 2 years. Thus, the family interventions appear to virtually eliminate the increased risk from high EE over these follow-up periods. Relapse rates from group interventions for relatives (36%) lay between those of family intervention and control treatments and did not significantly differ from either. However, close

TABLE 7.1 Relapse Outcomes from Family Intervention (FI)[a]

	FI (%)	Group interventions for relatives (%)	Individual treatment for patients (%)
		0–9 months	
Leff et al. (1982)	8	—	50*
Falloon et al. (1982)	6	—	44**
Köttgen et al. (1984)	—	33[b]	50 n.s.
Hogarty et al. (1986)[c]	10	—	28 n.s.
Tarrier et al. (1988)	12	—	48*[d]
Leff et al. (1989)	8	36 n.s.[e]	—
Vaughan et al. (1989)	—	41	65 n.s.[f]
Median across studies	8	36	49
		0–24 months	
Leff et al. (1985)	40	—	78 n.s.[g]
Falloon et al. (1985)	17	—	83***
Hogarty et al. (1987)	32	—	66 n.s.
Tarrier et al. (1989)	33	—	59 n.s.
Leff et al. (1990)	33	36 n.s.	—
Median across studies	33	36	72

Note. From *Schizophrenia: An Overview and Practical Handbook* by D. J. Kavanagh, 1992b, London: Chapman & Hall. Copyright 1992 by Chapman & Hall. Adapted by permission. Recomputed significance of the group comparison using Fischer z or X^2 tests: n.s. $p > .05$ *$p < .05$ **$p < .01$ ***$p < .001$
[a]This table only includes studies that preselected for high EE households or ones that showed significant interpersonal problems.
[b]The intervention consisted of separate groups for relatives and sufferers.
[c]At 12 months, the relapse rates were 19% (FI), 41% (individual), $p < .05$.
[d]The control group included families who received a brief education program. There were no significant differences between the outcomes of education and routine treatment.
[e]Patients from families who attended at least one group session had 17% relapses.
[f]Relapse rates include subjects who were symptomatic at discharge. If these subjects were excluded, the rates were: 25% (relatives group) and 64% (control group).
[g]These figures count suicides as relapses but exclude subjects who stopped medication. The rates across the full sample were 50% (FI) and 75% (routine), n.s.

examination of these results shows that much of the reduced effect is because of problems in ensuring consistent attendance at these groups (e.g., Leff et al., 1989).

Effects from family intervention are not limited to relapse. A differential effect on employment, performance of household tasks, and decision making can also be observed (Falloon, McGill, Boyd, & Pederson, 1987). In addition, Falloon and Pederson (1985) reported that families who received family intervention had less disruption of their activities, fewer health problems, and less subjective burden than those who did not.

Table 7.1 does not include the outcome of family interventions that are applied without preselection for high EE. These studies have typically shown less powerful effects for family intervention (Goldstein et al., 1978; Hogarty, Goldberg, & Collaborative Study Group, 1973; Hogarty, Goldberg, Schooler, Ulrich, & Collaborative Study Group, 1974; Hogarty et al., 1979). For example, Hogarty et al. (1979) failed to obtain a significantly superior outcome from a combination of family and individual casework than from routine surveillance.

Table 7.1 also omits social-skills interventions that are applied to individual patients. These interventions result in medians of 21% relapses over 9 months and 46% over 2 years (Hogarty et al., 1986; Hogarty, Anderson, & Reiss, 1987; Wallace & Liberman, 1985). Particulary powerful effects may be obtained by an intervention that combines family sessions with a social-skills intervention for patients that focuses on prevention and resolution of family conflict by changing the patients' own behavior. In Hogarty et al. (1986), such an intervention resulted in 0% relapses in 9 months, and 25% over 2 years.

There are substantial similarities between the family programs in the successful studies. They all begin during an episode of schizophrenia, when families are often highly motivated to accept assistance. They all include some education about the disorder and provide practical suggestions for its management within the family, so that relatives can control their own stress and avoid high EE responses. Usually families are trained in systematic goal setting and problem-solving procedures. Most sessions are typically held in the home, although some positive results have been obtained with inpatient variants of the approach (Glick et al., 1985; Liberman, Wallace, Falloon, & Vaughn, 1981).

The effects of family intervention cannot be explained by obvious methodological problems. Clients in the family and individual conditions had comparable levels of pretreatment problems and refusals or dropouts (Kavanagh, 1992b). While not all of the studies used blind assessments of symptoms, the outcome of at least some of them (Falloon et al., 1982; Tarrier et al., 1988; Leff et al., 1989) were all confirmed by blind assessments. Nor can the amount of ingested medication account for the effects. While family intervention may improve adherence to medication, subjects receiving the family intervention require a lower dosage of prescribed neuroleptics (Falloon et al., 1985). As a result, their ingested dosage is actually lower than that of control subjects.

At this stage, it is not clear which aspects of the family intervention are producing the effect or precisely what the mechanism may be. We do know that brief interventions that simply give information about the disorder and its treatment have little effect beyond a short-term increase in knowledge (Smith & Birchwood, 1987; Cozolino Goldstein, Nuechterlein, West, & Snyder, 1988; Tarrier et al., 1988). These results suggest that a brief didactic program is insufficient to impact on critical treatment aims, although it may provide an informational basis for other strategies.

The theoretical basis of the family intervention suggests that the basis for the effects may be a change in negative interactions within the family. A family approach can produce greater reductions in EE than routine treatment (Tarrier et al., 1988), although the differential changes are mainly in criticism rather than emotional overinvolvement. Excellent outcomes can be observed in the cases where EE does become low over the course of the intervention (Hogarty et al., 1986; Leff et al., 1989). However, the changes in EE could be a consequence of greater improvements in symptoms or skills during the intervention rather than the primary mechanism for its effects. Also, reductions in EE may not be essential for positive outcomes when a family intervention is combined with training for patients in avoiding conflict and settling disputes (Hogarty et al., 1986). When EE remains high, sufferers may be able to moderate its effects by reducing contact with their relatives (Vaughn & Leff, 1976a). However, reductions in contact time after a family intervention are usually associated with increased involvement by sufferers or their relatives in leisure activities, employment, or day programs (Leff, Kuipers, Berkowitz, Eberlein-Fries, & Sturgeon, 1982). Some subjects in an individual intervention also reduce contact, but in their case it often reflects a tendency to withdraw from others (Leff et al., 1982). It is not clear whether it is reduction in contact per se or some other effect of the activities that may be contributing to the family intervention results.

An alternative mechanism for the effects is that the family interventions assist in heading off symptomatic exacerbations before they become severe, by increasing the family's awareness of schizophrenic symptoms (see the section on monitoring early warning signs) and improving the member's ability to react more appropriately to symptoms. Suggestive evidence in favor of this hypothesis is provided by Falloon et al. (1982). In their study, the overall rate of symptom exacerbations was similar across treatments, but subjects in the family intervention program had fewer major episodes.

Anderson, Reiss and Hogarty (1986), Falloon, Boyd, and McGill (1984) and Kavanagh, Piatkowska, Manicavasagar, O'Halloran, and Clark (1991) provide detailed descriptions of family interventions. The approach of Kavanagh et al. (1991) includes multiple components:

- Assessment and engagement
- Interactive education and symptom monitoring

- Basic communication training
- Goal setting
- Problem solving
- Behavioral self-management and symptom control
- Stress management
- Maintenance of change

Their program aims not only to reduce conflict and intrusive interactions within the family but also to develop a coalition with family members in supporting the client's efforts to maintain medication adherence, track and control symptoms, and develop other behavioral skills. The program is therefore seen as much more than a program for high EE: Instead, it is viewed as an intervention that supports the maintenance of treatment gains across the board. Special attention is paid to ensure that the family sessions themselves do not prove distressing for clients or other family members, by encouraging a focus on positive changes, discouraging labeling and blaming, and providing "time out" as necessary.

The approach applied cognitive and behavioral strategies that are tailored to the specific schizophrenic symptoms and to the capabilities and concerns of family members as they are identified in behavioral analyses. The approach emphasizes current knowledge and achievements, it encourages sufferers to model functional behaviors, and it fosters realistic optimism about the future. To increase maintenance and generalization, the concepts are applied to a range of issues and progressive steps to self-management are encouraged.

In an ongoing treatment trial conducted by Kavanagh et al. (1988), the program is delivered in approximately ten sessions over the first 6 months. The sessions are initially held weekly and are gradually reduced in frequency. They are followed by three monthly sessions for at least another 18 months. These sessions review the material in the program and apply it to new issues. Each session is about 2 hours in length (including rest breaks) and is usually held in the family home. Two family trainers usually participate in the sessions and provide peer consultation and ensure continuity when one is unable to attend.

Until now, interventions such as these focused on nuclear families, but approximately one third of patients are discharged to live in nonfamilial settings (MacMillan, Gold, Crow, Johnson, & Johnstone, 1986). It is plausible that EE-related behaviors may be important in these settings as well. For example, staff and coresidents can be highly critical (Herzog, 1988), and informal observation suggests that increased symptoms are often preceded by an interpersonal crisis within the residence. If the EE results are generalizable to other living groups, perhaps we could apply an intervention like the one described above to these settings. A preliminary study by Higson and Kavanagh (1988) showed that a 10–12-session program did have a short-term impact on criticism within hostels for schizophrenic sufferers. While a more extensive evaluation is required, the study suggested that modified family intervention programs might be productively applied to hostels or group homes.

Although family interventions have great potential in schizophrenia, at present they have one important limitation. Despite their focus on RP, the programs themselves have not demonstrated very strong maintenance of treatment gains. The best 2-year results were obtained by Falloon et al. (1985), who continued to have monthly sessions throughout the study period. Relatively poor maintenance is shown by interventions that have no continuing sessions at all (e.g., Vaughan et al., 1992). It seems that the interventions for this population may require some continuing contact if their beneficial effects are to be maintained.

MAINTENANCE OF HEALTH CARE BEHAVIORS BY STAFF

Much of the literature on the treatment of schizophrenia involves the evaluation of special trials. A critical challenge is the maintenance of the health care behaviors of treating clinicians within standard health care settings. For most sufferers this is a long-term disorder that requires a sustained and systematic approach to its problems. What is needed most of all are individuals and treatment teams who will consistently maintain programs over long periods in the face of often very small incremental gains and periodic relapses. What is also needed is a health care system that will provide consistent services, which inevitably will be costly, and continue to deliver them in the face of pressure for cost minimization. In support of the services is the dramatic reduction in costs that can be achieved by cutting the frequency of inpatient treatment (Goldberg, 1991).

During the family intervention trial of Kavanagh et al. (1988), a number of requirements for sustained maintenance of health care behaviors were highlighted. Overall, the trial demonstrated the difficulty in systematically applying a comprehensive cognitive–behavioral approach to maintenance within standard community health settings.

Support by the Center and Availability of Staff

The invervention needs to be supported by the health service administration through the provision of establishment positions and the rapid replacement of staff who leave. If the intervention is delivered after normal working hours (as in the family or crisis interventions) overtime or time in lieu needs to be easily accessible. Trained clinicians who are willing to undertake work after business hours are required, and they need priority access to appropriate referrals. The intervention behaviors need to be consistent with the overall demands of their position (e.g., their case load and status) and with the expectations of other staff. Other staff members need to be sympathetic to the theoretical and service delivery models being applied and take the intervention into account when making other treatment decisions (e.g., medication dosage).

Effective Training and Consultation

As in the training of clients, the training of health staff needs to include realistic skills practice across the range of client and family problems that may be experienced. Even though the intervention in Kavanagh et al. (1988) included 35 hours of workshop training, some therapists found the skills difficult to acquire when they did not have detailed professional training in behavioral skills or were used to working within different theoretical orientations. To address this issue, consultants were selected and these clinicians were given additional training both in the behavioral family intervention skills and in consultation practice. They then delivered assistance to trainers in each center and acted as advocates for the intervention in case conferences and other staff meetings.

Continued Incentives for High Quality of Practice

Each service needs to develop specific and comprehensive treatment guidelines that are responsive to the needs and preferences of the client and family population in the area. They also need to institute rigorous, comprehensive, and independent assessments at regular intervals, including a close inquiry into apparent failures and successes in treatment. These procedures can help to ensure that standards in the service do not begin to slip. Case reviews also provide a mechanism for delivering incentives to staff for high-quality work. However, the service also needs to address the costs that individual staff are facing in delivering particular services, and particularly those delivered after hours.

It is salutary to note that the maintenance problems that are encountered with staff are similar to the issues that emerge when we consider the maintenance of clients' behaviors. Without attention to factors such as these, services will be sporadic and unsystematic, and as a consequence, the gains of schizophrenic sufferers and their families will be short-lived.

CONCLUSION

Kraepelin's (1896) view that a progressive impairment is universal in schizophrenia is no longer current. But substantial risks of relapse and functional impairment persist. There are a range of treatments available to improve the long-term prospects of people with schizophrenia. However, each of these has limited long-term efficacy. Part of the problem is that we are dealing with a biological disorder that, for all but approximately 20% of sufferers, will have periods of symptomatic exacerbation regardless of the intervention used. When a mild exacerbation of symptoms does occur, it will be considerably more difficult for sufferers to apply the cognitive–behavioral skills they have learned. There is a need for continued and often lifelong vigilance because the risk of functional deterioration and severe exacerbation may always be there. This is a difficult challenge for any intervention to meet. A partial solution may be to train people in the environment to assist sufferers to moderate environmental demands according to their fluctuating capabilities, and to offer prompts, rewards, and problem-solving assistance when requested. The schizophrenic literature has gone further than substance abuse work in training families to offer assistance without becoming more critical or intrusive. What it may not yet have achieved is maintenance of these supportive behaviors and the generalization of the support to the wide range of potential problems that may be encountered by the person with schizophrenia.

REFERENCES

American Psychiatric Association. (1980). Effects of antipsychotic drugs: Tardive dyskinesia [Task Force Report]. *American Journal of Psychiatry, 37,* 1163–1171.

Anderson, C. M., Reiss, D. J., & Hogarty, G. E. (1986). *Schizophrenia and the family: A practitioner's guide to psychoeducation and management.* New York: Guilford Press.

Andreason, N. C., & Olsen, S. (1982). Negative and positive schizophrenia, definition and validation. *Archives of General Psychiatry, 39,* 789–793.

Andrews, G. (1991). The cost of schizophrenia revisited. *Schizophrenia Bulletin, 17,* 389–394.

Angermeyer, M. C., Goldstein, J. M., & Kuehn, L. (1989). Gender differences in schizophrenia: Rehospitalization and community survival. *Psychological Medicine, 19,* 365–382.

Angst, J. (1988). European long-term followup studies of schizophrenia. *Schizophrenia Bulletin, 14,* 501–513.

Anthony, W. A., & Liberman, R. P. (1986). The practice of psychiatric rehabilitation. *Schizophrenia Bulletin, 12,* 542–559.

Asarnow, R. F., Marder, S. R., Mintz, J., Van Putten, T., & Zimmerman, K. E. (1988). Differential effect of low and conventional doses of fluphenazine on schizophrenic outpatients with good or poor information processing abilities. *Archives of General Psychiatry, 45,* 822–826.

Avison, W. R., & Speechley, K. N. (1987). The discharged psychiatric patient: A review of social, social–psychological, and psychiatric correlates of outcome. *American Journal of Psychiatry, 144,* 10–18.

Ayllon, T., & Azrin, N. (1968). *The token economy: A motivational system for therapy and rehabiliation.* New York: Appleton-Century-Crofts.

Bandura, A. (1986). *Social foundations of thought and action: A social cognitive theory.* Englewood Cliffs, NJ: Prentice-Hall.

Barofsky, I., & Connelly, C. E. (1983). Problems in providing effective care for the chronic psychiatric patient. In I. Barofsky & R. D. Budson (Eds.), *The chronic psychiatric patient in the community: Principles of treatment* (pp. 83–119). New York: SP Medical and Scientific.

Bartels, S. J., Drake, R. E., Wallach, M. A., & Freeman, D. H. (1991). Characteristic hostility in schizophrenic outpatients. *Schizophrenia Bulletin, 17,* 163–171.

Beard, J. H., Malamud, T. J., & Rossman, E. (1978). Psychiatric rehabilitation and long-term rehospitalization rates: The findings of two research studies. *Schizophrenia Bulletin, 4,* 622–635.

Bebbington, P., & Kuipers, L. (1992). Life events and social factors. In D. J. Kavanagh (Ed.), *Schizoprenia: An overview and practical handbook* (pp. 126–144). London: Chapman & Hall.

Bennett, D. H. (1980). The chronic psychiatric patient today. *Journal of the Royal Society of Medicine, 73,* 301–303.

Bentall, R. P. (1992). The classification of schizophrenia. In D. J. Kavanagh (Ed.), *Schizophrenia: An overview and practical handbook* (pp. 23–44). London: Chapman & Hall.

Birchwood, M., Hallett, S. E., & Preston, M. C. (1988). *Schizophrenia: An integrated approach to research and treatment.* London: Longman.

Birchwood, M., Smith, J., Macmillan, F., Hogg, B., Prasad, R., Harvey, C., & Bering, S. (1989). Predicting relapse in schizophrenia: The development and implementation of an early signs monitoring system using patients and families as observers. *Psychological Medicine, 19,* 649–656.

Bland, R. C., & Orn, H. (1978). 14-year outcome in schizophrenia. *Acta Psychiatrica Scandinavica, 58,* 327–338.

Boczkowski, J., Zeichner, A., & De Santo, N. (1985). Neuroleptic compliance among chronic schizophrenic outpatients: An intervention outcome report. *Journal of Consulting and Clinical Psychology, 53,* 666–671.

Braun, P., Kochansky, G., Shapiro, R., Greenberg, S., Gudeman, J. E., Johnson, S., & Shore, M. F. (1981). Overview: Deinstitutionalization of psychiatric patients, a critical review of outcome studies. *American Journal of Psychiatry, 138,* 736–749.

Breier, A., Schreiber, J. L., Dyer, J., & Pickar, D. (1991). National Institute of Mental Health longitudinal study of chronic schizophrenia. *Archives of General Psychiatry, 48,* 239–246.

Brown, G. W., & Birley, J. L. T. (1968). Crises and life changes and the onset of schizophrenia. *Journal of Health and Social Behaviour, 9,* 203–214.

Brown, G. W., Birley, J. L. T., & Wing, J. K. (1972). Influence of family life on the course of schizophrenic disorders: A replication. *British Journal of Psychiatry, 121,* 241–258.

Caldwell, C. B., & Gottesman, I. I. (1990). Schizophrenics kill themselves too. *Schizophrenia Bulletin, 16,* 571–589.

Cannon, T. D., Mednick, S. A., & Parnas, J. (1990). Antecedents of predominantly negative- and predominantly positive-symptom schizophrenia in a high-risk population. *Archives of General Psychiatry, 47,* 622–632.

Carone, B. J., Harrow, M., & Westermeyer, J. F. (1991). Posthospital course and outcome in schizophrenia. *Archives of General Psychiatry, 48,* 247–253.

Carpenter, W. T., Heinrichs, D. W., & Alphs, L. D. (1985). Treatment of negative symptoms. *Schizophrenia Bulletin, 11,* 441–452.

Caton, C. L., Koh, S. P., Fleiss, J. L., Barrow, S., & Goldstein, J. M. (1985). Rehospitalization in chronic schizophrenia. *Journal of Nervous and Mental Disease, 173,* 139–148.

Cole, J. O., & Davis, J. M. (1969). Antipsychotic drugs. In L. Bellack & L. Loeb (Eds.), *The schizophrenic syndrome* (pp. 478–568). New York: Grune & Stratton.

Cooper, J., & Sartorius, N. (1977). Cultural and temporal variations in schizophrenia: A speculation on the importance of industrialisation. *British Journal of Psychiatry, 130,* 50–55.

Cozolino, L. J., Goldstein, M. J., Nuechterlein, K. H., West, K. L., & Snyder, K. S. (1988). The impact of education about schizophrenia on relatives varying in levels of expressed emotion. *Schizophrenia Bulletin, 14,* 675–685.

Creer, C., & Wing, J. (1974). *Schizophrenia at home.* Surbiton, Surrey: Schizophrenia Fellowship.

Crow, T. J. (1980). Molecular pathology of schizophrenia: More than one disease process. *British Medical Journal, 280,* 66–68.

Crow, T. J. (1985). The two-syndrome concept: Origins and current status. *Schizophrenia Bulletin, 11,* 471–485.

Curson, D. A., Barnes, T. R. E., Bamber, R. W., Platt, S. D., Hirsch, S. R., & Duffy, J. D. (1985). Long-term depot maintenance of chronic schizophrenic outpatients. *British Journal of Psychiatry, 146,* 464–480.

Davis, J. (1975). Overview: Maintenance therapy in psychiatry: I. Schizophrenia. *American Journal of Psychiatry, 132,* 1237–1245.

Dixon, L., Haas, G., Weiden, P., Sweeney, J., & Frances, A. (1991). Drug abuse in schizophrenic patients: Clinical correlates and reasons for use. *American Journal of Psychiatry, 148,* 224–230.

Dollfus, S., & Petit, M. (1991). Essai d'evaluation de l'efficacité des neuroléptiques sur le devenir des schizophrenies. *Encephalé, 17,* 247–253.

Drake, R. E., & Sederer, L. I. (1986). The adverse effects of intensive treatment of chronic schizophrenia. *Comprehensive Psychiatry, 27,* 313–326.

Eckman, T. A., Liberman, R. P., Phipps, C. C., & Blair, K. E. (1990). Teaching medication management skills to schizophrenic patients. *Journal of Clinical Psychopharmacology, 10*, 33–38.

El-Islam, M. F. (1979). A better outlook for schizophrenics living in extended families. *British Journal of Psychiatry, 135*, 343–347.

El-Islam, M. F. (1982). Rehabiliation of schizophrenics by the extended family. *Acta Psychiatrica Scandinavia, 65*, 112–119.

Fairweather, G. W. (1964). *Social psychology in treating mental illness: An experimental approach*. New York: Wiley.

Falloon, I. R. H., Boyd, J. L., & McGill, C. W. (1984). *Family care of schizophrenia*. New York: Guilford Press.

Falloon, I. R. H., Boyd, J. L., McGill, C. W., Razani, J., Moss, H. B., & Gilderman, A. M. (1982). Family management in the prevention of exacerbations of schizophrenia: A controlled study. *New England Journal of Medicine, 306*, 1437–1440.

Falloon, I. R. H., Boyd, J. L., McGill, C. W., Williamson, M., Razani, J., Moss, H. B., Gilderman, A. M., & Simpson, G. M. (1985). Family management in the prevention of morbidity of schizophrenia: Clinical outcome of a two-year longitudinal study. *Archives of General Psychiatry, 42*, 887–896.

Falloon, I. R. H., Marshall, G. N., Boyd, J. L., Razani, J., & Wood-Siverio, C. (1983). Editorial. Relapse in schizophrenia: A review of the concept and its definitions. *Psychological Medicine, 13*, 469–477.

Falloon, I. R. H., McGill, C. W., Boyd, J. L., & Pederson, J. (1987). Family management in the prevention of morbidity of schizophrenia: Social outcome of a two-year longitudinal study. *Psychological Medicine, 17*, 59–66.

Falloon, I. R. H., & Pederson, J. (1985). Family management in the prevention of morbidity of schizophrenia: The adjustment of the family unit. *British Journal of Psychiatry, 147*, 156–163.

Falloon, I. R. H., & Talbot, R. E. (1981). Persistent auditory hallucinations: Coping mechanisms and implications for management. *Psychological Medicine, 11*, 329–339.

Falloon, I. R. H., Watt, D. C., & Shepherd, M. (1978). A comparative controlled trial of pimozide and fluphenazine deconoate in the continuation therapy of schizophrenia. *Psychological Medicine, 8*, 59–70.

Fenton, W. S., & McGlashan, T. H. (1987). Prognostic scale for schizophrenia. *Schizophrenia Bulletin, 13*, 277–286.

Fremming, K. H. (1951). The expectation of mental infirmity in a sample of the Danish population. *Occasional Papers on Eugenics, 7*, London: Cassell.

Gaebel, W., & Pietzcker, A. (1987). Prospective study of course of illness in schizophrenia: Part II. Prediction of outcome. *Schizophrenia Bulletin, 13*, 299–306.

Gibbons, J. S., Horn, S. H., Powell, J. M., & Gibbons, J. L. (1984). Schizophrenic patients and their families. A survey in a psychiatric service based on a DGH unit. *British Journal of Psychiatry, 144*, 70–77.

Glazer, W. M. (1984). Depot fluphenazine: Risk/benefit ratio. *Journal of Clinical Psychiatry, 45*, 28–35.

Glick, I. A., Clarkin, J. F., Spencer, J. H., Haas, G. L. Lewis, A. B., Peyser, J.,

De Mane, N., Good-Ellis, M., Harris, E., & Lestelle, V. (1985). A controlled evaluation of inpatient family education. *Archives of General Psychiatry, 42,* 882–886.

Goldberg, D. (1991). Cost-effectiveness studies in the treatment of schizophrenia: A review. *Schizophrenia Bulletin, 17,* 453–459.

Goldberg, D. P., Bridges, K., Cooper, W., Hyde, C., Sterling, C., & Wyatt, R. (1985). Douglas House: A new type of hostel ward for chronic psychiatric patients. *British Journal of Psychiatry, 147,* 383–388.

Goldberg, S. C., Schooler, N. R., Hogarty, G. E., & Roper, M. (1977). Prediction of relapse in schizoprenic outpatients treated by drug and sociotherapy. *Archives of General Psychiatry, 34,* 171–184.

Goldstein, M. J., & Kreisman, D. (1988). Gender, family environment and schizophrenia. *Psychological Medicine, 18,* 861–872.

Goldstein, M. J., Rodnick, E. H., Evans, J. R., May, P. R. A., & Steinberg, M. R. (1978). Drug and family therapy in the aftercare of acute schizophrenics. *Archives of General Psychiatry, 35,* 1169–1177.

Gureje, O. (1991). Gender and schizophrenia: Age at onset and sociodemographic attributes. *Acta Psychiatrica Scandinavica, 83,* 402–405.

Halford, K., & Hayes, R. L. (1992). Social skills training with schizophrenic patients. In D. J. Kavanagh (Ed.), *Schizophrenia: An overview and practical handbook* (pp. 374–392). London: Chapman & Hall.

Harris, T. O. (1987). Recent developments in the study of life events in relation to psychiatric and physical disorders. In B. Cooper (Ed.), *Psychiatric epidemiology: Progress and prospects* (pp. 81–102). London: Croom Helm.

Haynes, R. B. (1979). Determinants of compliance: The disease and the mechanics of treatment. In R. B. Haynes, D. W. Taylor, & D. L. Sackett (Eds.), *Compliance in health care* (pp. 49–62). Baltimore: Johns Hopkins University Press.

Herz, M., & Melville, C. (1980). Relapse in schizophrenia. *American Journal of Psychiatry, 137,* 801–812.

Herzog, T. (1988, November 18–19). Nurses, patients and relatives: A study of family patterns on psychiatric wards. In C. L. Cazzullo & G. Invernizzi (Eds.), *Family intervention in schizophrenia: Experiences and orientations in Europe* (pp. 407–423). Proceedings of a conference held in Milan.

Higson, M., & Kavanagh, D. J. (1988). A hostel-based psychoeducational intervention for schizophrenia: Programme development and preliminary findings. *Behaviour Change, 5,* 85–89.

Hogarty, G. E. (1984). Depot neuroleptics: The relevance of psychosocial factors—A United States perspective. *Journal of Clinical Psychiatry, 45,* 36–42.

Hogarty, G. E., Anderson, C. M., & Reiss, D. J. (1987). Family psychoeducation, social skills training and medication in schizophrenia: The long and the short of it. *Psychopharmacology Bulletin, 23,* 12–13.

Hogarty, G. E., Anderson, C. M., Reiss, D. J., Kornblith, S. J., Greenwald, D. P., Javan, C. D., & Madonia, M. J. (1986). Family psychoeducation, social skills training and maintenance chemotherapy in the aftercare treatment of schizophrenia. 1. One-year effects of a controlled study on relapse and expressed emotion. *Archives of General Psychiatry, 43,* 633–642.

Hogarty, G. E., Goldberg, S., & Collaborative Study Group. (1973). Drug and sociotherapy in the aftercare of schizophrenic patients. *Archives of General Psychiatry, 28,* 54–64.

Hogarty, G. E., Goldberg, S., Schooler, N. R., Ulrich, R., & Collaborative Study Group. (1974). Drug and sociotherapy in the aftercare of schizophrenic patients: II. Two-year relapse rates. *Archives of General Psychiatry, 31,* 603–608.

Hogarty, G. E., Schooler, N. R., Ulrich, R., Mussare, F., Ferro, P., & Herron, E. (1979). Fluphenazine and social therapy in the aftercare of schizophrenic patients: Relapse analyses of a two-year controlled study of fluphenazine deconoate and fluphenazine hydrochloride. *Archives of General Psychiatry, 36,* 1283–1294.

Hoult, J. (1986). The community care of the acutely mentally ill. *British Journal of Psychiatry, 149,* 137–144.

Jackson, H., & Edwards, J. (1992). Social networks and social support in schizophrenia: Correlates and assessment. In D. J. Kavanagh (Ed.), *Schizophrenia: An overview and practical handbook* (pp. 275–292). London: Chapman & Hall.

Jackson, H. J., Minas, I. H., Burgess, P. M., Joshua, S. D., Charisiou, J., & Campbell, I. M. (1989). Negative symptoms and social skills performance in schizophrenia. *Schizophrenia Research, 2,* 457–463.

Johnson, D. A. W. (1981a). Studies of depressive symptoms in schizophrenia. I. The prevalence of depression and its possible causes. *British Journal of Psychiatry, 139,* 89–93.

Johnson, D. A. W. (1981b). Studies of depressive symptoms in schizophrenia. II. A two-year longitudinal study of symptoms. *British Journal of Psychiatry, 139,* 93–96.

Johnson, D. A. W. (1984). Observations on the use of long-acting depot neuroleptic injections in the maintenance therapy of schizophrenia. *Journal of Clinical Psychiatry, 45,* 13–21.

Johnson, D. A. W., & Freeman, H. (1973). Drug defaulting by patients on long-acting phenothiazines. *Psychological Medicine, 3,* 115–119.

Johnson, D. A. W., Pasterski, G., Ludlow, J. M., Street, K., & Taylor, R. D. W. (1983). The discontinuance of maintenance neuroleptic therapy in chronic schizophrenic patients: Drug and social consequences. *Acta Psychiatrica Scandinavica, 67,* 339–352.

Johnstone, E. C., Owens, D. G. C., Gold, A., Crow, T., & Macmillan, J. F. (1984). Schizophrenic patients discharged from hospital—A follow-up study. *British Journal of Psychiatry, 145,* 586–590.

Jolly, A. G., Hirsch, S. R., Morrison, E., McRink, A., & Wilson, L. (1990). Trial of brief neuroleptic prophylaxis for selected schizophrenic outpatients: Clinical and social outcome at two years. *British Medical Journal, 301,* 837–842.

Jonsson, H., & Nyman, A. K. (1991). Predicting long-term outcome in schizophrenia. *Acta Psychiatrica Scandinavica, 83,* 342–46.

Kane, J. M. (1984). The use of depot neuroleptics. Clinical experience in the United States. *Journal of Clinical Psychiatry, 45,* 5–12.

Kane, J. M. (1989). Schizophrenia: Somatic treatment. In H. I. Kaplan & B. J.

Sadock (Eds.), *Comprehensive textbook of psychiatry* (pp. 777–792). Baltimore: Williams & Wilkins.

Katschnig, H. (Ed.). (1986). *Life events and psychiatric disorders: Controversial issues*. Cambridge: Cambridge University Press.

Kavanagh, D. J. (1992a). Recent developments in expressed emotion and schizophrenia. *British Journal of Psychiatry, 160*, 601–620.

Kavanagh, D. J. (1992b). Family interventions for schizophrenia. In D. J. Kavanagh (Ed.), *Schizophrenia: An overview and practical handbook* (pp. 407–423). London: Chapman & Hall.

Kavanagh, D. J., Piatkowska, O., Manicavasagar, V. O'Halloran, P., & Clark, D. (1991). *Living with schizophrenia: A cognitive–behavioural intervention for individuals and families*. University of Sydney, Sydney.

Kavanagh, D. J., Tennant, C. C., Rosen, A., Piatkowska, O., Manicavasagar, V., & O'Halloran, P. (1988). *Prevention of relapse in schizophrenia*. Research and Development Grant, Australian Department of Health.

Kazdin, A. E. (1982). The token economy: A decade later. *Journal of Applied Behavioral Analysis, 15*, 431–445.

Kingdon, D. G., & Turkington, D. (1991). The use of cognitive–behavior therapy with a normalizing rationale in schizophrenia. Preliminary report. *The Journal of Nervous and Mental Disease, 179*, 207–211.

Kokes, R. F., Strauss, J. S., & Klorman, R. (1977). Premorbid adjustment in schizophrenia: Concepts, measures, and implications. Part II. Measuring premorbid adjustment: The instruments and their development. *Schizophrenia Bulletin, 3*, 186–213.

Köttgen, C., Sonnichsen, I., Mollenhauer, K., & Jurth, R. (1984). Group therapy with families of schizophrenic patients: Results of the Hamburg Camberwell Family Interview Study III. *International Journal of Family Psychiatry, 5*, 83–94.

Kraepelin, E. (1896). Dementia praecox. In J. Cutting & M. Shepherd (Eds.), (1987). *The clinical roots of the schizophrenia concept* (pp. 13–24). Cambridge: Cambridge University Press.

Leff, J., Berkowitz, R., Shavit, N., Strachan, A., Glass, I., & Vaughn, C. (1989). A trial of family therapy v. A relatives group for schizophrenia. *British Journal of Psychiatry, 154*, 58–66.

Leff, J., Berkowitz, R., Shavit, N., Strachan, A., Glass, I., & Vaughn, C. (1990). A trial of family therapy versus a relatives group for schizophrenia: Two-year follow-up. *British Journal of Psychiatry, 157*, 571–577.

Leff, J., Kuipers, L., Berkowitz, R., Eberlein-Fries, R., & Sturgeon, D. (1982). A controlled trial of intervention in the families of schizophrenic patients. *British Journal of Psychiatry, 141*, 121–134.

Leff, J., Kuipers, L., Berkowitz, R., & Sturgeon, D. (1985). A controlled trial of social intervention in the families of schizophrenic patients: Two-year follow-up. *British Journal of Psychiatry, 146*, 594–600.

Lewine, R. R. J. (1988). Gender and schizophrenia. In M. T. Tsuang & J. C. Simpson (Eds.), *Handbook of schizophrenia. Volume 3. Nosology, epidemiology and genetics of schizophrenia* (pp. 379–397). Amsterdam: Elsevier.

Ley, P. (1979). The psychology of compliance. In D. J. Oborne, M. M.

Gruneberg, & F. R. Eiser (Eds.), *Research in psychology and medicine* (pp. 187–195). London: Academic Press.

Ley, P. (1982). Giving information to patients. In J. R. Eiser (Ed.), *Social psychology and behavioral medicine* (pp. 49–62). New York: John Wiley.

Liberman, R. P., Wallace, C. J., Falloon, I. R. H., & Vaughn, C. E. (1981). Interpersonal problem-solving therapy for schizophrenics and their families. *Comprehensive Psychiatry, 22,* 627–630.

Lipton, F. R., Cohen, C. I., Fischer, E., & Katz, S. E. (1981). Schizophrenia: A network crisis. *Schizophrenia Bulletin, 7,* 144–151.

MacMillan, J. F., Gold, A., Crow, T. J., Johnson, A. L., & Johnstone, E. C. (1986). The Northwick Park study of first episodes of schizophrenia. IV. Expressed emotion and relapse. *British Journal of Psychiatry, 148,* 133–143.

Malla, A. K., Cortese, L., Shaw, T. S., & Ginsberg, B. (1990). Life events and relapse in schizophrenia. A one-year prospective study. *Social Psychiatry and Psychiatric Epidemiology, 25,* 221–224.

Mantonakis, J. E., Jemos, J. J., Christodoulou, G. N., & Lykouras, E. P. (1982). Short-term social prognosis of schizophrenia. *Acta Psychiatrica Scandinavica, 66,* 306–310.

Marder, S. R. (1986). Depot neuroleptics: Side effects and safety. *Journal of Clinical Psychopharmacology, 6,* 24s–29s.

Marder, S. R. (1992). Pharmacological treatment of schizophrenia. In D. J. Kavanagh (Ed.), *Schizophrenia: An overview and practical handbook* (pp. 325–38). London: Chapman & Hall.

Marder, S. R., Van Putten, T., Mintz, J., Lebell, M., McKenzie, J., & May, P. R. A. (1987). Low and conventional dose maintenance therapy with fluphenazine decanoate: Two-year outcome. *Archives of General Psychiatry, 44,* 518–521.

McEvoy, J. P., Howe, A. C., & Hogarty, G. E. (1984). Differences in the nature of relapse and subsequent inpatient course between medication-compliant and noncompliant schizophrenic patients. *The Journal of Nervous and Mental Disease, 172,* 412–416.

McGlashan, T. H. (1988). A selective review of recent American long-term follow-up studies of schizophrenia. *Schizophrenia Bulletin, 14,* 515–542.

McGuire, T. G. (1991). Measuring the economic costs of schizophrenia. *Schizophrenia Bulletin, 17,* 375–388.

Mischel, W. (1968). *Personality and assessment.* New York: Wiley.

Möller, H. J., Schmid-Bode, W., Wittchen, H. U., & Zerssen, D. V. (1986). Outcome and prediction of outcome in schizophrenia: Results from the literature and from two personal studies. In M. J. Goldstein, I. Hand, & K. Hahlweg (Eds.), *Treatment of schizophrenia: Family assessment and intervention* (pp. 11–24). Berlin: Springer-Verlag.

Monahan, J. (1981). *The clinical prediction of violent behavior.* Maryland: United States Department of Health and Human Services.

Mueser, K. T., Yarnold, P. R., Levinson, D. F., Singh, H., Bellack, A. S., Kee, K., Morrison, R. L., & Wadalam, K. G. (1990). Prevalence of substance abuse in schizophrenia: Demographic and clinical correlates. *Schizophrenia Bulletin, 16,* 31–56.

Novaco, R. W. (1985). Anger and its therapeutic regulation. In M. Chesney & R. Rosenman (Eds.), *Anger and hostility in cardiovascular disorders* (pp. 203–226). Washington, DC: Hemisphere.

Nuechterlein, K. H., & Dawson, M. E. (1984). A heuristic vulnerability-stress model of schizophrenic eposides. *Schizophrenia Bulletin, 10,* 300–312.

Objordsmoen, S. (1991). Long-term clinical outcome of schizophrenia with special reference to gender differences. *Acta Psychiatrica Scandinavica, 83,* 307–313.

Parker, G., Johnston, P., & Hayward, L. (1988). Parental "expressed emotion" as a predictor of schizophrenic relapse. *Archives of General Psychiatry, 45,* 806–813.

Patterson, G. R. (1982). *Coercive family process.* Eugene, OR: Castilia.

Paul, G. L., & Lentz, R. J. (1977). *Psychosocial treatment of chronic mental patients: Milieu versus social learning programs.* Cambridge, MA: Harvard University Press.

Piatkowska, O., & Farnill, D. (1992). Medication—Compliance or alliance? In D. J. Kavanagh (Ed.), *Schizophrenia: An overview and practical handbook* (pp. 339–355). London: Chapman & Hall.

Rajkumar, S., & Thara, R. (1989). Factors affecting relapse in schizophrenia. *Schizophrenia Research, 2,* 403–409.

Safferman, A., Lieberman, J. A., Kane, J. M., Szymanski, S., & Kinon, B. (1991). Update on the clinical efficacy and side effects of clozapine. *Schizophrenia Bulletin, 17,* 247–261.

Salokangas, R. K. R., Palo-Oja, T., & Ojanen, M. (1991). The need for social support among out-patients suffering from functional psychosis. *Psychological Medicine, 21,* 209–217.

Salokangas, R. K. R., & Stengard, E. (1990). Gender and short-term outcome in schizophrenia. *Schizophrenia Research, 3,* 333–345.

Sanders, D. H. (1972). Innovative environments in the community: A life for the chronic patient. *Schizophrenia Bulletin, 1,* 49–59.

Schneider, B. J. (1982). Electrodermal activity and therapeutic response to neuroleptic treatment in chronic schizophrenic in-patients. *Psychological Medicine, 12,* 607–613.

Seltzer, A., Roncari, I., & Garfinkel, P. (1980). Effect of patient education on patient compliance. *Canadian Journal of Psychiatry, 25,* 638–645.

Shepherd, G. (1991). Foreword. Psychiatric rehabilitation in the 1990s. In F. N. Watts & D. H. Bennett (Eds.), *Theory and practice of psychiatric rehabilitation* (pp. xiii–xlviii), Chichester: John Wiley.

Siris, S. G. (1991). Diagnosis of secondary depression in schizophrenia: Implications for DSM-IV. *Schizophrenia Bulletin, 17,* 75–98.

Smith, J. V., & Birchwood, M. J. (1987). Specific and non-specific effects of educational intervention with families living with a schizophrenic relative. *British Journal of Psychiatry, 150,* 645–652.

Smith, J. V., & Birchwood, M. J. (1990). Relatives and patients as partners in the management of schizophrenia: The development of a service model. *British Journal of Psychiatry, 156,* 654–660.

Stein, L. I., & Test, M. A. (1985). *The training in community living model: A decade of experience*. San Francisco: Jossey-Bass.

Strauss, J. S., & Carpenter, W. T. (1977). The prediction of outcome in schizophrenia: III. Five-year outcome and its predictors. *Archives of General Psychiatry, 34,* 159–163.

Strauss, J. S., & Carpenter, W. T. (1978). The prognosis of schizophrenia: Rationale for a multidimensional concept. *Schizophrenia Bulletin, 4,* 56–67.

Subotnik, K. L., & Nuechterlein, K. H. (1988). Prodromal signs and symptoms of schizophrenic relapse. *Journal of Abnormal Psychology, 97,* 405–412.

Tarrier, N. (1987). An investigation of residual psychotic symptoms in discharged schizophrenic patients. *British Journal of Clinical Psychology, 26,* 141–143.

Tarrier, N. (1992). Psychological treatment of positive schizophrenic symptoms. In D. J. Kavanagh (Ed.), *Schizophrenia: An overview and practical handbook* (pp. 356–373). London: Chapman & Hall.

Tarrier, N., Barrowclough, C., Vaughn, C., Bamrah, J. S., Porceddu, K., Watts, S., & Freeman, H. (1988). The community management of schizophrenia: A controlled trial of a behavioural intervention with families to reduce relapse. *British Journal of Psychiatry, 153,* 532–542.

Tarrier, N., Barrowclough, C., Vaughn, C., Bamrah, J. S., Porceddu, K., Watts, S., & Freeman, H. (1989). Community management of schizophrenia: A two-year follow-up of a behavioural intervention with families. *British Journal of Psychiatry, 154,* 625–628.

Tennant, C. (1985). Stress and schizophrenia: A review. *Integrative Psychiatry, 3,* 248–255.

Van Putten, T., May, P. R. A., & Marder, S. R. (1984). Akathisia with haloperidol and thiothixene. *Archives of General Psychiatry, 41,* 1036–1039.

Vaughan, K., Doyle, M., McConaghy, N., Blaszczynski, A., Fox, A., & Tarrier, N. (1992). The Sydney intervention trial: A controlled trial of relatives' counselling to reduce schizophrenic relapse. *Social Psychiatry and Psychiatric Epidemiology, 27,* 16–21.

Vaughn, C., & Leff, J. (1976a). The influence of family and social factors on the course of psychiatric illness. *British Journal of Psychiatry, 129,* 125–137.

Verghese, A., John, J. K., Rajkumar, S., Richard, J., Sethi, B. B., & Trivedi, J. K. (1989). Factors associated with the course and outcome of schizophrenia in India. Results of a two-year multicentre follow-up study. *British Journal of Psychiatry, 154,* 499–503.

Wallace, C. J., Donahoe, C. P., & Boone, S. E. (1988). Schizophrenia. In M. Hersen (Ed.), *Pharmacological and behavioral treatment: An integrative approach*. New York: Wiley.

Wallace, C. J., & Liberman, R. P. (1985). Social skills training for patients with schizophrenia: A controlled clinical trial. *Psychiatry Research, 15,* 239–247.

Warner, R. (1983). Recovery from schizophrenia in the third world. *Psychiatry, 46,* 197–212.

Watt, D. C., Katz, K., & Shepherd, M. (1983). The natural history of schizophrenia: A 5-year prospective follow-up of a representative sample of schizophrenics by means of a standardized clinical and social assessment. *Psychological Medicine, 13,* 603–670.

Waxler, N. (1979). Is outcome for schizophrenia better in nonindustrial societies? The case of Sri Lanka. *The Journal of Nervous and Mental Disease, 167,* 144–158.

West, D. (1990). *Cognitive–behaviour therapy in the treatment of post-psychotic depression in schizophrenia.* Unpublished master's thesis, University of Sydney, Sydney.

Westermeyer, J. F., Harrow, M., & Marengo, J. T. (1991). Risk for suicide in schizophrenia and other psychotic and nonpsychotic disorders. *The Journal of Nervous and Mental Disease, 179,* 259–266.

Wiedl, K. H., & Schötner, B. (1991). Coping with symptoms related to schizophrenia. *Schizophrenia Bulletin, 17,* 525–538.

Wing, J. K., & Brown, G. W. (1970). *Institutionalism and schizophrenia.* London: Cambridge University Press.

World Health Organization. (1979). *Schizophrenia: An international follow-up study.* New York: Wiley.

Wykes, T. (1983). A follow-up of "new" long-stay patients in Camberwell 1977–1982. *Psychological Medicine, 13,* 659–662.

Yesavage, J. (1983). Inpatient violence and the schizophrenic patient. *Acta Psychiatrica Scandinavica, 67,* 353–357.

Young, J. L., Zonana, H. V., & Shepler, L. (1986). Medication noncompliance in schizophrenia: Codification and update. *Bulletin of the American Academy of Psychiatry and Law, 14,* 105–122.

Zubin, J., & Spring, B. (1977). Vulnerability: A new view of schizophrenia. *Journal of Abnormal Psychology, 86,* 103–126.

CHAPTER 8

PANIC DISORDER AND PANIC DISORDER WITH AGORAPHOBIA

Timothy A. Brown
David H. Barlow
THE UNIVERSITY AT ALBANY,
STATE UNIVERSITY OF NEW YORK

In the last several years, substantial advances have been achieved in the development and refinement of cognitive–behavioral treatments of panic disorder (PD) and panic disorder with agoraphobia (PDA) (cf. Barlow, 1988; Brown, Hertz, & Barlow, 1992). For instance, until recently, behavioral treatments for PDA largely consisted of exposure-based interventions targeting agoraphobic avoidance. On the whole, these treatments did not address panic directly, although a reduction in panic attack frequency was often observed following successful exposure-based treatment. Nevertheless, in the last 5 years, cognitive–behavioral treatments aimed directly at panic reduction have been developed and evaluated. As this chapter shows, these treatments have been highly successful in effecting clinically significant change in panic patients.

What is also immediately evident from a review of the extant literature is that many patients with PD or PDA, while showing a favorable response, still display significant residual symptomatology or do not fully maintain their gains after treatment. In this chapter, we review findings pertaining to patterns and predictors of long-term clinical outcome following cognitive–behavioral treatment of PD and PDA. In addition, findings from the pharmacological treatment literature are discussed since these treatments represent the most widely researched alternative treatment of PD and PDA. These findings are contrasted to the long-term results from cognitive–behavioral treatment trials. Rates of relapse and/or rates of success (e.g., percentage panic free) at follow-up for the key studies discussed in subsequent sections are presented in Table 8.1. As can be

TABLE 8.1. Summary of Relapse Rates for Pharmacological and Psychosocial Treatments of PD and PDA

Study	Treatment(s)	Group(s)	Follow-up type and interval	Follow-up findings
Pharmacological and combined pharmacological/psychosocial treatment studies				
Zitrin et al., 1983	IMI+SE[a], IMI+ST, PLA+SE	PDA (n = 46)[b]	FU (24 mos.)	31%, 19%, 14% relapsed in the IMI+ST, IMI+SE, PLA+SE groups, respectively
Telch et al., 1985	IMI, IMI+SE, PLA+SE	PDA (n = 27)	FU (4 mos.)	11%, 77%, 11% of IMI, IMI+SE, PLA+SE groups panic free, respectively; IMI+SE superior to other groups on measures of avoidance and other symptoms
Mavissakalian & Michelson, 1986	IMI+SE, IMI+PP, PLA+SE, PLA+PP	PDA (n = 47)	FU (1, 6, 12, 24 mos.)	At 24 mos, rates of relapse were 17%, 38%, 14%, and 0% for the IMI+SE, IMI+PP, PLA+SE, PLA+PP groups, respectively
Mellman & Uhde, 1986	AZ	PD, PDA (n = 8)	DC (varied)	100% returned to pretreatment symptom levels following DC
Sheehan, 1986	IMI, PZ, AZ, PLA	PD, PDA (n = ?)	FU (12 mos.)	70% relapsed
Fyer et al., 1987	AZ	PD (n = 17)	DC (1 mo.)	88% relapsed during DC period
Fyer, 1988	IMI	PDA (n = 14)	DC FU (1–6 mos.)	43% panicked in response to lactate following DC
Pecknold et al., 1988	AZ, PLA	PD, PDA (n = 54)	DC (1 mo.) FU (2 wks.)	47% of treatment completers dropped from study during DC and FU phase; 90% relapsed following DC
Cognitive–Behavioral Treatment Studies				
Arnow et al., 1985	SP+COMM, SP+PMR	PDA (n = 24)	FU (8 mos.)	No composite measures of endstate status provided; SP+COMM superior to SP+PMR on measures of situational exposure

Study	Treatment	Sample	Follow-up	Results
Clark et al., 1985	BRT	PD, PDA ($n = 18$)	FU (6, 24 mos.)	At 24 mos, 100% of PDs were panic free; percent panic free of PDAs not provided[c]
Jansson et al., 1986	SE, AR	PDA ($n = 32$)	FU (7, 15 mos.)	At 15 mos, 71% of SE group and 83% of AR group classified as treatment responders; only 1 relapse noted[d]
Cerny et al., 1987	SP, SE	PDA ($n = 28$)	FU (12, 24 mos.)	At 24 mos, 87% of SP group and 46% of SE group classified as treatment responders
Öst, 1988	AR, PMR	PD ($n = 12$)	FU (19 mos.)	100% of AR group panic free; 25% of PMR group panic free
Michelson et al., 1989	SE, SE+CR, SE+PMR	PDA ($n = 74$)	FU (3 mos.)	65%, 88%, and 47% of the SE, SE+CR, and SE+PMR groups met high endstate status, respectively
Sokol et al., 1989	CR	PDA ($n = 26$)	FU (3 mos.)	77% panic free
Côté et al., 1990	CR+BRT	PD ($n = 21$)	FU (6 mos.)	90% panic free
Newman et al., 1990	CR	PD, PDA ($n = 43$)	FU (12 mos.)	87% panic free
Craske et al., 1991	PMR, CR+IE, CR+IE+PMR	PD ($n = 34$)	FU (6, 24 mos.)	At 24 mos., 56%, 87%, 60% of PMR, CR+IE, CR+IE+PMR groups were panic free, respectively; 50% met high endstate status

Note. PD = panic disorder; PDA = panic disorder with agoraphobia; FU = follow-up; DC = discontinuation; IMI = imipramine; AZ = alprazolam; PLA = placebo; PZ = phenelzine; SE = situational exposure; ST = supportive therapy; PP = programmed practice; SP = spouse-assisted exposure; COMM = communication skills training; BRT = breathing retraining; AR = applied relaxation; PMR = progressive muscle relaxation; CR = cognitive restructuring; IE = interoceptive exposure.

[a]Exposure consisted of imaginal exposure in this study.

[b]Ns reflect number of subjects available for follow-up analysis.

[c]PDAs' panic frequency continued to be below pretreatment levels.

[d]All patients were provided self-exposure instructions during the follow-up period.

193

readily noted in Table 8.1, pharmacological and psychosocial treatment studies differ considerably with regard to the metric relied on for evaluating the long-term clinical effects of treatment. Moreover, as will become evident, little work has been done specifically on the development and evaluation of methods for promoting treatment gain generalization and maintenance. Therefore, we conclude this chapter with suggestions for future research.

LONG-TERM CLINICAL OUTCOME OF PHARMACOLOGICAL TREATMENTS

Few studies have examined systematically the long-term clinical outcome from pharmacological treatments for PD and PDA. Of the studies that do exist, long-term results have been most frequently reported following clinical trials of alprazolam and imipramine. These studies are the focus of this section of the chapter. Nevertheless, in addition to the paucity of extant findings, research on long-term clinical outcome of pharmacological treatments has been hindered by several methodological difficulties including the fact that the definition of "relapse" in these studies is rarely well specified (cf. Telch, Tearnan, & Taylor, 1983).

In the drug treatment literature, the term "discontinuation" typically refers to the period during medication tapering; "follow-up" denotes the period after discontinuation has been completed. Similarly, the term "relapse" represents the reemergence of the disorder following its successful amelioration during treatment; "withdrawal symptoms" refer to the specific iatrogenic effects of the process of discontinuation; "rebound panics" refer to a recurrence of panics of a severity greater than was experienced prior to treatment (cf. Fyer, 1988).

With regard to alprazolam, the few studies reporting follow-up results after treatment of PD and PDA are not optimistic. For instance, clinical status immediately following withdrawal from an 8-week trial of alprazolam for PD and PDA was examined in the large-scale, cross-national study sponsored by Upjohn (Pecknold, Swinson, Kuch, & Lewis, 1988). Interpretation of the results of this study is hindered because 47% of subjects completing the treatment trial dropped out of the study prior to completing the discontinuation and 2-week follow-up phase. Nevertheless, after the 4-week discontinuation period, up to 90% of subjects treated with alprazolam relapsed, with 28% reporting rebound panic attacks. Rebound and withdrawal effects diminished by the end of the follow-up period such that subjects who received alprazolam were no longer different from placebo subjects.

Similarly, Fyer et al. (1987) examined the effects of discontinuation in 17 of 30 PD patients treated with alprazolam. Only 4 patients completed discontinuation in accordance with the period specified in the protocol (30 days); 4 additional patients successfully reached a zero dosage in 7 to 13 weeks by slowing the tapering rate. The remaining 9 patients either refused to withdraw or required adjunctive medication prior to consenting to alprazolam discontinuation. During discontinuation, Fyer et al. (1987) reported that 15 of the 17 patients relapsed; in 7 patients, relapse was rated as severe. In addition, 14 of the 17 patients reported withdrawal symptoms with 9 patients considered to have experienced a clinically significant withdrawal syndrome.

Concordant findings have been reported by Mellman and Uhde (1986) who found that all of their small sample of PD and PDA patients (n = 8) returned to pretreatment symptom levels following alprazolam discontinuation. Similarly, Sheehan (1986) reported that over 70% of subjects receiving either imipramine, phenelzine, alprazolam, or placebo relapsed within 1 year of discontinuation.

Studies examining the long-term outcome of imipramine trials have been somewhat more favorable, although the majority have examined the efficacy of imipramine delivered in combination with some form of psychosocial treatment (Agras, Telch, Taylor, Roth, & Brouillard, 1990; Mavissakalian & Michelson, 1986; Telch, Agras, Taylor, Roth, & Gallen, 1985; Zitrin, Klein, Woerner, & Ross, 1983). For example, Zitrin et al. (1983) examined the efficacy of imipramine combined with either behavioral therapy (imaginal exposure) or supportive therapy in a large sample of PDAs and "mixed phobics" (e.g., PD patients). "Relapse" was defined as the return of agoraphobic avoidance. Relapse rates across the 2-year follow-up period for PDAs were 31% for imipramine plus supportive therapy, 19% for imipramine plus behavioral therapy, and 14% for behavioral therapy plus placebo.

In another study examining the additive effects of imipramine to exposure therapy, Mavissakalian and Michelson (1986) randomly assigned 77 PDA patients to one of four conditions in accordance with a 2 × 2 design (therapist-assisted exposure vs. programmed practice; imipramine vs. placebo). Although posttreatment results favored exposure, imipramine, or their combination over programmed practice alone, 2-year follow-up results (N = 47) revealed deterioration among imipramine-treated patients, whereas behaviorally treated patients tended to evidence treatment gain maintenance and further improvement.

In one of the few studies to evaluate the effects of imipramine in the treatment of PDA in the absence of *in vivo* exposure, Telch et al. (1985) compared imipramine plus antiexposure instructions, imipramine plus exposure, and placebo plus exposure in 37 PDA patients. After 8 weeks, patients in the imipramine plus antiexposure condition evidenced negligible improvement on panic, phobic avoidance, and anxiety, although a reduction in depressed mood was observed. In contrast, patients in the exposure conditions, with or without imipramine, showed marked improvement on these measures. At the 4-month follow-up, the imipramine plus exposure condition continued to show superior gains relative to the other conditions. Although imipramine did seem to potentiate *in vivo* exposure, certain caveats were observed including its rates of refusal (20%) and dropout (17%–23%). Moreover, observed relapse rates in the literature averaging 35%–40% reflect additional potential obstacles in the treatment of PDA with imipramine (cf. Michelson & Marchione, 1991).

Finally, Fyer (1988) reported rates of panic response to sodium lactate infusions in 14 PDA patients posttreatment and 1 to 6 months following imipramine treatment. Although none of the 14 subjects panicked during the infusion posttreatment, 43% did so at a later point following imipramine discontinuation.

LONG-TERM CLINICAL OUTCOME OF PSYCHOSOCIAL TREATMENTS

As is the case with the pharmacological treatments, there is a paucity of follow-up studies in the psychosocial treatment literature of PDA, and particularly PD.

Panic Disorder with Agoraphobia

Reviews of the extant treatment literature indicate that 60%–75% of patients completing a cognitive–behavioral treatment program for PDA respond in a clinically significant manner (Barlow, 1988; Clum, 1989; Jansson & Öst, 1982; Michelson & Marchione, 1991). Nevertheless, as is the case with pharmacological treatment studies, these figures are less impressive when dropouts are considered in the analyses or when considering the fact that 25%–40% of patients fail to show a significant treatment response. In addition, whereas the majority of patients do benefit from treatment, many are left with residual symptomatology (e.g., anticipatory anxiety, mild avoidance). Despite these caveats, results of controlled studies examining long-term clinical outcome following PDA treatment indicate that of the patients who do respond, the majority maintain their treatment gains or show continued improvement across the follow-up period.

For example, Michelson, Marchione, and Greenwald (1989) reported the results of a comparative outcome study examining three treat-

ment conditions: graduated exposure (GE), GE plus cognitive restructuring (GE + CR), and GE plus relaxation training (GE + RT) in 92 PDA
patients. Patients in all conditions received instructions for self-exposure
(programmed practice) as well. Of the 74 patients completing treatment,
the percentage of patients achieving high endstate status at posttreatment
was 86%, 73%, and 65% for the GE + CT, GE + RT, and GE only
conditions, respectively. At a 3-month follow-up, the percentage of
patients meeting high endstate criteria was 87.5%, 47%, and 65%, for
these three conditions, respectively. Analysis of clinical response over a
longer follow-up interval is currently under way. Michelson and Marchione (1991), in their recent review of the PDA treatment literature,
state that the GE + CT protocol has been the most effective treatment
that they have devised over the past decade of development and evaluation of a variety of pharmacological, cognitive, and behavioral interventions at their center.

In one of the more extensive follow-up studies that has been conducted to date, Jansson, Jerremalm, and Öst (1986) presented the results
of a 7- to 15-month follow-up of 32 PDA patients treated with *in vivo*
exposure or applied relaxation. During the follow-up period, all patients
were given self-exposure instructions. Although both groups evidenced
clinically significant improvement rates comparable to other PDA treatment outcome studies, these rates significantly increased across both
follow-up periods. For example, whereas 59% of patients treated with *in
vivo* exposure were improved to a clinically significant degree posttreatment, this percentage increased to 65% and 71% at the 7- and 15-month
assessments, respectively. Similarly, in the applied relaxation group, the
percentage of clinically significant responders posttreatment was 58%,
increasing to 67% and 83% at the 7- and 15-month assessments, respectively. Only one relapse was recorded. In light of the encouraging result
of continued improvement in many of the subjects in their study, the
authors concluded that treatment protocols for PDA should contain a
maintenance program of self-exposure of at least 6 months to ensure
continued improvement or maintenance of treatment gains. Despite this
clinically sound recommendation, the issue whether the inclusion of a
maintenance program along with lines of Jansson et al.'s (1986) contributes to enhanced long-term functioning awaits controlled investigation.

Although most cognitive–behavioral researchers concur that some
form of therapeutic exposure is a necessary ingredient in the treatment of
PDA, the fact that a significant minority of patients do not evidence
clinically significant improvement has led researchers to examine various
modifications in the delivery of exposure in an effort to increase the
proportion of patients achieving meaningful benefit. One of the most

extensively studied variations of the exposure format is the inclusion of the patient's spouse in treatment. The development of spouse-assisted exposure treatment arose partly from findings, albeit often inconsistent and/or contradictory, suggesting that (1) marital satisfaction is a significant predictor of treatment response (e.g., Milton & Hafner, 1979; Monteiro, Marks, & Ramm, 1985), and (2) successful PDA treatment may result in increases in marital discord (e.g., Milton & Hafner, 1979). Despite the fact that reviews of the extant literature note that research on the role of relationship issues and PDA symptomatology and response to treatment has often produced inconsistent findings (e.g., Arrindell, Emmelkamp, & Sanderman, 1986; Kleiner & Marshall, 1985), spouse-assisted approaches to PDA treatment have a number of potential advantages. First, spousal involvement may facilitate between-session practice and practice following the active treatment phase. Moreover, such practice may enhance generalization of treatment effects since this format allows for therapeutic exposure within the patient's home environment and mitigates the possibility of dependence on the therapist. Second, in cases where marital discord may potentially affect treatment response as either a pretreatment predictor or a consequence of successful treatment of PDA symptomatology, the inclusion of spouses in treatment allows for the potential resolution of these difficulties if they arise. Possibly as a result of these features, this treatment has produced dropout rates lower than those observed in other exposure-based approaches (Arnow, Taylor, Agras, & Telch, 1985; Barlow, O'Brien, & Last, 1984; Jannoun, Munby, Catalan, & Gelder, 1980; Mathews, Teasdale, Munby, Johnston, & Shaw, 1977).

In a study comparing 14 PDAs treated in a spouse-assisted program involving 12 sessions of cognitive restructuring and self-initiated exposure with 14 patients treated in an identical format but without their spouse, Barlow et al. (1984) found that the spouse-assisted group contained a significantly greater number of treatment responders posttreatment (86%) than in the nonspousal group (43%). Interestingly, there was a nonsignificant trend for the treatment responder group to engage in a greater number of between-session practices than nonresponders. In a follow-up study of these patients, Cerny, Barlow, Craske, and Himadi (1987) found that the spousal group evidenced an increasingly more positive response than the nonspousal group at 1- and 2-year follow-ups, augmenting the between-group differences observed posttreatment. The fact that PDA patients treated in the spouse-assisted format continued to improve across the follow-up period is consistent with several other studies showing enhanced long-term functioning in patients treated with their spouses or significant others (Hand, Lamontagne, & Marks, 1974; Jannoun et al., 1980; Mathews et al., 1977; Munby & Johnston, 1980).

In another well-controlled study pertaining to the inclusion of spouses in the treatment of PDA, Arnow et al. (1985) evaluated the issue whether the provision of a communications skills training package as an additional treatment component would significantly enhance treatment gains derived from a standard spouse-assisted exposure protocol. Twenty-four PDA patients underwent 4 weeks of spouse-assisted exposure after which they were divided into two matched groups according to their change scores on behavioral measures of agoraphobia. One group received the 8-week communications training package focusing on communication patterns that may have potentially maintained PDA symptomatology. The other group received 8 weeks of couples relaxation training. At both posttreatment and at an 8-month follow-up, patients treated in the communications training condition showed a significantly greater response than the relaxation group on measures of agoraphobic symptomatology. Unfortunately, composite measures of treatment responder and high endstate functioning status were not provided in this study. It is also important to note that based on pretreatment measures, most of the subjects in Arnow et al. (1985) evidenced good marital adjustment from the outset of the study.

Panic Disorder

Of the few existing studies examining long-term clinical functioning following psychosocial treatment of PD with no or minimal agoraphobic avoidance, most are based on uncontrolled trials. Of course, these treatments differ in nature from most of the PDA treatments discussed previously because treatments for PD without agoraphobic avoidance are designed specifically for the amelioration of panic rather than avoidance. Hence, the paucity of well-controlled follow-up studies is because cognitive–behavioral researchers have only recently directed their efforts toward designing and evaluating panic-control treatments, an area that had previously been addressed solely by pharmacological treatments.

Nevertheless, initial findings indicate that cognitive–behavioral treatments are quite effective in producing significant and durable changes in panic frequency and associated symptomatology. For example, Clark, Salkovskis, and Chalkley (1985) described maintenance of treatment gains for up to 2 years in 18 panickers after a brief cognitive–behavioral intervention, particularly in panickers who experienced nonsituational panic attacks. However, their subject sample was restricted to panickers who experienced hyperventilation symptoms, and hence the generalizability of the results is potentially limited. Sokol, Beck, and Clark (1989) implemented cognitive–behavioral panic-control procedures for 28 subjects with PDA. Of the 26 who completed treatment, all were panic free posttreatment, as were the 20 patients assessed at the 3-month follow-up. Similarly, Newman, Beck, Beck, and Tran (1990) compared the differential effectiveness of cognitive therapy in a mixed sample of 43 PD and PDA patients on the basis of presence–absence of current medication use (antidepressant, antianxiety). Following a 12–16-week active treatment phase, panic-free status was observed in 83% and 84% of medicated and nonmedicated patients, respectively. At the 12-month follow-up, 87% of both groups were panic free. Thus, medication status did not have an adverse impact on short- and long-term clinical outcome following cognitive therapy. Interestingly, only 35% of medication subjects were still using medications on either a daily or a PRN basis posttreatment. At the 12-month follow-up, this percentage had increased to 53%, although only 33% were using medication on a daily basis.

In one of the few controlled investigations of the follow-up effects of nonpharmacological treatment specifically targeting panic, Öst (1988) compared the efficacy of progressive muscle relaxation and applied relaxation in 16 patients with PD. Subjects were followed for an average of 19 months. All members of the applied relaxation group were panic free posttreatment and at follow-up assessment. Furthermore, of the 12 subjects available at follow-up, 100% of the applied relaxation group were defined as improved to a clinically significant degree in contrast to only 25% of the progressive muscle relaxation group.

In the only other controlled study of the long-term effects of behavioral treatment of PD published to date, Craske, Brown, and Barlow (1991) recently reported the 2-year follow-up results of an outcome study conducted by Barlow, Craske, Cerny, and Klosko (1989). In the earlier report, the following treatment conditions were compared: applied progressive muscle relaxation, interoceptive exposure plus cognitive restructuring, the combination of relaxation with exposure and cognitive restructuring, and a wait-list control. Posttreatment, more than 85% of patients in the two groups containing exposure and cognitive restructuring were panic free. In contrast, the relaxation condition was associated with greater reductions on measures of general anxiety but also with greater attrition (33%). Although subjects in the two conditions receiving exposure and cognitive restructuring were more improved on measures of panic than relaxation-treated subjects, since the latter group evidenced greater reductions in general anxiety, overall equivalence in outcome was observed. That is, composite measures of responder status and endstate functioning status showed that all three active treatment conditions yielded proportionally more responders and high endstate functioners than the wait-list group, but differences among the three active conditions were not apparent.

Craske et al. (1991) hypothesized that since more subjects in the relaxation group continued to panic posttreatment in Barlow et al. (1989), group differences might become more apparent over the follow-up period. Indeed, at the 24-month follow-up, when dropouts during the active treatment phase were included in the analyses and were presumed to be continuing to panic, observed panic-free rates were 81% for the exposure plus cognitive restructuring condition, in contrast to 43% and 36% for the combination and relaxation conditions, respectively. On the majority of the remaining variables (e.g., general anxiety, depression) patients evidenced treatment gain maintenance or continued improvement. Craske et al. (1991) speculated that a dilution effect, or perhaps a detrimental effect of the addition of relaxation procedures, accounted for the lower success of the combination condition in comparison to the exposure plus cognitive restructuring group.

In another recent outcome study involving cognitive–behavioral panic-control treatments, Côté et al. (1990) compared the efficacy of 17-week therapist-directed and minimal-therapist-contact treatments in 21 PD patients without agoraphobic avoidance. Posttreatment, over 82% of patients in both conditions were panic free; indeed, between-group differences were negligible posttreatment, indicating minimal-therapist-contact procedures to be a viable form of treatment for PD. Relevant to this chapter, 90% of patients were panic free at a 6-month follow-up assessment. These improvements were associated with a reduction in medication intake as well.

Whereas these results compare quite favorably to the findings from the few studies reporting follow-up results of pharmacological treatments, certain caveats should be noted. For example, although more than 80% of patients treated using cognitive restructuring and exposure were panic free at a 24-month follow-up in Craske et al. (1991), it was observed that only 50% of the cognitive plus exposure subjects met criteria for high endstate status at this period. This finding partly reflects the fact that while the majority of these subjects were panic free, some continued to evidence mild agoraphobic avoidance. Thus, the authors concluded that this feature may need to be targeted separately in treatment since the elimination of panic may not ensure the amelioration of agoraphobic avoidance. In addition, these findings lend support to earlier assertions (e.g., Barlow, 1988) that reliance on panic-free status as the central measure of treatment outcome may be an overly optimistic indicator of treatment success since patients free of panic posttreatment may often evidence other significant symptomatology (e.g., avoidance, general anxiety). Thus, additional indices of long-term functioning should be reported as well (e.g., operationally defined endstate status variables).

Summary of Pharmacological and
Psychosocial Treatment Studies

In evaluating the comparative efficacy of pharmacological and psychosocial approaches to PD and PDA treatment, recent reviews have frequently focused on three major indices of outcome: rates of dropouts, rates of success (e.g., treatment responder, endstate status), and rates of relapse (e.g., Clum, 1989; Michelson & Marchione, 1991). However, these endeavors are frequently hindered by the fact that dropout and relapse rates are often not provided, and composite measures of clinically significant change are often not calculated. Whereas the primary focus of this chapter is long-term clinical functioning following treatment, evaluation of a treatment's ability to achieve durable results (e.g., proportion of relapses, high endstate functioners) cannot be made without consideration of the effects produced by the intervention during the active treatment phase (e.g., dropouts, rates of success). This point is underscored by the observation that pharmacological and psychosocial treatment studies have differed considerably with regard to the index relied on to reflect long-term clinical outcome, with drug studies more apt to report rates of relapse and psychosocial studies rates of success (e.g., percent of panic-free or high endstate subjects). Thus, comparisons of the long-term efficacy of drug and psychosocial treatments are hindered since these indices do not reflect opposite sides of the same coin. For instance, rates of success at follow-up involve calculation of the proportion of the entire sample of treated subjects meeting this criterion; in the calculation of relapse rates, only subjects evidencing favorable clinical response posttreatment are considered.

Nevertheless, the conclusions generated from reviews of the extant literature generally concur that although the majority of patients do receive clinically significant benefits from cognitive–behavioral treatments for PD and PDA, many continue to display significant symptomatology. Although there are relatively few studies examining the efficacy of cognitive–behavioral packages specifically targeting panic, recent reviewers (e.g., Clum, 1989) have tentatively concluded that these treatments are more effective than previously existing treatments for PDA (e.g., in vivo exposure) in terms of success rates, dropout rates, and perhaps rates of relapse (cf. Michelson & Marchione, 1991). Dropout rates in cognitive–behavioral treatment trials are generally in the 10%–20% range, although certain formats have produced lower rates (i.e., spouse-assisted treatment) and others, higher rates (e.g., massed, intensive exposure) (cf. Jansson & Öst, 1982). In contrast, pharmacological treatments often are associated with higher rates of attrition, particularly those using tricyclic antidepressants such as imipramine. However, as noted earlier, evaluation of the tricyclics in the treatment of PD and PDA has proven difficult given the preponderance of studies delivering these medications in combination with a psychosocial treatment such as exposure. Nevertheless, several studies are currently under way and/or nearing completion that have addressed the comparative short- and long-term efficacy of imipramine only and cognitive–behavioral approaches to the treatment of PD (e.g., Clark et al., 1990).

In contrast, although the high-potency benzodiazepines (e.g., alprazolam) often produce fewer dropouts than other commonly used medications such as imipramine, discontinuation has been associated with high rates of relapse and rebound panic, leading to some controversy among psychopharmacologists over whether discontinuation of medication should even be attempted (e.g., Sheehan, 1986). On the other hand, a few studies have produced findings indicating that although not an explicit goal of treatment, cognitive–behavioral interventions may be associated with a reduction in medication intake (Côté et al., 1990; Newman et al., 1990), even with benzodiazepines (Barlow, Rapee, & Brown, in press; Butler, Fennell, Robson, & Gelder, 1991), a drug notorious for its resiliency to discontinuation (Schweizer & Rickels, 1991).

Furthermore, whereas some data indicate that the addition of imipramine to behavioral therapy may enhance treatment outcome, there is some evidence that the addition of benzodiazepines may interfere with behavioral treatment efficacy. For example, Clum (1989) estimated that the success rate for behavioral therapy alone in the treatment of panic was 71% (83% for PD; 61% for PDA); however, these rates were reduced to 28% and 57% when behavioral therapy was delivered in tandem with placebos and benzodiazepines, respectively.

PREDICTORS OF LONG-TERM OUTCOME: REVIEW AND DIRECTIONS FOR FUTURE RESEARCH

Given the dearth of controlled follow-up studies of cognitive–behavioral treatments of PD and PDA, it follows that data pertaining to predictors of long-term clinical functioning are lacking as well. Although cognitive–behavioral researchers have become more interested in the evaluation of predictors of short- and long-term clinical outcome in recent years (cf. Foa & Emmelkamp, 1983), there are numerous methodological difficulties that have arisen impeding advancement in this area. Chambless and Gracely (1988) noted several methodological limitations: (1) the preponderant use of small sample sizes in treatment trials reduces statistical power thereby resulting in nonsignificant findings and/or unstable results; (2) marked variability in instruments used to a measure similar variables, as well as marked variability in the criteria used to define treatment responder or endstate status hinders comparison of extant findings across studies; and (3) the statistical procedures used to evaluate potential predictors and methods of reporting these analyses are frequently inadequate (e.g., failure to report significant predictors in correlational form so that the clinical significance of predictors can be evaluated).

Many of the problems noted by Chambless and Gracely (1988) are exacerbated if one is examining predictors of clinical status across long follow-up intervals due to the increasing likelihood of subject attrition. In addition to reducing the power of statistical tests of predictors, the possibility of differential attrition must be addressed since this factor may potentially confound the validity of the analyses (e.g., selection bias—unavailability of low-functioning subjects at follow-up may restrict the range of outcome scores, thereby reducing the chance of finding valid predictors). Furthermore, many patients receive additional treatment during the follow-up phase. Frequently, follow-up studies fail to assess this factor or do not adequately take into account the impact that additional treatment may have had when interpreting the significance of follow-up results.

Partially as a result of the aforementioned issues, as well as other factors, research concerning the prediction of long-term clinical functioning following cognitive–behavioral treatment of PD and PDA has failed to explicate reliable predictors of outcome. For instance, research examining the role of marital satisfaction as a predictor of treatment response in PDA has produced inconsistent findings, with some studies finding a relationship between pretreatment marital adjustment and treatment success (e.g., Chambless & Gracely, 1988; Milton & Hafner, 1979) and others finding this factor to be independent of treatment response (e.g., Himadi, Cerny, Barlow, Cohen, & O'Brien, 1986). Moreover, some studies have found that general social adjustment at pretreatment, rather than marital adjustment per se, may be predictive of clinical functioning posttreatment and at long-term follow-up (Arrindell et al., 1986; Fischer, Hand, Angenendt, Buttner-Westphal, & Manecke, 1988; Lelliott, Marks, Monteiro, Tsakiris, & Noshirvani, 1987). Irrespective of whether marital factors play a considerable role in PDA, several studies have produced converging evidence for the clinical benefit of spouse-assisted exposure therapy both in the short and the long term (Barlow et al., 1984; Hand et al., 1974; Jannoun et al., 1980; Mathews et al., 1977; Munby & Johnston, 1980). Although there is evidence from well-controlled studies that directly targeting marital-related issues may augment the effects of exposure-based treatments (e.g., Arnow et al., 1985), the superior results of spouse-assisted treatments could be largely attributable to the factors described earlier, namely, the facilitation of frequent *in vivo* exposure in the natural environment both during and after the active treatment phase. Indeed, Sinnott, Jones, Scott-Fordham, and Woodward (1981) reported that PDAs taken from the same neighborhood and treated in a group evidenced superior functioning on many outcome measures than did a group comprising PDAs from diverse geographical areas who presumably did not meet, socialize, or generally support each other during and after treatment.

Thus, spouse-assisted treatments may be associated with more favorable long-term outcome since they contain an ingredient facilitating posttreatment practice of fear-reducing exercises, a factor that has been widely linked to the decreased likelihood of return of fear (cf. Rachman, 1989). This position is bolstered further by the superior follow-up results of Jansson et al. (1986), who incorporated a formal self-exposure element in the posttreatment phase. In light of these findings, it is somewhat surprising that this form of maintenance program has not yet been examined in a controlled fashion.

Moreover, with the emergence of self-help treatment manuals detailing the latest advances in panic and PDA management (e.g., Barlow & Craske, 1989), a useful future endeavor would be to evaluate the extent to which the provision of such manuals to clients during and/or following treatment facilitates treatment gain maintenance and/or continued improvement. The success of minimal-therapist-contact procedures in the treatment of PD (Côté et al., 1990) and PDA (Ghosh & Marks, 1987; Jannoun et al., 1980; Mathews et al., 1977; McNamee, O'Sullivan, Lelliott, & Marks, 1989) highlights the potential utility of this approach to augmenting posttreatment functioning across the long term. In addition, further evaluation of the processes by which gains are maintained would complement this endeavor. For example, does extent of posttreatment practice relate to degree of maintenance and improvement?

Another variable that has been associated with long-term functioning following PDA treatment is the extent and severity of life stressors during the follow-up period. For example, Burns, Thorpe, and Cavallaro (1986), in their 8-year follow-up study of 18 of 32 PDA patients originally treated with exposure, found that most of their sample experienced brief setbacks at some point during the follow-up period. In many instances, these temporary setbacks were precipitated by the emergence of a life stressor such as interpersonal loss. The authors noted that their findings were limited by the fact that there were differences between follow-up completers and noncompleters on measures of treatment response, an issue requiring attention, yet infrequently acknowledged, in follow-up studies. Given the role of stressful life events in the emergence of initial panics and exacerbation of existing symptomatology (Last, Barlow, & O'Brien, 1984; Pollard, Pollard, & Corn, 1989; Rapee, Litwin, & Barlow, 1990), this is certainly an area worthy of further study. Additionally, methods for relapse prevention (RP) in response to stressful life events following treatment would be another useful research endeavor (cf. Marlatt & Gordon, 1985).

Exposure-based treatments of PDA, which specifically address agoraphobic avoidance, nonetheless have been associated with a reduction of panic in many cases as well. However, exposure-based treatments do not universally result in the cessation of panic; conversely, treatments designed specifically for panic management may not always lead to reductions in agoraphobic avoidance, even in milder forms (Craske et al., 1991). Moreover, panic frequency and extent of avoidance are weakly correlated at best (Craske, Rapee, & Barlow, 1988). These observations, in tandem with the consistent finding that PDA and PD patients receiving meaningful benefit from treatment may continue to display residual symptomatology, suggest that future research should be directed at evaluating treatment packages containing both exposure and the newly developed panic-control treatments. There is always the risk that a multi-component treatment package will produce a dilution effect where the delivery of its components is more efficacious in isolation than in their combination due to compromises in their treatment integrity (cf. Craske et al., 1991; Margraf, 1989). Nevertheless, initial findings from combination treatment trials have produced encouraging results in the treatment of PDA (e.g., Michelson et al., 1989).

Although several studies indicate that successful treatment of PD and PDA via cognitive–behavioral procedures leads to a reduction or cessation of medication intake in patients taking medications pretreatment (e.g., Côté et al., 1990; Newman et al., 1990), medication withdrawal is rarely targeted in psychosocial treatment outcome studies. Indeed, a stipulation often implemented in these studies is for subjects to maintain their pretreatment levels of medication throughout the active treatment phase (and sometimes through follow-up) so that any changes observed in subjects can be attributed to the treatment's being evaluated rather than to the adjustments in medication intake. Given that medication discontinuation is frequently associated with relapse and rebound panic, another important avenue for future research is developing methods of facilitating successful withdrawal from medications, particularly the benzodiazepines. In this arena, utilization of panic-control techniques (e.g., Barlow et al., 1989) may be a particularly efficacious adjunct to a medication discontinuation schedule as a means of alleviating anxiety associated with withdrawal symptomatology.

Another underresearched variable that has the potential to contribute significantly to long-term posttreatment functioning in PD and PDA patients is the presence and/or type of comorbid diagnoses. One of the reasons for the lack of research on the rates and impact of comorbidity is the existence of hierarchical exclusionary rules present in diagnostic classification systems prior to DSM-III-R (American Psychiatric Association, 1987). Nevertheless, recent studies indicate that the majority of patients with PD and PDA carry at least one additional diagnosis as well (de Ruiter, Rijken, Garssen, van Schaik, & Kraaimaat, 1989; Sanderson, Di Nardo, Rapee, & Barlow, 1990). These high rates of comorbidity may have substantial implications in terms of short- and long-term responsiveness to treatment. Although the data are quite sparse in this area to date, one comorbid pattern that has been examined is that of PD and PDA with or without an accompanying mood disorder. These findings suggest that PD patients with comorbid major depression display greater psychopathology (Coryell et al., 1988; Lesser et al., 1988), are less likely to respond to "conventional antidepressants" (Grunhaus, 1988) and placebo therapy (Coryell & Noyes, 1988), and are less likely to recover over a 2-year period (Coryell et al., 1988) than are PD patients without major depression. Although a few studies suggest that levels of self-reported depression (e.g., Beck Depression Inventory scores) are associated with a poorer response to cognitive–behavioral treatments of PD and PDA (Jansson & Öst, 1982), the impact of comorbid diagnoses on response to psychosocial treatments of PD and PDA awaits further investigation.

CONCLUSION

The development and evaluation of maintenance and RP strategies in the long-term treatment of PD and PDA are important for two reasons. First, it is only recently that we have had successful treatments for psychological disorders, making the issue of maintaining and enhancing these therapeutic gains an important one. Second, anxiety disorders, including PD and PDA, are chronic conditions that may manifest periodic exacerbations and remissions (Barlow, 1988). Therefore, any therapeutic benefit immediately following treatment is potentially short-lived and must be followed over a longer period. Only then may we be confident that the treatment is more effective than a palliative that may create as many problems as it solves.

   This chapter addresses only a few of the substantive and methodological issues surrounding the study of long-term treatment effectiveness. As we discover new, more effective and more powerful treatments, these issues will be increasingly more salient.

REFERENCES

Agras, W. S., Telch, M. J., Taylor, C. B., Roth, W. T., & Brouillard, M. E. (1990). *Imipramine and exposure therapy in agoraphobia: The type of exposure may matter*. Manuscript submitted for publication.

American Psychiatric Association. (1987). *Diagnostic and statistical manual of mental disorders* (3rd ed., rev.). Washington, DC: Author.

Arnow, B. A., Taylor, C. B., Agras, W. S., & Telch, M. J. (1985). Enhancing agoraphobia treatment outcome by changing couple communication patterns. *Behavior Therapy, 16,* 452–467.

Arrindell, W. A., Emmelkamp, P. M. G., & Sanderman, R. (1986). Marital quality and general life adjustment in relation to treatment outcome in agoraphobia. *Advances in Behaviour Research and Therapy, 8,* 139–185.

Barlow, D. H. (1988). *Anxiety and its disorders: The nature and treatment of anxiety and panic*. New York: Guilford Press.

Barlow, D. H., & Craske, M. G. (1989). *Mastery of your anxiety and panic*. Albany, NY: Graywind Publications.

Barlow, D. H., Craske, M. G., Cerny, J. A., & Klosko, J. S. (1989). Behavioral treatment of panic disorder. *Behavior Therapy, 20,* 261–282.

Barlow, D. H., O'Brien, G. T., & Last, C. G. (1984). Couples treatment of agoraphobia. *Behavior Therapy, 15,* 41–58.

Barlow, D. H., Rapee, R. M., & Brown, T. A. (in press). Behavioral treatment of generalized anxiety disorder. *Behavior Therapy*.

Brown, T. A., Hertz, R. M., & Barlow, D. H. (1992). New developments in cognitive–behavioral treatment of anxiety disorders. In A. Tasman (Ed.), *American Psychiatric Press review of psychiatry* (Vol. 11, 285–306). Washington, DC: American Psychiatric Press.

Burns, L. E., Thorpe, G. L., & Cavallaro, L. A. (1986). Agoraphobia eight years after behavioral treatment: A follow-up study with interview, self-report, and behavioral data. *Behavior Therapy, 17,* 580–591.

Butler, G., Fennell, M., Robson, P., & Gelder, M. (1991). Comparison of behavior therapy and cognitive–behavior therapy in the treatment of generalized anxiety disorder. *Journal of Consulting and Clinical Psychology, 59,* 167–175.

Cerny, J. A., Barlow, D. H., Craske, M. G., & Himadi, W. G. (1987). Couples treatment of agoraphobia: A two-year follow-up. *Behavior Therapy, 18,* 401–415.

Chambless, D. L., & Gracely, E. J. (1988). Prediction of outcome following *in vivo* exposure treatment of agoraphobia. In I. Hand & H. U. Wittchen (Eds.), *Panic and phobias: Treatments and variables affecting course and outcome* (pp. 209–220). Berlin: Springer-Verlag.

Clark, D. M., Gelder, M. G., Salkovskis, P. M., Hackmann, A., Middleton, H., & Anastasiades, P. (1990, May). *Cognitive therapy for panic: Comparative efficacy*. Paper presented at the meeting of the American Psychiatric Association, New York, NY.

Clark, D. M., Salkovskis, P. M., & Chalkley, A. J. (1985). Respiratory control as a treatment for panic attacks. *Journal of Behavior Therapy and Experimental Psychiatry, 16,* 23–30.

Clum, G. A. (1989). Psychological interventions vs. drugs in the treatment of panic. *Behavior Therapy, 20,* 429–457.

Coryell, W., Endicott, J., Andreasen, N. C., Keller, M. B., Clayton, P. J., Hirschfeld, R. M. A., Scheftner, W. A., & Winokur, G. (1988). Depression and panic attacks: The significance of overlap as reflected in follow-up and family study data. *American Journal of Psychiatry, 145,* 293–300.

Coryell, W., & Noyes, R. (1988). Placebo response in panic disorder. *American Journal of Psychiatry, 145,* 1138–1140.

Côté, G., Gauthier, J. G., Laberge, B., Fillion, L., Cormier, H., & Plamondon, J. (1990, November). *Clinic-based vs. home-based treatment with minimal therapist contact for panic disorder.* Paper presented at the meeting of the Association for Advancement of Behavior Therapy, San Francisco, CA.

Craske, M. G., Brown, T. A., & Barlow, D. H. (1991). Behavioral treatment of panic: A two-year follow-up. *Behavior Therapy, 22,* 289–304.

Craske, M. G., Rapee, R. M., & Barlow, D. H. (1988). The significance of panic expectancy for individual patterns of avoidance. *Behavior Therapy, 19,* 577–592.

de Ruiter, C., Rijken, H., Garssen, B., van Schaik, A., & Kraaimaat, F. (1989). Comorbidity among the anxiety disorders. *Journal of Anxiety Disorders, 3,* 57–68.

Fischer, M., Hand, I., Angenendt, H., Buttner-Westphal, H., & Manecke, C. (1988). Failures in exposure treatment of agoraphobia: Evaluation and prediction. In I. Hand & H. U. Wittchen (Eds.), *Panic and phobias: Treatments and variables affecting course and outcome* (pp. 195–208). Berlin: Springer-Verlag.

Foa, E. B., & Emmelkamp, P. M. G. (1983). *Failures in behavior therapy.* New York: Wiley.

Fyer, A. J. (1988). Effects of discontinuation of antipanic medication. In I. Hand & H. U. Wittchen (Eds.), *Panic and phobias: Treatments and variables affecting course and outcome* (pp. 47–53). Berlin: Springer-Verlag.

Fyer, A., Liebowitz, M., Gorman, J., Campeas, R., Levin, A., Davies, S., Goetz, D., & Klein, D. (1987). Discontinuation of alprazolam treatment in panic patients. *American Journal of Psychiatry, 144,* 303–308.

Ghosh, A., & Marks, I. M. (1987). Self-directed exposure for agoraphobia: A controlled trial. *Behavior Therapy, 18,* 3–16.

Grunhaus, L. (1988). Clinical and psychobiological characteristics of simultaneous panic disorder and major depression. *American Journal of Psychiatry, 145,* 1214–1221.

Hand, I., Lamontagne, Y., & Marks, I. M. (1974). Group exposure (flooding) *in vivo* for agoraphobics. *British Journal of Psychiatry, 124,* 588–602.

Himadi, W. G., Cerny, J. A., Barlow, D. H., Cohen, S., & O'Brien, G. T. (1986). The relationship of marital adjustment to agoraphobia treatment outcome. *Behaviour Research and Therapy, 24,* 107–115.

Jannoun, L., Munby, M., Catalan, J., & Gelder, M. (1980). A home-based treatment programme for agoraphobia: Replication and controlled evaluation. *Behavior Therapy, 11,* 294–305.

Jansson, L., Jerremalm, A., & Öst, L. G. (1986). Follow-up of agoraphobic patients treated with exposure *in vivo* or applied relaxation. *British Journal of Psychiatry, 149,* 486–490.

Jansson, L., & Öst, L. G. (1982). Behavioral treatments for agoraphobia: An evaluative review. *Clinical Psychology Review, 2,* 311–337.

Kleiner, L., & Marshall, W. L. (1985). Relationship difficulties and agoraphobia. *Clinical Psychology Review, 5,* 581–595.

Last, C. G., Barlow, D. H., & O'Brien, G. T. (1984). Precipitants of agoraphobia: Role of stressful life events. *Psychological Reports, 54,* 567–570.

Lelliott, P. T., Marks, I. M., Monteiro, W. O., Tsakiris, F., & Noshirvani, H. (1987). Agoraphobics five years after imipramine and exposure. *Journal of Nervous and Mental Disease, 175,* 599–

Lesser, I. M., Rubin, R. T., Pecknold, J. C., Rifkin, A., Swinson, R. P., Lydiard, R. B., Burrows, G. D., Noyes, R., & DuPont, R. L. (1988). Secondary depression in panic disorder. *Archives of General Psychiatry, 45,* 437–443.

Margraf, J. (1989, June). *Comparative efficacy of cognitive, exposure, and combined treatments for panic disorder.* Paper presented at the World Congress of Cognitive Therapy, Oxford, England.

Marlatt, G. A., & Gordon, J. R. (Eds.). (1985). *Relapse prevention: Maintenance strategies in the treatment of addictive behaviors.* New York: Guilford Press.

Mathews, A., Teasdale, J., Munby, M., Johnston, D., & Shaw, P. (1977). A home-based treatment program for agoraphobia. *Behavior Therapy, 8,* 915–924.

Mavissakalian, M., & Michelson, L. (1986). Two-year follow-up of exposure and imipramine treatment of agoraphobia. *American Journal of Psychiatry, 143,* 1106–1112.

McNamee, G., O'Sullivan, G., Lellott, P., & Marks, I. (1989). Telephone-guided treatment for housebound agoraphobics with panic disorder: Exposure vs. relaxation. *Behavior Therapy, 20,* 490–497.

Mellman, T. A., & Uhde, T. W. (1986). Withdrawal syndrome with gradual tapering of alprazolam. *American Journal of Psychiatry, 143,* 1464–1466.

Michelson, L. K., & Marchione, K. (1991). Behavioral, cognitive, and pharmacological treatments of panic disorder with agoraphobia: Critique and synthesis. *Journal of Consulting and Clinical Psychology, 59,* 100–114.

Michelson, L. K., Marchione, K., & Greenwald, M. (1989, November). Cognitive–behavioral treatments of panic disorder with agoraphobia: A comparative outcome investigation. In L. Michelson (Chair), *Emerging issues in assessment and treatment of anxiety disorders.* Symposium conducted at the meeting of the Association for Advancement of Behavior Therapy, Washington, DC.

Milton, F., & Hafner, J. (1979). The outcome of behavior therapy for agoraphobia in relation to marital adjustment. *Archives of General Psychiatry, 36,* 807–811.

Monteiro, W., Marks, I. M., & Ramm, E. (1985). Marital adjustment and treatment outcome in agoraphobia. *British Journal of Psychiatry, 146,* 383–390.

Munby, J., & Johnston, D. W. (1980). Agoraphobia: The long-term follow-up of behavioural treatment. *British Journal of Psychiatry, 137,* 418–427.

Newman, C. F., Beck, J. S., Beck, A. T., & Tran, G. Q. (1990, November). *Efficacy of cognitive therapy in reducing panic attacks and medication.* Paper presented at the meeting of the Association for Advancement of Behavior Therapy, San Francisco, CA.

Öst, L. G. (1988). Applied relaxation in the treatment of panic disorder. *Behaviour Research and Therapy, 26,* 13–22.

Pecknold, J. C., Swinson, R. P., Kuch, K., & Lewis, C. P. (1988). Alprazolam in panic disorder and agoraphobia: Results from a multicenter trial: III. Discontinuation effects. *Archives of General Psychiatry, 45,* 429–436.

Pollard, C. A., Pollard, H. J., & Corn, K. J. (1989). Panic onset and major life events in the lives of agoraphobics: A test of contiguity. *Journal of Abnormal Psychology, 98,* 318–321.

Rachman, S. (1989). The return of fear: Review and prospect. *Clinical Psychology Review, 9,* 147–168.

Rapee, R. M., Litwin, E. M., & Barlow, D. H. (1990). Life events in panic disorder: A comparison study. *American Journal of Psychiatry, 147,* 640–644.

Salkovskis, P. M., Jones, D. R. O., & Clark, D. M. (1986). Respiratory control in the treatment of panic attacks: Replication and extension with concurrent measurement of behaviour and pCO_2. *British Journal of Psychiatry, 148,* 526–532.

Sanderson, W. C., Di Nardo, P. A., Rapee, R. M., & Barlow, D. H. (1990). Syndrome comorbidity in patients diagnosed with a DSM-III-R anxiety disorder. *Journal of Abnormal Psychology, 99,* 308–312.

Schweizer, E., & Rickels, K. (1991). Pharmacotherapy of generalized anxiety disorder. In R. M. Rapee & D. H. Barlow (Eds.), *Chronic anxiety, generalized anxiety disorder, and mixed anxiety depression* (pp. 172–186). New York: Guilford Press.

Sheehan, D. (1986, April). *One-year follow-up of patients with panic disorder and withdrawal from long-term anti-panic medications.* Paper presented at the UpJohn Panic Disorder Biological Research Workshop, Washington, DC.

Sinnott, A., Jones, R. B., Scott-Fordham, A., & Woodward, R. (1981). Augmentation of *in vivo* exposure treatment of agoraphobia by the formation of neighborhood self-help groups. *Behaviour Research and Therapy, 19,* 339–347.

Sokol, L., Beck, A. T., & Clark, D. A. (1989, June). *A controlled treatment trial of cognitive therapy for panic disorder.* Paper presented at the World Congress of Cognitive Therapy, Oxford, England.

Telch, M. J., Agras, W. S., Taylor, C. B., Roth, W. T., & Gallen, C. C. (1985). Combined pharmacological and behavioral treatment for agoraphobia. *Behaviour Research and Therapy, 23,* 325–335.

Telch, M. J., Tearnan, B. H., & Taylor, C. B. (1983). Antidepressant medication in the treatment of agoraphobia: A critical review. *Behaviour Research and Therapy, 21,* 505–517.

Zitrin, C. M., Klein, D. F., Woerner, M. G., & Ross, D. C. (1983). Treatment of phobias: I. Comparison of imipramine and placebo. *Archives of General Psychiatry, 40,* 125–138.

CHAPTER 9

OBSESSIVE–COMPULSIVE DISORDERS

Paul M. G. Emmelkamp
Jan Kloek
Eric Blaauw
UNIVERSITY OF GRONINGEN

O bsessive–compulsive disorder (OCD) is among the most difficult problems to treat and it is especially in this area that behavioral research has made significant advances. Exposure *in vivo* and response prevention are effective with a substantial number of obsessive–compulsive patients (see, e.g., Emmelkamp, 1982, 1991; Marks, 1987; Steketee & Cleere, 1990). This treatment exposes patients to stimuli that trigger obsessions and urges to ritualize but prevents them from performing the rituals.

The value of prolonged exposure *in vivo* and response prevention was suggested by uncontrolled studies by Meyer and his colleagues (Meyer, 1966; Meyer, Levy, & Schnurer, 1974). The essence of their treatment approach, which at the time was called "apotrepic therapy," is response prevention, modeling, and exposure *in vivo*. The treatment involves several stages. After a behavioral analysis, nurses were instructed to prevent the patient from carrying out his/her rituals. Exposure *in vivo* was introduced as soon as the total elimination of rituals under supervision was achieved. The therapist increased the stress by confronting the patient with situations that normally triggered obsessive rituals. During this stage of treatment, modeling was employed. With modeling, the therapist first demonstrated what the patient had to do afterward. For example, the therapist touched contaminated objects such as underwear and encouraged the patient to imitate this behavior. When patients could tolerate the most difficult situations, supervision was gradually diminished.

Meyer et al. (1974) reported the results of his program with 15 patients. Most patients showed a marked reduction of compulsive behavior. Since then, a number of controlled studies have investigated the' components of this therapeutic package, the results of which are briefly summarized.

There is no need to elicit high anxiety during treatment since gradual exposure *in vivo* is equally as effective as flooding *in vivo* (Boersma, Den Hengst, Dekker, & Emmelkamp, 1976; Marks, Hodgson, & Rachman, 1975). Since gradual exposure evokes less tension and is easier for the patient to carry out by himself/herself, it is preferred to flooding. Further, modeling does not seem to enhance treatment effectiveness (Boersma et al., 1976; Rachman, Marks, & Hodgson, 1973).

Although treatment by exposure and response prevention was originally applied when the patient was hospitalized, treatment can also be administered by the patient in his/her natural environment. Such home-based treatment is not only cost effective (van de Hout, Emmelkamp, Kraaykamp, & Griez, 1988), but may also result in superior maintenance of treatment-produced change (Emmelkamp & Kraanen, 1977; Emmelkamp, van Linden van den Heuvell, Rüphan, & Sanderman, 1989).

Both exposure to distressing stimuli and response prevention of the ritual are essential components. To date, only one controlled between-group study of this issue has been reported (Foa, Steketee, & Milby, 1980). Eight obsessive–compulsive patients served as subjects. Patients were randomly assigned to two treatment conditions: (1) exposure alone followed by exposure and response prevention and (2) response prevention alone followed by the combined treatment. Exposure led to more anxiety reduction but less improvement of rituals. The reverse was found for response prevention. When the combined treatment was applied at the second period, the differences between the groups on anxiety and ritualistic behavior disappeared.

DEFINITION OF "RELAPSE"

It is important to make a distinction between relapse and failure. Failure in the treatment of OCD can be defined as a lack of noticeable change after adequate treatment. Relapse can be defined as a noticeable change in the negative direction (worsening) after an initially more or less successful treatment. However, this definition is not without problems in the case of OCD, relating to the goals of treatment. Many obsessive–

compulsive patients have more than one obsessive–compulsive problem. To complicate matters further, they often have additional problems as well. For example, an obsessive–compulsive patient may suffer not only from an extensive washing ritual, but also from checking rituals and harming obsessions around killing his/her baby. In addition, the patient may be quite depressed and have marital problems. How many of these problems should be solved before we can speak of successful treatment? In the same vein, relapse is not absolute. The patient described above may have received adequate treatment for his/her rituals, harming obsessions, depressed mood, and marital problems, leading to improved functioning in all these areas. If he/she starts ritualizing again after some time, we call this a relapse, but what do we call it if he/she does not relapse with respect to ritualizing but becomes severely depressed and maritally distressed? Another problem relates to how little change in the negative direction qualifies a patient as having had a relapse. Thus, as is the case with failures during treatment, relapse is relative. Improvements can be maintained in one or more areas, whereas the patient may relapse in other areas. Further, such a relapse may range from a slight worsening to a 100% relapse.

Given this definitional problem, it is not surprising that there are no figures of relapse rate reported in the literature. While a substantial number of follow-up studies have been conducted (O'Sullivan & Marks, 1990), they do not usually provide information with respect to the number of patients who relapsed. The general picture is that 70%–80% of obsessive–compulsive patients who completed trials of exposure therapy remained improved up to 6 years. Follow-up studies after cognitive therapy are lacking. In the case of antidepressants, relapse is the rule rather than the exception when medication is discontinued.

THE RELAPSE MODEL

The list of potential factors associated with relapse in OCD patients is rather long, including environmental factors, interpersonal factors, personality characteristics, coping resources, social support, and mood disturbances. A cognitive–behavioral model of the relapse process in obsessive–compulsive patients is presented in Figure 9.1. It assumes that individuals freely make a choice whether to give in to the urge to ritualize. Although patients may have become symptom free, sooner or later they will be confronted with stressful situations that pose a threat to their sense of control. Such stressful situations may involve major stressors like the loss of job, divorce, or death, but they also consist of an

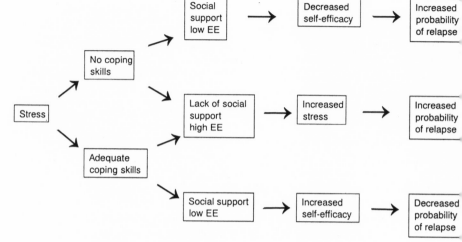

FIGURE 9.1. Relapse model in obsessive–compulsive disorder.

accumulation of daily hassles with which a patient is unable to cope. The model assumes an important role for a number of mediating factors: coping style of the patient, social support, and expressed emotion of significant others. A number of other variables are presumably also relevant, including personality characteristics, overvalued ideation, and mood disturbances, but these have not been included in the model.

In the model, the more stress an individual experiences, the less coping skills he/she has, the more he/she lacks an adequate social support system, the more he/she is exposed to high levels of expressed emotion, the more likely he/she will relapse.

Initial giving in to urges may lead to a process that is comparable to the abstinence violation effect in substance abusers (Marlatt & Gordon, 1980). As noted by Marlatt and Gordon (1985): "The category of addictive behaviors may be expanded to include any compulsive habit pattern in which the individual seeks a state of immediate gratification" (p. 4). Substance abuse and obsessive–compulsive behavior can both be seen as a problem in impulse control, in which the individual feels that he/she has no control over his/her behavior. The cause of relapse in OCD is often attributed to personal weakness or a chronic disease, which may actually offer an excuse for further ritualizing. If obsessive–compulsive patients see their ritualizing as the result of a disease, they may be more likely to engage in ritualizing rather than trying to get some control over their urges.

Life Events and Daily Hassles

The influence of life events on psychopathology, especially depression, is now well established (Brown & Harris, 1978; Dohrenwend & Dohrenwend, 1981; Dohrenwend, Shrout, Link, Skodol, & Martin, 1986; Finlay-Jones & Brown, 1981; Shrout et al., 1989). The fact that most individuals do not develop psychopathology when confronted with stressful events has led to the diathesis stress model, which holds that life events will only affect people who already have a preexisting vulnerability, either biologically or psychosocially determined. More recently, attention has been given to the role of chronic stress and daily hassles in the development of psychopathology. Given the fact that both life events and daily hassles have been found to be related to the onset of psychopathology, it seems quite plausible that these factors are also related to relapse.

Coping Style

Coping styles of patients with anxiety disorders have hardly been investigated. In other areas, particularly the field of health psychology, coping strategies are the center of attention for researchers. For example, a number of studies have shown that coping strategies may be related to the course of malignant cancer (e.g., Temoshok et al., 1985). It is predicted here that inadequate coping strategies are related to relapse in obsessive–compulsive patients. The fact that individuals react differently to stressful events may be accounted for by individual differences in registration and interpretation as well as in coping styles. It is our clinical impression that the coping of obsessive–compulsive patients is often characterizied by (1) denial, (2) avoidance of problems, and (3) tension reduction.

Whereas with normal persons *denial* is usually only temporary, with obsessive–compulsive patients the emotional processing may stagnate at this stage. A common characteristic of the defense mechanism of obsessive–compulsive patients is that a significant stressful event is not forgotten but deprived of its affect. This fits with psychoanalytical notions holding that the most important defense mechanisms in obsessional neurosis are undoing, displacement, reaction formation, and isolation of content and affect (Nagera, 1976). Another prevalent coping strategy of obsessive–compulsives is *avoidance of problems* rather than confronting them and solving them. Finally, most obsessive–compulsives hold that tension is intolerable and that something should be done about it. This coping style has been labeled "*tension reduction.*"

Social Support and Expressed Emotion

The role of an adequate social support system has also to be stressed. Social support may be defined as the expression of positive affect, giving the person the impression that he/she is loved, cared for, and valued; offering practical assistance (e.g., advice or information); and providing material assistance. There are now a number of studies that show that social support is related to mental health. Brown and Harris (1978) and Henderson, Byrne, and Duncan-Jones (1981) found that social support has a stress-buffering role. Krantz and Moos (1988) and Goering, Masylenki, Lancee, and Freeman (1983) found that lack of social support was associated with poor treatment outcome and relapse, but this has not yet been investigated with obsessive–compulsive patients.

While social support has been found to be associated with adjustment, negative support (conflictual relationships) may be negatively associated with adjustment. Studies of expressed emotion are therefore also important. Leff and Vaughn (1985) found that the level of hostile criticism from the spouse strongly predicted patient relapse in depressed patients. Similarly, Hooley, Orley, and Teasdale (1986) found that criticism of the spouse predicted relapse in depressed patients. It should be noted that social support is not an absolute phenomenon. The obsessive–compulsive behavior may have also its negative effects on the patient's social network, causing support and tolerance for the obsessive–compulsive behavior progressively to decrease.

OTHER FACTORS RELATED TO RELAPSE

Overvalued Ideation

Foa (1979) proposed that patients who strongly believe that their fears are realistic and that their rituals prevent the occurrence of actual disasters fail to benefit from treatment. Consequently, Rachman (1983) supposed that overvalued ideation may also be related to relapse after treatment: "As things stand at present . . . we can do little further than going beyond the somewhat pessimistic prediction that the presence of a significant overvalued idea associated with, or part of, an obsessional disorder is predictive of long-term failure, even if temporary improvements can be achieved" (p. 46). While such beliefs may make a person particularly vulnerable to relapse and thus may be causally related to relapse, it may also be the case that these irrational beliefs are one of the manifestations of relapse; that is, that the irrational beliefs are merely epiphenomena or "symptoms" of the OCD. Alternatively, overvalued ideation may be particularly prevalent among obsessive–compulsive patients with schizotypal features.

Personality Disorders

The part played by personality disorders also deserves some attention. Many obsessive–compulsive patients not only suffer from OCD but also qualify for one or more personality disorders. Early researchers of obsessive–compulsive neurosis often failed to distinguish OCD from obsessive personality traits. According to Black (1974), 71% of patients with OCD are characterized by compulsive personality traits. The frequency of personality disorders among obsessive–compulsives is high. In a number of studies (Joffe, Swinson, & Regan, 1988; Rasmussen & Tsuang, 1986; Jenike, Baer, Minichiello, Schwartz, & Garey, 1986; Mavissakalian, Hamann, & Jones, 1990a, 1990b; Steketee, 1990), a wide range of personality disorders were found, most patients having mixed personality disorder with avoidant, dependent, histrionic, and passive–aggressive features. In one study (Jenike et al., 1986), one third of the patients also had a schizotypal personality disorder, but this was lower in the other studies (see also Stanley, Turner, & Borden, 1990). Steketee (1990) found no relationship between schizotypal, dependent, histrionic, and avoidant personality disorder and treatment outcome. Moreover, these personality disorders were also not found to be related to relapse. Only passive–aggressive traits distinguished relapsers from maintainers. Other studies, however, found that schizotypal (Jenike et al., 1986; Minichiello, Baer, & Jenike, 1987), histrionic (Rasmussen & Tsuang, 1986), and borderline (Hermesh, Shahar, & Munitz, 1987; Rasmussen & Tsuang, 1986) personality disorders were associated with poorer treatment outcome of behavioral and drug treatment.

Depression

Mood disturbance is another factor that may make a former obsessive–compulsive patient vulnerable to relapse. There is a clear relationship between depression and OCD. Many obsessive–compulsive patients have suffered from a major depressive episode or are concurrently suffering from a major depression (Foa, Steketee, Kozak, & Dugger, 1986; Rachman & Hodgson, 1980; Rasmussen & Tsuang, 1986; Yaryura Tobias & Neziroglu, 1983). It is now well established that over half of the individuals who experience major depression will experience another depressive episode within 2 years (Keller, 1985). The relationship between depression and OCD makes it clear that depressed obsessive–

compulsive patients are presumably more susceptible to relapse than persons who have never had an episode of major depression.

According to Horowitz (1986), intrusive thoughts are common reactions to stressful events. While this is a transient period in the emotional processing of a stressful event for normal persons, a number of obsessive–compulsives do not habituate to these intrusive thoughts, presumably because of their high arousal level (Rachman, 1983), thus making relapse more likely. Disturbance of mood may aggravate the problem. First, it may prevent habituation of intrusive thoughts. Second, when a patient is depressed he/she will less likely be in a position to fight against the urges to ritualize.

STUDY INTO FACTORS ASSOCIATED WITH RELAPSE

Patients from a study in which the effects of a standardized exposure program were compared with individualized treatment were asked to participate in a follow-up study approximately 2 years after treatment (range 9 months to 37 months). They completed self-ratings and were interviewed by a clinical psychologist (J.K.). Of the original 22 patients, all but one participated in the follow-up study.

Measures

At follow-up, patients completed, among others, the following measures that had also been completed before and at the end of the treatment:

Anxiety/Discomfort Scale. The patient rated five obsessive–compulsive targets on 0–8 scales for anxiety/discomfort.
Self-rating Depression Scale (SDS) (Zung, 1965).

At follow-up the following measures were added:

Social Support Inventory (SSI) (van Sonderen, 1991). This questionnaire lists 49 items reflecting emotional or practical aspects of social support and results in two scores: (1) how frequently the patient received social support and (2) how satisfied he/she was with the received social support. In this study, only the frequency data are used.
Level of Expressed Emotion (LEE) (Gerlsma, van der Lubbe, & van Nieuwenhuizen, 1991). This is a 33-question self-report questionnaire that measures the perceived label of expressed emotion of the significant other (usually the partner).

Daily Hassles (Appelo, 1988). This is an inventory that lists 40 items reflecting daily hassles occurring in the last 2 weeks. We assume daily hassles experienced in this period are representative of the daily hassles an individual would regularly experience.

In addition, patients were interviewed at follow-up with respect to significant *life events* that occurred in the last 2 years. A structured interview was held concerning the occurrence of 36 life events during the last 2 years. Patients indicated (1) whether a life event had occurred and (2) the interference of the event on a 1-to-5 scale. The assessor tried to establish the exact date/period that the life event occurred. In addition, the patient indicated on a time scale (ranging from end of treatment to follow-up) the severity of the obsessive–compulsive complaints.

At the pretest, patients filled out the *Utrechtse Coping List* (UCL) (Schreurs, van de Willige, Tellegen, & Brosschot, 1988). The following three subscales are particularly relevant for obsessive–compulsives and were used in the present study: (1) denial, (2) avoidance of problems, and (3) tension reduction.

Results

To study the relationship between coping style and outcome at follow-up Pearsonian correlational analyses were conducted. Coping did not predict success of treatment at follow-up: distress reduction ($r = .03$); avoidance of problems ($r = .17$); and denial ($r = .03$). None of these coefficients were statistically significant. However, a substantial relationship was found between coping strategies and relapse at follow-up: distress reduction ($r = .44$); avoidance of problems ($r = .55$); (denial, $r = .44$), all of which were statistically significant ($p < .02$). Further, the following psychosocial variables also significantly predicted relapse at follow-up: life events ($r = 36; p < .05$); daily hassles ($r = .49, p < .01$); and expressed emotion ($r = .44, p < .02$). Frequency of received social support did not significantly predict relapse ($r = .24$).

In addition to regression analyses, we also present individual data for relapse cases. If we define relapse as a significant deterioration at follow-up of more than 20% relative to status at the posttest, the number of relapsed patients are as follows: On the anxiety/discomfort scale, $n = 6$; and on depressed mood (SDS), $n = 5$. Remarkably, only two of the relapsed cases on the target rituals were also relapsed with respect to depressed mood, which means that for three other patients deterioration of mood did not lead to a relapse with respect to the rituals.

For each of the patients who relapsed with respect to his/her OCD, the following data are listed: target rituals (anxiety/discomfort); depressed mood (SDS); daily hassles (higher scores indicating more stress); social support (higher scores indicating more support); expressed emotion (higher scores indicating more negative expressed emotion); and life events (higher scores indicating more stress associated with life events).

Relapse Number 1

Anxiety/discomfort	pre = 26; post = 8; follow-up = 14
Depressed mood	pre = 63; post = 45; follow-up = 46
Daily hassles	= 15 (group mean = 20.0, SD = 19.7)
Social support	= 123 (group mean = 89.1, SD = 16.4)
Expressed emotion	= 60 (group mean = 55.8, SD = 16.9)
Life events	= 22 (group mean = 26.2, SD = 14.7)

The patient is a 38-year-old female with contamination fears and washing rituals. She has been treated with exposure *in vivo* and assertiveness training. Results at follow-up show only a partial relapse; the patient has many fewer rituals than at the start of the treatment. The improvement of her depressed mood has been maintained. The patient experiences relatively few daily hassles. Social support is more than adequate. Negative expressed emotions (from her partner) are not remarkably high. Although the patient had experienced a number of life events, these were clearly not related to fluctuations in her obsessive–compulsive problems. In sum, the (partial) relapse in this case cannot be explained in terms of stress, lack of social support, or negative expressed emotions.

Relapse Number 2

Anxiety/discomfort	pre = 29; post = 9; follow-up = 24
Depressed mood	pre = 49; post = 32; follow-up = 54
Daily hassles	= 11
Social support	= 78
Expressed emotion	= 77
Life events	= 0

The patient is a 30-year-old male with checking rituals. He has been treated with cognitive therapy and exposure *in vivo*. Results at follow-up show a clear relapse; the patient has as many rituals as at the start of the treatment. There is also a significant relapse in depressed mood. The patient experiences relatively few daily hassles. Social support is less than adequate. The level of negative expressed emotions (from his mother) is high. The patient has not experienced major life events. The increase in obsessive–compulsive problems was not found to be related to external stressors. Presumably, personality features (dependency and overvalued ideas) and stress related to lack of close friends, combined with a over-critical mother, are primarily responsible for the gradual deterioration of both the rituals and the depressed mood.

Relapse Number 3

Anxiety/discomfort	pre = 31; post = 4; follow-up = 30
Depressed mood	pre = 64; post = 50; follow-up = 60
Daily hassles	= 28
Social support	= 77
Expressed emotion	= 82
Life events	= 16

The patient is a 40-year-old female with checking rituals and agoraphobia. She has been treated with exposure *in vivo*. Results at follow-up show a clear relapse both with respect to her obsessive–compulsive problems, agoraphobia, and depressed mood. The patient experiences relatively many daily hassles. Social support is less than adequate. The level of negative expressed emotions (from her partner) is remarkably high. The patient had experienced relatively little stress as a result of major life events and the stress did not seem to be related to the gradual increase in the obsessive–compulsive problems. In sum, the gradual relapse in this case can be explained in terms of continuous daily stress, lack of social support, and high levels of negative expressed emotions by her partner.

Relapse Number 4

Anxiety/discomfort	pre = 29; post = 1; follow-up = 8
Depressed mood	pre = 44; post = 31; follow-up = 40
Daily hassles	= 1
Social support	= 93
Expressed emotion	= 46
Life events	= 20

The patient is a 43-year-old female with cleaning and washing rituals. She has been treated with exposure *in vivo*, cognitive therapy, and assertiveness training. Results at follow-up show only a marginal relapse; the patient has many fewer rituals than at the start of the treatment. She is slightly more depressed than at the end of treatment. The patient experiences no stress as a result of daily hassles. Social support is adequate. The level of negative expressed emotions (from her partner) is low. Although the patient had experienced some major life events, these were inversely related to her obsessive–compulsive problems. In sum, although this patient formally qualifies for relapse status, she actually functions quite well.

Relapse Number 5

Anxiety/discomfort	pre = 40; post = 9; follow-up = 32
Depressed mood	pre = 58; post = 61; follow-up = 73
Daily hassles	= 83
Social support	= 88
Expressed emotion	= 96
Life events	= 45

The patient is a 34-year-old female with checking and washing rituals. She has been treated with exposure *in vivo*. Results at follow-up show a clear relapse, not only with respect to her rituals but also with respect to her depressed mood. At follow-up she is severely depressed, even more depressed than at the start of the treatment. The patient experiences a great deal of stress as a result of daily hassles. Social support is adequate. The level of negative expressed emotions (from her partner) is extremely high. The patient had experienced much stress as a result of major life events. In this case, stress as a result of life events appeared to be related to fluctuations in her obsessive–compulsive problems. In sum, extreme levels of stress and an overcritical partner seem to be responsible for the relapse in this case.

Relapse Number 6

Anxiety/discomfort	pre = 27; post = 15; follow-up = 24
Depressed mood	pre = 54; post = 48; follow-up = 43
Daily hassles	= 14
Social support	= 119
Expressed emotion	= 39
Life events	= 56

The patient is a 28-year-old male with checking rituals. He has been treated with cognitive therapy. Results at follow-up show a clear relapse; the patient has as many rituals as at the start of the treatment. There is no relapse in depressed mood. The patient experiences relatively few daily hassles. Social support is more than adequate. The level of negative expressed emotions (from his partner) is low. The patient has experienced a number of major life events. There is no relationship between experienced stress as a result of major life events and relapse. The increase in obsessive–compulsive problems is not related to external stressors. The patient himself attributed the relapse to the failure of cognitive therapy. Alternatively, personality features of this patient (dependency) may also account for the relapse.

RELAPSE PREVENTION

Presumably the ability to remain free from rituals after treatment is a rare outcome. Thus, it is therapeutically wise to prepare the patient for a possible relapse and to teach him/her how to deal with that relapse. Therefore, it is important to challenge inadequate attributions of responsibility for the development of a potential lapse and its solution.

Arranging the conditions for relapse prevention (RP) is an important task at the end of therapy. One approach is to relabel relapses during treatment as positive opportunities to practice the techniques the patient has acquired. Dependent patients in particular perceive the termination of therapy as threatening and try to find a way to continue by displaying numerous relapses. Emphasizing self-efficacy and gradually minimizing the role of the therapist may prove to be a fruitful strategy in these cases.

There are a number of other strategies the therapist may consider in RP in obsessive–compulsive patients, including providing booster sessions; involving the patient's partner in the treatment; dealing with related problems like social anxiety, unassertiveness, and inadequate expression of emotions; dealing with underlying depression; and challenging irrational cognitions and teaching problem solving.

Booster Sessions

The use of booster sessions has long been advocated as a maintenance strategy in behavioral therapy. With disorders other than OCD, booster maintenance sessions have been found to be moderately successful in maintaining treatment-induced behavioral change (Whisman, 1990). Marks et al. (1975) reported beneficial effects of booster sessions conducted in groups with patients who had been treated individually with exposure *in vivo* and response prevention, but no data were provided. Two other uncontrolled studies (Hand & Tichatzky, 1979; Enright, 1991) in which obsessive–compulsives have been treated in groups have been reported. The groups dealt with obsessive–compulsive problems as well as with additional problems in order to prevent relapse. Since both studies were uncontrolled, no conclusion can be drawn with respect to the value of group treatment. Generally, the results are less than those typically found with exposure *in vivo* and response prevention conducted on an individual basis. Given the low prevalence of relapse in OCD, booster sessions conducted in groups do not seem worthwhile. However, individual booster sessions on a regular basis for patients who are at risk for relapse are recommended.

Involving the Partner of the Patient

Although there is little evidence that spouse-aided therapy is more effective than treatment of the patient alone (Emmelkamp & de Lange, 1983; Emmelkamp, de Haan, & Hoogduin, 1990), this does not preclude the possibility that spousal involvement may prevent relapse. Given the fact that the patient's partner has received a detailed rationale of the exposure principle, it is likely that he/she may assist the patient in difficult periods after the treatment has ended. Apart from cooperation in exposing the patient and preventing him/her from ritualizing during stressful periods, the social support offered by the partner may also be important in dealing with the patient's reactions after a significant stressor or in times of an exaggeration of daily hassles.

In cases of marital distress with partners who are characterized by a high level of expressed negative emotions, it may be worthwhile to include the partner in the therapy. There is now a growing body of evidence suggesting that communications training is helpful for couples in conflict (Emmelkamp, Van der Helm, MacGillavry, & Van Zanten, 1984). In couples treatment, the therapist may teach the patient appropriately assertive behavior and work with the partner to shape more effective responses, such as empathic listening skills.

Social Anxiety and Unassertiveness

A significant proportion of obsessive–compulsive patients are also socially anxious or phobic or have difficulty being assertive (Emmelkamp, 1983). These problems usually do not improve as a result of treatment for OCD and have to be dealt with more directly. When social anxiety is related to a lack of social skills, an appropriate goal of therapy is to assist patients to acquire adequate skills in order to teach them how to deal more adequately with interpersonal stress in the hope of preventing relapse. For example, when obsessive–compulsive patients are unassertive, assertiveness training may be included in the treatment program. The aim of such training is to equip the patient with skills that will facilitate better interpersonal relations and increase resistance to relapse after treatment ends. Social-skills training or assertiveness training may be given either in groups or individually. The format chosen depends on the characteristics of the individual patient and the availability of group therapy. When patients are too anxious to benefit from treatment conducted in groups, or when they have extreme skills deficits, the best option is to start with individual training and switch to a group when the patient is ready. Individual assertiveness or social-skills training may have the advantage of providing a more comprehensive program adapted to the individual needs of the patients.

The need for assertiveness or social-skills training is indicated when the patient's anxiety is at least partly due to a lack of interpersonal skills. When social anxiety is not due to a lack of skills, other approaches may be more appropriate, such as exposure procedures and/or cognitive therapy (Emmelkamp, Mersch, Vissia, & Van der Helm, 1985; Scholing & Emmelkamp, 1990). Cognitive methods are also indicated when nonassertive behavior is a result of irrational beliefs or fear of the consequences of assertive behavior. (For a more detailed discussion of the management of social phobia, see Scholing & Emmelkamp, 1990).

Another important approach in assertiveness training, especially for patients who have a strong interdependent relationship with their parents, is to teach patients to handle conflict and express their feelings in those relationships. Family conflicts may be a significant factor maintaining obsessive–compulsive problems, and increased assertiveness skills may help the patient to deal with these conflicts more adequately.

Little research has been done on the effectiveness of assertiveness training for patients with OCD, although there have been some suggestions in the earlier behavioral literature that obsessive–compulsives could be treated by assertiveness training (Walton & Mather, 1963; Wolpe, 1958). Emmelkamp (1983) reported two case studies in which assertiveness training was found to be effective in reducing obsessive–compulsive problems. Further positive results of assertiveness training were found in a study by Emmelkamp and van der Heyden (1980) with patients with harming obsessions. Assertiveness training led to a more adequate handling of aggression and hence to a reduction of the harming obsessions. It should be noted that in all these studies, only short-term effects were assessed. Although it is likely that assertiveness training will help a number of obsessive–compulsives to cope more effectively with interpersonal stress and so may reduce the probability of relapse, this has not yet been evaluated.

In some cases, patients are unable to differentiate among various emotions. For example, they actually may be very angry but experience their feelings as anxiety rather than anger. When patients have difficulty coping with their anger, emotional expression training may be of help. In this approach, patients are systematically trained to express their feelings more directly. In addition, rational–emotive therapy may be used when patients have the irrational belief that they must never be angry. Some patients are afraid of any sign of conflict or aggression and go to extreme lengths to avoid such exposure. For these cases, systematic exposure to situations involving conflict or aggression may be a worthwhile therapeutic strategy. This can be done either imaginally or *in vivo* by means of role play.

Depression

When depression is associated with OCD, a careful history should be taken to investigate whether the obsessive–compulsive problems are primary or secondary to the depression or unrelated. Most patients are able to discriminate between these emotional states and use different words for their description. Many of our patients are quite capable of delineating the relationship between the two. Often patients with OCD lead a very restricted life, resulting in a depressed mood that can be considered secondary to the anxiety disorder. In these cases the depression often lifts after treatment of the obsessive–compulsive problems, and no further measures dealing with the depressive symptoms are necessary. In some patients the (originally secondary) depression evolves to become the major complaint after the patient has become disabled by the obsessive–compulsive problems. Functional analysis may then indicate starting with treatment of the depression, rather than the OCD, to mobilize the patient.

If the patient is still depressed at the end of treatment, he/she is particularly vulnerable for relapse. In such cases, additional interventions are indicated. In depression, certain cognitive patterns or schemata are activated (Beck, Rush, Shaw, & Emery, 1979) that structure patients' interpretations of themselves, their situation, and the world as a whole. In these cases, cognitive treatment approaches, aiming to identify and change the patient's assumptions, and cognitive schemata that support stereotypical negative thinking may give full relief. (For more details on this challenging approach, see Beck et al., 1979).

Behavioral approaches for depression have been found to be as effective as cognitive therapy (Emmelkamp, 1992). In cognitively less amenable patients, behavioral approaches to depression are the treatment of choice to increase positive reinforcement and reduce depression. Typically, nonobsessional activities that the patient has enjoyed in the past but in which the person does not currently engage are given as homework assignments. Apparently easy activities are chosen first; the most difficult tasks are assigned in later sessions.

Of course, prescribing antidepressant drugs may be considered. While some psychopharmacological agents such as clomipramine and fluvoxamine may be of some help with depressed obsessive–compulsive patients (Emmelkamp, Bouman, & Scholing, 1992), it should be emphasized that giving a patient a medication is in itself a complex act. One potential and often neglected side effect of taking medication is that it may reduce the self-efficacy of the patient. It may increase dependency and allow the patient to take a passive role. When considering medication, it is important to deal with the attributions patients hold. Many obsessive–compulsives who hold that ritualizing is a disease have this idea reinforced by the prescription of a medication.

Cognitive Therapy and Problem Solving

Cognitive coping skills may also be prophylactic in preventing future relapse. Two studies (Emmelkamp et al., 1988; Emmelkamp & Beens, 1991) have been reported that demonstrate the effectiveness of rational–emotive therapy with obsessive–compulsive patients. However, since these studies were not designed to investigate the long-term effects of cognitive therapy with obsessive–compulsive patients, conclusions with respect to RP are precluded.

Another strategy that may help prevent relapse is teaching problem solving. Kleiner, Marshall, and Spevack (1987) developed a problem-solving skills program for patients with panic disorder with agoraphobia. The main goals of this program were to increase the patient's awareness of ongoing interpersonal problems, to develop an awareness of the effects of those problems on the phobia, and to teach basic skills (including assertiveness skills) to deal with those problems. Patients who had received treatment combining *in vivo* exposure with problem solving improved significantly after 12 treatment sessions. Subjects in the *in vivo* exposure-alone condition either failed to show further gains at follow-up or relapsed, whereas the group receiving training in problem solving showed further improvement at the 6-month follow-up. Interestingly, the latter also showed a significant shift in locus of control toward more internal control. It seems worthwhile to study whether problem solving has something to offer to obsessive–compulsive patients.

CONCLUSION

Research in the area of relapse in obsessive–compulsives is in an embryonic state. In this chapter, many factors have been suggested that may be related to relapse (e.g., stress, coping skills, social support, and expressed emotion), and some evidence was provided that these factors indeed are related to relapse in obsessive–compulsive patients. Only frequency of received social support was not found to be related to relapse. We hope that the model presented here will inspire other researchers to test the predictions made. The model will be difficult to test because of the interactive nature of the variables, but it can serve as a useful guide to examining the role of each variable and the interactions between them.

As has been suggested before (Emmelkamp, 1982), a functional analysis of the problem behaviors is an essential condition with difficult patients and might be very important in guiding treatment strategies to prevent relapse. Unfortunately, only one controlled study (Emmelkamp, 1992) with respect to the functional behavioral analysis and treatment of obsessive–compulsive patients has been conducted to date, and the results did not support the idea that idiosyncratic treatment based on such an analysis is superior to exposure *in vivo* and response prevention. A great deal of additional research is needed on how best to deal with obsessive–compulsive patients presenting with multiple problems in order to prevent relapse. But as clinicians we are not in the position to wait until future research provides some of the answers on effective RP. For most obsessive–compulsive patients who also have related or underlying problems, presumably a plan in which various problems are tackled sequentially will be the most fruitful. The therapist should begin with the intervention that is likely to show the most rapid results, to boost the patient's motivation and hope, and in most cases, this will be exposure *in vivo* and response prevention.

REFERENCES

Appelo, M. T. (1988). *De ontwikkeling van de D.O.L.: Dagelijkse ongemakken bij psychiatrische en niet-psychiatrische patiënten*. Unpublished manuscript, University of Groningen, Department of Psychiatry.

Black, A. (1974). The natural history of obsessional neurosis. In H. R. Beech (Ed.), *Obsessional states*. London: Methuen.

Beck, A. T., Rush, A. J., Shaw, B. F., & Emery, G. (1979). *Cognitive therapy of depression*. New York: Guilford Press.

Boersma, K., Den Hengst, S., Dekker, J., & Emmelkamp, P. M. G. (1976). Exposure and response prevention in the natural environment: A comparison with obsessive–compulsive patients. *Behaviour Research and Therapy, 14*, 19–24.

Brown, G. W., & Harris, T. (1978). *Social origins of depression: A study of psychiatric disorder in women*. London: Tavistock.

Dohrenwend, B. S., & Dohrenwend, B. P. (1981). Social and cultural influences on psychopathology. *Annual Review of Psychology, 25*, 417–452.

Dohrenwend, B. P., Shrout, P. E., Link, B. G., Martin, J. L., & Skodol, A. E. (1986). Overview and initial results from a risk-factor study of depression and schizophrenia. In J. E. Barrett (Ed.), *Mental disorders in the community: Progress and challenge* (pp. 184–215). New York: Guilford Press.

Emmelkamp, P. M. G. (1982). *Phobic and obsessive–compulsive disorders: Theory, research and practice.* New York: Plenum Press.

Emmelkamp, P. M. G. (1983). Recent developments in the behavioural treatment of obsessive–compulsive patients. In J. C. Boulougouris (Ed.), *Learning theory approaches to psychiatry* (pp. 119–128). New York: Wiley.

Emmelkamp, P. M. G. (1986). Behavior therapy with adults. In S. Garfield & A. Bergin (Eds.), *Handbook of psychotherapy and behavior change* (pp. 383–442). New York: Wiley.

Emmelkamp, P. M. G. (1991). Obsessive–compulsive disorder: The contribution of an experimental clinical approach. In A. Ehlers, W. Fiegenbaum, I. Florin, & J. Margraf (Eds.), *Perspectives and promises of clinical psychology* (pp. 149–156).

Emmelkamp, P. M. G. (1992). Behaviour therapy in the fin du siècle. In J. Cottraux, P. Legeron, & E. Mollard (Eds.), *Which psychotherapies in year 2000.* Lisse: Swets & Zeitlinger.

Emmelkamp, P. M. G., & Beens, H. (1991). Cognitive therapy with obsessive–compulsive disorder: A comparative evaluation. *Behaviour Research and Therapy, 29,* 293–300.

Emmelkamp, P. M. G., Bouman, T. K., & Scholing, A. (1991). *Anxiety, phobias and obsessive–compulsive disorders: A clinical guide.* London: Wiley.

Emmelkamp, P. M. G., de Haan, E., & Hoogduin, C. A. L. (1990). Marital adjustment and obsessive–compulsive disorder. *British Journal of Psychiatry, 156,* 55–60.

Emmelkamp, P. M. G., & de Lange, I. (1983). Spouse involvement in the treatment of obsessive–compulsive patients. *Behaviour Research and Therapy, 21,* 341–346.

Emmelkamp, P. M. G., & Kraanen, J. (1977). Therapist controlled exposure *in vivo* versus self-controlled exposure *in vivo*: A comparison with obsessive–compulsive patients. *Behaviour Research and Therapy, 15,* 491–495.

Emmelkamp, P. M. G., Mersch, P. P. A., Vissia, E., & van der Helm, M. (1985). Social phobia: A comparative evaluation of cognitive and behavioral interventions. *Behaviour Research and Therapy, 23,* 365–369.

Emmelkamp, P., Van der Helm, M., MacGillavry, D., & Van Zanten, B. (1984). Marital therapy with clinically distressed couples: A comparative evaluation of system–theoretic, contingency-contracting, and communication skills approaches. In K. Hahlweg & N. Jacobson (Eds.), *Marital interaction: Analysis & Modification* (pp. 36–52). New York: Guilford Press.

Emmelkamp, P. M. G., & van der Heyden, H. (1980). Treatment of harming obsessions. *Behavioural Analysis and Modification, 4,* 28–35.

Emmelkamp, P. M. G., van Linden van den Heuvell, G., Rüphan, M., & Sanderman, R. (1989). Home-based treatment of obsessive–compulsive patients: Intersession interval and therapist involvement. *Behaviour Research and Therapy, 27,* 89–93.

Emmelkamp, P. M. G., Visser, S., & Hoekstra, R. (1988). Cognitive therapy vs.

exposure in treatment of obsessive–compulsives. *Cognitive Research and Therapy, 12,* 103–114.

Enright, S. J. (1991). Group treatment for obsessive–compulsive disorder: An evaluation. *Behavioural Psychotherapy, 19,* 183–192.

Finlay-Jones, R. A., & Brown, G. W. (1981). Types of stressful life events and the onset of anxiety and depressive disorders. *Psychological Medicine, 11,* 803–815.

Foa, E. B. (1979). Failures in treating obsessive–compulsives. *Behaviour Research and Therapy, 17,* 169–176.

Foa, E. B., Steketee, G. S., Kozak, M. J., & Dugger, D. (1986). Imipramine and placebo in the treatment of obsessive–compulsives: Their effects on depression and on obsessional symptoms. *Psychopharmacology Bulletin, 23,* 8–11.

Foa, E. B., Steketee, G., & Milby, J. B. (1980). Differential effects of exposure and response prevention in obsessive–compulsive washers. *Behaviour Research and Therapy, 18,* 449–455.

Gerlsma, C., van der Lubbe, P. M., & van Nieuwenhuizen, C. (in press). Factor analysis of the LEE scale, a questionnaire intended to measure perceived expressed emotion. *British Journal of Psychiatry.*

Goering, P., Masylenki, D., Lancee, W., & Freeman, S. J. (1983). Social support and posthospital outcome for depressed women. *Canadian Journal of Psychiatry, 28,* 612–618.

Hand, I., & Tichatzky, M. (1979). Behavioural group therapy for obsessions and compulsions. In P. O. Sjoden, S. Bates, & W. S. Dockens (Eds.), *Trends in behavior therapy* (pp. 269–297). New York: Academic Press.

Henderson, S., Byrne, D. G., & Duncan-Jones, P. (1981). *Neurosis and the social environment.* Sydney: Academic Press.

Hermesh, H., Shahar, A., & Munitz, H. (1987). Obsessive–compulsive disorder and borderline personality disorder. *American Journal of Psychiatry, 44,* 120–121.

Hooley, J. M., Orley, J., & Teasdale, J. D. (1986). Levels of expressed emotion and relapse in depressed patients. *British Journal of Psychology, 148,* 642–647.

Horowitz, M. J. (1986). *Stress response syndromes* (2nd ed.). New Jersey: Jason Aronson.

Jenike, M. A., Baer, L., Minichiello, W. E., Schwartz, C. E., & Carey, R. J. (1986). Concomitant obsessive–compulsive disorder and schizotypal personality disorder. *American Journal of Psychiatry, 143,* 530–532.

Joffe, R. T., Swinson, R. P., & Regan, J. J. (1988). Personality features of obsessive–compulsive disorder. *American Journal of Psychiatry, 145,* 1127–1129.

Keller, M. B. (1985). Chronic and recurrent affective disorders: Incidence, course, and influencing factors. *Advances in Biochemistry and Psychopharmacology, 40,* 111–120.

Kleiner, L., Marshall, W. L., & Spevack, M. (1987). Training in problem-solving and exposure treatment for agoraphobics with panic attacks. *Journal of Anxiety Disorders, 1,* 219–238.

Krantz, S. E., & Moos, R. H. (1988). Risk factors at intake predict nonremission among depressed patients. *Journal of Consulting and Clinical Psychology*, 56, 863–869.

Leff, J. P., & Vaughn, C. (1985). *Expressed emotions in families*. New York: Guilford Press.

Marks, I. M. (1987). *Fears, phobias, and rituals*. New York: Oxford University Press.

Marks, I. M., Hodgson, R. J., & Rachman, S. (1975). Treatment of chronic obsessive–compulsive neurosis by *in vivo* exposure. *British Journal of Psychiatry*, 127, 349–364.

Marlatt, G. A., & Gordon, J. R. (1980). Determinants of relapse: Implications for the maintenance of behavior change. In P. O. Davidson & S. M. Davidson (Eds.), *Behavioral medicine: Changing health lifestyles*. New York: Brunner/Mazel.

Marlatt, G. A., & Gordon, J. R. (Eds.). (1985). *Relapse prevention: Maintenance strategies in the treatment of addictive behaviors*. New York: Guilford Press.

Mavissakalian, M., Hamann, M. S., & Jones, B. (1990a). A comparison of DSM-III personality disorders in panic/agoraphobia and obsessive–compulsive disorder. *Comprehensive Psychiatry*, 31, 238–244.

Mavissakalian, M., Hamann, M. S., & Jones, B. (1990b). Correlates of DSM-III personality disorders in obsessive–compulsive disorder. *Comprehensive Psychiatry*, 31, 481–489.

Meyer, V. (1966). Modification of expectations in cases with obsessional rituals. *Behaviour Research and Therapy*, 4, 273–280.

Meyer, V., Levy, R., & Schnurer, A. (1974). The behavioural treatment of obsessive–compulsive disorder. In H. R. Beech (Ed.), *Obsessional states* (pp. 233–258). London: Methuen.

Minichiello, W. E., Baer, L., & Jenike, M. A. (1987). Schizotypal personality disorder: A poor prognostic indicator for behavior therapy in the treatment of obsessive–compulsive disorder. *Journal of Anxiety Disorder*, 1, 273–276.

Nagera, H. (1976). *Obsessional neurosis: Developmental psychopathology*. New York: Jason Aronson.

O'Sullivan, G., & Marks, I. (1990). Long-term outcome of phobic and obsessive–compulsive disorders after treatment. In R. Noyes, M. Roth, & G. D. Burrows (Eds.), *Handbook of anxiety* (Vol. 4). Amsterdam: Elsevier.

Rachman, S. (1983). Obstacles to the successful treatment of obsessions. In E. B. Foa & P. M. G. Emmelkamp (Eds.), *Failures in behavior therapy* (pp. 35–57). New York: Wiley.

Rachman, S., & Hodgson, R. (1980). *Obsessions and compulsions*. Englewood Cliffs, NJ: Prentice-Hall.

Rachman, S., Marks, I., & Hodgson, R. (1973). The treatment of chronic obsessive–compulsive neurosis. *Behaviour Research and Therapy*, 9, 237–247.

Rasmussen, S. A., & Tsuang, M. T. (1986). Clinical characteristics and family history in DSM-III obsessive–compulsive disorder. *American Journal of Psychiatry*, 144, 121–122.

Scholing, A., & Emmelkamp, P. M. G. (1990). Social phobia: Nature and treatment. In H. Leitenberg (Ed.), *Handbook of social and evaluation anxiety* (pp. 269–324). New York: Plenum Press.

Shrout, P. E., Link, B. G. Dohrenwend, B. P., Skodol, A. E., Stueve, A., & Mirotznik, J. (1989). Characterizing life events as risk factors for depression: The role of fateful loss events. *Journal of Abnormal Psychology, 98,* 460–467.

Schreurs, P. J. G., van de Willige, G., Tellegen, P., & Brosschot, J. F. (1988). *De Utrechtse coping lijst. Omgaan met problemen en gebeurtenissen. Handleiding.* Lisse: Swets & Zeitlinger.

Stanley, M. A., Turner, S. M., & Borden, J. W. (1990). Schizotypal features in obsessive–compulsive disorder. *Comprehensive Psychiatry, 31,* 511–518.

Steketee, G. (1990). Personality traits and disorders in obsessive–compulsives. *Journal of Anxiety Disorders, 4,* 351–364.

Steketee, G., & Cleere, L. (1990). Obsessional–compulsive disorder. In A. S. Bellack, M. Hersen, & E. Kazdin (Eds.), *International handbook of behavior modification and therapy* (2nd ed., pp. 307–332). New York: Plenum Press.

Temoshok, L., Heller, B. W., Sagebiel, R. W., Blois, M. S., Sweet, D. M., DiClemente, R. J., & Gold, M. L. (1985). The relationship of psychosocial factors to prognostic indicators in cutaneous malignant melanoma. *Journal of Psychosomatic Research, 29,* 139–153.

van de Hout, M., Emmelkamp, P. M. G., Kraaykamp, J., & Griez, E. (1988). Behavioural treatment of obsessive–compulsives: Inpatient versus outpatient. *Behaviour Research and Therapy, 26,* 331–332.

van Sonderen, E. (1991). *Het meten van sociale steun.* Unpublished doctoral dissertation, University of Groningen, The Netherlands.

Visser, S., Hoekstra, R. J., & Emmelkamp, P. M. G. (1992). Follow-up study on behavioural treatment of obsessive–compulsive disorders. In W. Fiegenbaum, I. Floring, A. Ehlers, & J. Margraf (Eds.), *Perspectives and promises of clinical psychology* (pp. 157–170). New York: Plenum Press.

Walton, D., & Mather, M. D. (1963). The application of learning principles to the treatment of obsessive–compulsive states in acute and chronic phases of the illness. *Behaviour Research and Therapy, 1,* 163–174.

Whisman, M. A. (1990). The efficacy of booster maintenance sessions in behavior therapy: Review and methodological critique. *Clinical Psychology Review, 10,* 155–170.

Wolpe, J. (1958). *Psychotherapy and reciprocal inhibition.* Stanford: Stanford University Press.

Yaryura Tobias, J. A., & Neziroglu, F. A. (1983). *Obsessive–compulsive disorders.* New York: Marcel Dekker.

Zung, W. W. K. (1965). A self-rating depression scale. *Archives of General Psychiatry, 12,* 63–70.

CHAPTER 10

SEXUAL DEVIANCE

W. L. Marshall
QUEEN'S UNIVERSITY

S. M. Hudson
UNIVERSITY OF CANTERBURY

T. Ward
ROLLESTON, NEW ZEALAND

Sexually deviant behavior has been traditionally subdivided into those sexual acts that differ with respect to the mode of gratification and with respect to the objects of sexual interest. The focus of this chapter, however, is the treatment of men who engage in sexual offenses that constitute one category of deviant acts. We further limit our focus to those offenders who either rape or sexually assault women, molest children, or expose their genitals to unwilling females (since they constitute at least 95% of offenders presenting at clinics).

There are other types of deviations, as opposed to offenses, such as fetishisms or tranvestisms, for which we suspect that similar (albeit somewhat briefer) treatment programs would be appropriate, and there are other types of offenders (e.g., frotteurs, obscene telephone callers, and voyeurs), but these men appear so infrequently at clinics that there is little information on their treatment to justify including them in this chapter. We will not use DSM-III-R (American Psychiatric Association, 1987) criteria to identify the problem behaviors because those criteria restrict the population in a way that does not match the typical application of treatment. Treatment programs have targeted sex offenders regardless of whether or not they can be said to have a sexual disorder according to DSM-III-R.

The definition of sexual abuse is a cultural phenomenon and as such suffers from drift. For example, homosexual behavior has until recently been defined both as a sexual deviation and an offense. Changes in legislation have forced the reconceptualization of this sexual orientation as simply a variation, and as such the law reflects similar changes in psychiatric classification. However, in stark contrast to sexual behavior between consenting adults of the same sex, the weight of evidence suggests that nonconsensual sexual contact and sex between adults and children both have significant harmful effects on the victims.

Sexually aggressive behavior appears to be multiply determined (Marshall & Barbaree, 1990a). It is likely that the physiological substrate supports the ready capacity to sexually aggress (Marshall, 1984), and that between individuals, variations in hormonal functioning potentiate this (Bradford, 1990). The need for socially created inhibitors is therefore critically important. The evidence suggests that poor parenting, especially involving inconsistent, harsh physical discipline in the absence of warmth and support, fails to implant the needed social controls and may fuse sex and aggression (Finkelhor, 1984). A paternalistic cultural tradition that sees women and children as objects for the sexual satisfaction of males is likely to be eagerly adopted by a vulnerable adolescent male to boost his sense of masculinity and self-esteem (Marshall & Barrett, 1990). These vulnerability factors interact with more transient situational elements such as intoxication, strong negative affect, a belief that he will not be caught, and the presence of a potential victim to determine the occurrence of a sexual assault (Marshall & Barbaree, 1990b).

COGNITIVE–BEHAVIORAL TREATMENT

Cognitive–behavioral treatment programs assume that sexual offending reflects at least some degree of sexual attraction to inappropriate partners or acts, often associated with a relative lack of appropriate arousal. These inappropriate arousal patterns and deviant sexual acts produce a broad range of cognitive distortions that serve to rationalize the antisocial behaviors. Many of these offenders also display deficits in social competence and daily living skills, which restrict access to appropriate partners and cause stress, which in turn increases the probability that the sexually deviant behavior will occur. The major aims, therefore, of treatment programs predicated on a cognitive–behavioral perspective are to eliminate cognitive distortions, normalize sexual preferences, enhance social functioning, and improve life management skills. All these goals are meant to reduce the probability of future offending, and in that sense these programs can be said to aim at relapse prevention (RP). However, in recent years additional components have been added to cognitive–

behavioral programs that are specifically meant to make the goal of RP more explicit and that provide specific components to reduce the chance of reoffending. These components were derived from Marlatt and Gordon's (1985) work on RP in the addiction field.

In order to best understand the application of RP procedures with sex offenders, we describe each component in the comprehensive programs we have developed in three different settings. The primary program that has served as the basis for these developments is our outpatient community-based program (Marshall & Barbaree, 1987, 1988). This program was adapted to operate within jails in Canada (Barbaree & Marshall, 1989) and New Zealand (Marshall, Johnston, Ward, Jones, & Hudson, 1991). Other similar programs operate within jails in the United States (Marques, Day, Nelson, & Miner, 1989; Pithers, Martin, & Cumming, 1989).

TRADITIONAL COMPONENTS

In this chapter, we describe the more traditional components of cognitive–behavioral programs rather briefly since they are detailed elsewhere (e.g., Marshall, Laws, & Barbaree, 1990). We emphasize the more recent additions specifically aimed at RP, although we stress that the total package of cognitive–behavioral treatment has always aimed at RP. The specific RP components are really meant to maintain and enhance the changes produced by the rest of the program and to ensure that the patient continues to utilize the skills he has learned once formal treatment is over.

Cognitive Distortions

Sex offenders distort the reality of their offending (Segal & Stermac, 1990). The processes involved in this distortion include denial, minimization, shifting of responsibility for the acts committed, distorted views of the victim's behavior and desires, and, finally, a belief that sexual offending does not harm the victim. These distortions are challenged and alternative views are offered. The benefits to the patient, which will result from his changing his views, are made clear, as are the costs of continuing to distort. Essentially we follow a "cognitive restructuring" approach in this component of treatment (Barbaree & Marshall, in press).

Sexual Behavior

As we noted, a number of sex offenders display deviant sexual preferences at laboratory testing, but it is important to note that far from all do.

Indeed, in our review of this literature (Marshall & Eccles, 1991), we concluded that for all types of sex offenders, the belief that deviant sexual preferences are fundamental is not empirically supported. In two large-scale evaluations of rapists, for example, Baxter, Barbaree, and Marshall (1986) and Marshall, Barbaree, Laws, and Baxter (1986) found that only 30% of them displayed either greater or equivalent arousal to rape cues than to consenting sex. In this respect they did not differ from nonoffenders. Similarly, Marshall, Payne, Barbaree, and Eccles (1991) could discern no differences between exhibitionists and matched nonoffenders in terms of their sexual arousal to either consenting intercourse or exhibiting. Among child molesters, there were more men who revealed deviant preferences, but even here less than 50% were either equally or more aroused by children than by adults (Barbaree & Marshall, 1986; Marshall, Barbaree, & Butt, 1988; Marshall, Barbaree, & Christophe, 1986). However, since some offenders do display deviant arousal, and since all of them are obviously prompted to act in a sexually deviant manner, it is necessary to implement procedures to reduce these tendencies whether or not they all appear as aberrant at laboratory assessment.

Four major techniques exist to modify sexual preferences. Electrical aversion typically involves the presentation of deviant stimuli during which a mild but unpleasant electric shock is delivered to the patient. Usually this procedure also uses "relief" stimuli (images of appropriate sex), which are not associated with shock (Abel, Levis, & Clancy, 1970; Marshall, 1973). There is little evidence supporting the use of this procedure (Quinsey & Marshall, 1983) and we have abandoned its use, even in those rare cases where deviant urges are frequent and impelling such that the man is at clear risk to reoffend while in outpatient treatment.

For these cases, we utilize one of three alternatives. Olfactory aversion (Maletzky, 1990) follows the same procedure as electrical aversion except that electric shock is replaced by a foul odor. This is sometimes effective in quickly eliminating deviant urges. Until recently we referred these patients for hormonal or antiandrogen treatment (Bradford, 1990), but presently Pearson, Barbaree, Southmayd, and Marshall (1992) are investigating the value of certain serotonergic drugs (e.g., buspirone) in bringing these impelling urges under control, and to date we have been pleased with the results of our single-case evaluations. The intention here, of course, is to use these drugs simply to reduce the urges to a level where the patient is no longer an immediate risk to the community and is able to profit from the rest of our program.

Masturbatory reconditioning procedures are in widespread use although the evidence supporting their value is weak (Laws & Marshall, 1991). Patients are instructed to imagine appropriate sexual acts while masturbating until they achieve orgasm. Immediately after orgasm they are to repeat aloud every variation they can imagine on their deviant theme so that by associating these deviant thoughts with a period of sexual refractoriness, their sexual provocativeness will extinguish (Marshall, 1979; Johnson, Hudson, & Marshall, in press).

We also assist offenders in constructing several imaginal approach sequences and corresponding negative consequences. For example, a nonfamilial child molester may imagine he is sitting at home bored. As a consequence of this boredom, he begins to think of sex with children and decides to drive to the local video arcade. He leaves his house, gets into his car, drives to the arcade, and seeks out a child. Once he has identified a vulnerable child, he approaches him/her, offers him/her some incentive (likely money to play the machines), and finally takes him/her for a ride in his car, where he enacts the offense. Several sequences such as this are written on one side of a pocket-sized card, and these cards are carried by the offender at all times. On the reverse of the card, he writes all the catastrophic consequences he typically thinks of *after* he has completed an offense. At least three times each day he is to read each of the approach sequences and stop at a point short of the terminal behavior, reverse the card, and read the consequences. This procedure, "covert sensitization," is meant to make clients aware of their typical approach sequences so that they can more readily abort the sequence at an early point. It is also intended to make them think of the consequences at an early point and to punish approaches by rehearsing the catastrophic consequences. This particular derivation of covert sensitization was adopted from the work of Annon and Robinson (1985).

Finally, since the world at large is replete with sights and sounds that evoke deviant thinking in these offenders, we have them carry a small vial of smelling salts to use as a self-administered punisher. Whenever they have a deviant thought, they are to open the vial, hold it below their nose, and rapidly inhale. This is experienced as aversive and not only punishes the thoughts but removes them, thereby allowing more constructive thoughts to be entertained (Hunt, 1985).

In addition to these procedures aimed at modifying deviant thoughts, we assist patients in identifying the needs they are attempting to meet by deviant sex. Sexual gratification is just one need that is met by engaging in sexual behavior. We attempt to have the offender realize that many of the other needs he is pursuing (which may be only vaguely understood) cannot be met by acting deviantly. For example, needs for affection and intimacy can hardly be satisfied by raping a woman, molesting a child, or exhibiting.

We also provide sex education, aimed not so much at expanding the patient's knowledge of the physiology and anatomy of sex but rather at reducing prudishness, changing pro-offending attitudes, and apprising the patient of the range of behaviors that are functionally related to the full enjoyment of sex with an adult partner.

Social Competence

Social competence involves a matrix of component skills and processes in the interpersonal (empathy, assertiveness, anger and anxiety management, and conversational skills) and relationship domains (particularly communication, conflict resolution, and intimacy skills). Sex offenders have been shown to be deficient in recognizing emotions in others (Hudson, Wales, Bakker, McLean, & Marshall, 1991) and they lack empathy (Finkelhor, 1984; Jones, Hudson, & Marshall, 1992). They are also less assertive (Segal & Marshall, 1985), more socially anxious (Gordon, Weisman, & Marshall, 1980), and less skilled in conversations (Stermac, Segal, & Gillis, 1990) than other men. It has recently been found that rapists, child molesters, and exhibitionists are socially lonely and lack intimacy in their lives (Garlic, 1991; Marshall & Seidman, 1991).

Our approach to treating these aspects of the problems of sex offenders involves modeling, role play, and feedback, and we conduct this aspect of treatment within a group context. Indeed, we do most of our treatment in groups, not only for reasons of economy but also because it maximizes the effectiveness of treatment by involving everyone as both patient and therapist.

Life Management

What are termed "life skills" in the rehabilitative literature are equally important to assess and ameliorate with sex offenders. For example deficits in health care, personal hygiene, and grooming serve to limit heterosexual opportunities. Similarly, lack of effective employment is a significant predictor of general recidivism (Riley, Hudson, & Anderson, 1991), and thus related skills such as literacy, budgeting, and job-search-and-secure skills are important. Also, the creative and balanced use of leisure is important, as is effective control over the use of intoxicants. While we deal with many of these issues in our group treatment, we also make extensive use of community resources. There is no point, for example, in our attempting to develop expertise in overcoming alcohol abuse when there are excellent local programs already available for this. Thus, our offenders frequently participate in other programs concurrent with their involvement with ours.

RP

Marlatt and Gordon (1985) were the first to formulate a view of the processes governing relapse among various types of addicts. Their conceptualization has proven remarkably valuable in the field of addictions, and the observed commonalities (presence of short-term satisfaction, delayed negative consequences, the probability of high personal and social costs, and difficulties maintaining behavioral change) with sexually aggressive behavior have resulted in these techniques being applied to sex offending (Pithers, Marques, Gibat, & Marlatt, 1983). RP procedures aim to enhance the client's self-management skills in order to maintain the initial behavioral change induced by therapy. It is absolutely essential, in this component of treatment, to constantly remind the client of the pertinent skills he has learned in the preceding components so that he can apply these to deal with relapse threats. He should also be told that in the event of the feeling that he is losing control, or that a relapse is imminent, he should immediately call the clinic and reenter treatment.

Accepting an RP view of sex offending does not imply acceptance of the addiction view of sexual behavior espoused by Carnes (1985). Viewed as an addiction, sexual offending can be understood as beyond the man's control. RP strategies, on the other hand, emphasize the offender's responsibility for his behavior and its management, rather than portraying him as the helpless recipient of treatment.

In the application of RP to sexual offenders, modifications have had to be made to the notions as they are applied to addictive behaviors. The fact that victims suffer at the hands of these offenders has necessitated the redefinition of both "lapse" and "relapse." For example, in treating nicotine addiction, defining a lapse as the first cigarette smoked and a relapse as a return to previous levels of smoking involves relatively little cost to anyone other than the smoker. For the sex offender, however, defining a lapse as the initial return to offending trivializes the consequences to the victim and suggests to the offender that a single abusive act is not problematic. Pithers (1990) has suggested that a lapse be construed as a fantasized deviant act whereas an overt offense constitutes a relapse. Hudson, Ward, and Marshall (in press) have argued that this is an incomplete analysis that may not maximize an RP approach. Our suggestion is that the concept of "lapse" be expanded to include considering plans to offend and entering a high-risk situation as well as deviant fantasizing. In addition, we think it is important to have the client understand that a single offense after treatment does not necessarily have to lead to a full return to prior rates of offending, while at the same time emphasizing the importance of avoiding even a single offense.

There is a conceptual difference between a single reoffense and a return to previous levels of offending. It is likely that this transition is mediated by a similar process (e.g., the abstinence violation effect) that mediates the lapse–relapse transition, and as such it also needs direct attention in treatment. This is especially important as offenders typically reoffend against more than one victim (Abel & Rouleau, 1990). Thus, we do not want clients to view reoffending as an all-or-none phenomenon. If they do reoffend, we want them to stop the process there and not let it escalate to more victims and perhaps more aggressive and intrusive behaviors.

Relapse processes may be understood as a chain of responses that include affect, cognitions, and behaviors. In some instances a negative emotional state may trigger the sequence; in others it may be a thought or a behavior that initiates the chain leading to a relapse. The types of emotional responses that may start the relapse process are many and varied and typically idiosyncratic. For example, one offender may typically respond to arguments with his partner by becoming angry, and he may deal with this anger by sexually assaulting a woman. For another offender, these arguments may make him depressed, which he may resolve by molesting a child. Other emotional states that typically trigger a relapse include loneliness, boredom, anxiety, or confusion. One particularly salient emotion is a feeling of deprivation. This may result from unsatisfactory sexual relations with a partner or it may arise when the man feels he is carrying too many responsibilities. In each case, these negative emotions lead to rationalizing processes, which justify deviant sexual fantasizing and lead to planning and executing a deviant act.

Cognitions that may prompt the unfolding of the relapse process include not only deviant sexual fantasies, but also rationalizations that either justify deviant behaviors (e.g., "It is not so bad really," or "When I offend, it does not really hurt the victim") or remove the man's sense of responsibility for his acts (e.g., "Its that bitch's fault for being out here all alone," "This kid wants me to have sex with her"). Deviant fantasizing may be prompted by internal states, such as sexual arousal, or the sight of a woman or child. When these deviant thoughts occur, they may trigger the "abstinence violation effect." If the offender has not experienced a deviant thought for some time, perhaps as a result of treatment or simply the exercise of self-control, when one does occur he may conclude that he is unable to control himself and is after all still a deviant. This gloomy conclusion characteristically leads to further catastrophizing, which induces those negative emotions that initiate the relapse process.

Sometimes behaviors rather than thoughts initiate the chain. The most common example is the use of intoxicants that reduce both inhibitions and treatment-induced constraints against offending. Also, setting high standards for accomplishments or allowing oneself to be chronically stressed, is a behavior that may lead to feelings of deprivation. Such feelings, as we have noted, may lead to a reoffense. Similarly, allowing events to unfold so that access to a victim occurs, or otherwise thoughtlessly putting himself in a high-risk situation, may permit the man's reoffense chain to begin. These latter types of behaviors are often referred to as "apparently irrelevant decisions," although they are rarely accidental mistakes. Once in a high-risk situation, the probability of deviant fantasizing occurring is markedly increased, and such thoughts may prompt the abstinence violation effect, leading to a reoffense.

In treatment, the offender must identify the emotions and cognitions that for him typically lead to the initiation of the relapse chain. He must be reminded of the skills he has learned to more effectively deal with these negative states so that he can avoid relapsing. Deviant fantasies, or lapses, should be seen as both inevitable and as opportunities to practice the procedures learned in treatment to deal with such thoughts. Behaviors that in the past have started the relapse process must be identified, and again the client is reminded to use his acquired skills both to reduce the probability of these behaviors occurring and to deal appropriately with them when they do occur. A good deal of time is spent in treatment, identifying apparently irrelevant decisions and understanding the abstinence violation effect. An excellent book on RP with sex offenders (Laws, 1989) provides detailed clinical insights into all these processes and offers clear suggestions for how they might be addressed in treatment.

Training the patient to recognize the factors, processes, and situations that put him at risk, is done within the usual context of the rest of the treatment program and has been described by Pithers (1990) as the "internal management" aspect of RP training. "External management," on the other hand, refers to the provision of some degree of supervisory control after discharge, although the precise form this takes has varied considerably. Prior to discharge from our treatment programs, we help each offender prepare a list of the factors, processes and situations that put him at risk. Attached to this is a list of the ways in which he can avoid the occurrence of these risks or deal with them in an appropriate manner when they cannot be avoided. He is to carry these lists with him at all times and periodically reread them to ensure that he remains at low risk. After release from the jail settings where we operate programs, each client is placed under the supervision of someone who is knowledgeable in RP processes and treatment strategies and who can assist the client in minimizing risk. If these supervisors recognize emerging problems, they can deal with them themselves, refer the client to a community treatment program, place him in a halfway house, or, in the worst case, return him to jail. Where possible, release from jail is made contingent upon the man's agreement to enter a further, albeit briefer, treatment program in a community setting. Unfortunately, governments rarely provide sufficient funds for all released offenders to enter such programs, but we have managed to get most of our clients into some form of postrelease treatment.

In his outpatient program, Abel (1987) employs an alternative strategy to the usual external management. Abel describes what he calls a "surveillance group." Four to five people, who are in regular contact with the offender, meet initially with the therapist to construct a list of risky and provocative situations for that particular individual, and they subsequently monitor the client's behavior and provide regular reports to the clinic. In yet another variation, Maletzky (1990) has clients return for regular "booster" sessions where they are reassessed and provided with whatever treatment seems necessary. As a final possible approach, Quinsey (1990) has recommended a draconian method of electronically monitoring the movements of released offenders, but fortunately no one has taken up his suggestion. While both Abel's and Maletzky's posttreatment procedures have obvious merits, the external management provided by Pithers (1990) and Marques (Marques et al., 1989) seems to be the strategy of choice, and outcome data from Pithers's program (Pithers & Cumming, 1989) are certainly encouraging.

REVIEW OF OUTCOME

Before examining the evidence concerning relapse in sex offenders, we briefly describe some of the methodological problems that are particularly troublesome in this area of study. Variations in selection criteria for entry into the treatment programs (Furby, Weinrott, & Blackshaw, 1989) constitute a major problem. Some institutions, and perhaps some community programs, attract only the most dangerous offenders, who are likely to be those most in need of treatment, whereas other programs employ restrictive selection criteria to allow inmates to enter. In fact, some of these latter programs express an eagerness to take only those at lowest risk to reoffend. This perhaps has some wisdom when attempting to gain credibility for a new program; that is, it reduces the probability of a dramatic failure, which might terminate the program, and it results in very low outcome recidivism. However, it not only reduces the generalizations we can make about the program's utility but also sets in place an approach that becomes hard to change. The sex offenders to whom we must give priority are those who are the most dangerous and who are going to be released eventually whether treated or not. The protection of innocent victims, not our own credibility, must be the number-one priority.

Length of follow-up, more appropriately seen as time at risk for reoffense, needs clear specification. Both Marshall and Barbaree (1988) and Soothill and his colleagues (Soothill & Gibbens, 1978; Soothill, Jack, & Gibbens, 1976) have shown that recidivism rates continue to increase for as long as these offenders are followed, at least up to 22 years. Our data revealed, for example, that of those offenders at risk for less than 2 years, only 8.8% reoffended, whereas this rose to 16.7% up to 4 years and 40.9% for periods longer than 4 years. Thereafter, however, the rate of increase appears to be near enough asymptotic. Thus, follow-up periods of less than 4 to 5 years seem unsatisfactory.

The third major problem is the adequacy of official records for determining the incidence of reoffending. Most studies acknowledge that these figures provide underestimates. Marshall and Barbaree (1988) were fortunate to be able to examine information held in the files of child protection agencies and local police stations. In these files, they found many instances of clear evidence of a reoffense but where the man was not charged. These unofficial data revealed recidivism rates that were, on average, 2½ times the rates revealed by an examination of the official police data set. However, interestingly, the proportionate increase did not differ for treated or untreated offenders, suggesting that while the official records are, indeed, an underestimate, this will not bias a comparison between a treated group and a no-treatment group; both will be distorted to the same degree. Hereafter, unless otherwise specified, we report recidivism data derived from official police records.

A final point is that there is no reason to expect all treatment approaches, in the hands of all therapists, to be equally effective with all types of offenders. For example, in our review of the evidence (Marshall, Jones, Ward, Johnston, & Barbaree, 1991), rapists and exhibitionists appear to profit less from treatment than do child molesters. Most people involved in the treatment of any kinds of problems would be surprised if psychoanalytical, behavioral, and medical approaches to treatment all produced the same results. There are so many variations on cognitive–behavioral approaches to the treatment of sex offenders, and even on the posttreatment strategies, that we can expect variations in outcome even within this one approach. While there is no evidence for the influence of therapist factors in the treatment of sex offenders, it seems reasonable to suppose that this may also be a source of variance in outcome studies.

. OUTCOME EVALUATIONS

We review treatment outcome studies under five headings: institutional programs with and without RP and community programs that do not have any elements of RP, that have just the internal management component, or that have both internal and external management components. We could have surveyed all treatment programs with and without RP, but that seems both unnecessary, since they are reviewed elsewhere (e.g.,

Marshall, Jones, et al., 1991), and inappropriate, since only behavioral programs actually aim at RP. That is, only behavioral programs explicitly train offenders in the skills meant to both reduce the likelihood of future offending and increase the capacity for meeting their needs in prosocial ways. Thus, this chapter if limited to behavioral or cognitive–behavioral programs for which there are adequate data to permit an appraisal.

Institutional Programs without RP

A program operating in a maximum security hospital in Ontario has been evaluated by Rice, Harris, and Quinsey (1990). This hospital houses sex offenders who have been found not guilty by reason of insanity or who are being assessed to determine their ability to stand trial. Obviously, these offenders are predominantly those who either have committed the most brutal crimes or have a long history of offending, or who in some other way appeared dangerous to the courts. Accordingly, we would expect them to receive extensive (in terms of both time in treatment and range of treatment components) and intensive treatment. Unfortunately, they received neither.

Treatment suitability for this program was assessed on the basis of laboratory-demonstrated deviant sexual arousal, and those deviant preferences were the prime targets for treatment. All offenders participating in this program received either electric aversion therapy or biofeedback training aimed at reducing deviant sexual interests. Approximately 30% of the 136 treated offenders also received heterosocial skills training and sex education. The treated patients were drawn from the long-term residents (i.e., those found not fit to plead or not guilty by reason of insanity), whereas the untreated comparison group was drawn from those on remand for a psychiatric assessment. Outcome data were presented on only 29 matched pairs of subjects (i.e., treated and untreated), and the resultant recidivism data were taken to suggest that the program had, if anything, an adverse effect. Thirty-seven percent of the treated group reoffended during the 7-year follow-up, in contrast to 31% of the controls. Given the nature of the treated population and the limited treatment program, this result is perhaps not surprising.

The most recent follow-up data (Leger, 1989) from a penitentiary-based treatment program similarly presents a discouraging picture. This program treats offenders over a 6-month period close to the end of their sentence. Clients were selected on the basis of deviant sexual preferences and their willingness to enter the program, so that a broad range of dangerousness is apparent prior to treatment. Until recently, this program did not have an explicit RP component, but otherwise it reflected, in terms of its content, a reasonably comprehensive cognitive–behavioral approach. Davidson (1984) had previously shown that 35% of similar untreated offenders released from Kingston Penitentiary reoffended over an 8-year follow-up period. Leger's (1989) appraisal of outcome revealed that 18% of the treated rapists and 20% of the treated child molesters reoffended within 3 to 12 years after release. These are not encouraging figures.

Institutional Programs with RP

Only Internal Management

We could identify only one institutional program having the internal management component that has provided outcome data. Gordon (1989) collected recidivism data over a 7-year period on 130 offenders released from his comprehensive treatment program. He reports a recidivism rate of 10% for a mixed group of treated sex offenders, which, given that his population is much the same as that housed in Leger's (1989) program, suggests a strong treatment effect.

Both Internal and External Management

One of the two best known RP programs has been described by Marques et al. (1989). In this program, offenders are not only exposed to a comprehensive program while in the institution, but are required to be both supervised on release by a person skilled in RP and involved, for 2 or more years after release, in a formal community treatment program. In one of their early reports of outcome, Marques et al. (1989) provided very encouraging data. Of 47 men who were at risk for an average of 12.7 months, only 8% had reoffended compared to 20% of the untreated volunteers ($N = 49$) and 21% of the nonvolunteers ($N = 42$). Although this appears to be impressive, the follow-up was not long and the men were still in treatment in the community. Furthermore, in her most recent report, Marques (1990) described a longer-term outcome for the treated offenders that no longer differed from that observed in the untreated men.

The other major RP program has been systematically evaluated by Pithers et al. (1989). In this program, comprehensive postrelease supervision and treatment if necessary continue until the end of the offender's parole (Pithers, 1990). Like, Marques's program, then, it is difficult to know just what the long-term outcome will be once all supervision and interventions are withdrawn. Nevertheless, in terms of reduced risk to the public, low recidivism figures for the treated offenders are impressive regardless of the level of professional involvement. However, the costs of operating such an elaborate program are another concern.

Of the 147 child molesters to graduate from Pithers's program, only 3% subsequently committed a sexual offense during a 6-year follow-up (Pithers & Cumming, 1989). Marshall, Jones, et al.'s (1991) reservations about the possible biases introduced by the selective entry requirements of this program notwithstanding, these data are remarkable and are substantially below what would normally be expected from similar offenders released from jail. By contrast, 15% of the 20 treated rapists reoffended during follow-up. This is not at all satisfactory and suggests, as do other data (see Marshall et al., 1991) that we need to reconceptualize the problems that beset rapists and alter our treatment approaches accordingly. Marshall (1992) has recently identified what he believes are the necessary changes to treatment to produce better outcome with rapists.

Community Programs without RP

Abel et al. (1988) describe an otherwise comprehensive program that has, as we noted earlier, a surveillance group for monitoring posttreatment functioning. However, since this involves supervision by nonprofessionals who are unskilled in RP management, we have decided to consider this program as lacking an external management component based on RP concepts. Similarly, in Abel et al.'s description of the program, there is no indication of any internal management training. Abel et al. (1988) report a 12.2% reoffense rate among their child molester sample ($N = 98$) over a 1-year follow-up, which suggests that if the follow-up were extended over several more years, the recidivism would be excessively high. High dropout rates among those most at risk to reoffend make these outcome data even less impressive.

Another reasonably comprehensive, community-based cognitive–behavioral program is that operated by Maletzky (1990). In his detailed description of this program, Maletzky makes no mention of RP training or external supervision, but he does have patients return on a regular basis after formal discharge to receive "booster sessions." Scrutiny of official police records has revealed very low recidivism rates for most types of offenders treated at this clinic. Over a 1- to 14-year follow-up period, only 12.7% of 1,719 treated heterosexual pedophiles reoffended, as did only 13.6% of 513 treated homosexual pedophiles. Even less (6.9%) of the 462 exhibitionists relapsed, but 26.5% of the 87 rapists failed to refrain from offending again. Once again we see that rapists are a problematic group.

Marshall and Barbaree (1988) reported treatment outcome for their early program with child molesters. While this early program covered many of the areas described in the section dealing with the traditional components of cognitive–behavioral programs, it had, at best, only a weak internal management component, and this was added only over the last year of the evaluated program. Our present program is both more comprehensive and includes internal management training, but we will have to wait another year to see whether these changes produce additional benefits.

Although Marshall and Barbaree (1988) originally reported data derived from unofficial records of police and child protection agencies, we describe the official police information here in order to make comparisons easier. Among the treated offenders, 7.5% of the heterosexual pedophiles, 5.5% of the homosexual pedophiles, and 2.9% of the incest offenders reoffended over the 4-year follow-up period. The corresponding recidivism figures for the untreated offenders were 17.9% for the heterosexual pedophiles, 19.2% for the homosexual pedophiles, and 7% for the incest offenders.

In their appraisal of treated and untreated exhibitionists, Marshall, Eccles, and Barbaree (1991) described two programs. The first had a limited focus and did not include any RP components. At that time, they construed exhibitionism as resulting from primarily disturbed sexual needs with associated deficits in social functioning. Outcome from this early program was encouraging but certainly not remarkable. Untreated exhibitionists displayed a recidivism rate of 23.8% over the 4-year follow-up, while only 17.8% of the treated men reoffended.

Community Programs with RP

In fact, a careful search of the literature failed to turn up any community programs that have both the internal and external management components of RP training and that provide satisfactory outcome data. Indeed, our own recent treatment of exhibitionists (Marshall, Jones, et al., 1991) appears to be the only community program with an internal management component that has provided clear outcome data. Treated exhibitionists in this recent program not only received training in internal management to avoid relapses but were also involved in more extensive social and interpersonal skills training and had far less emphasis given to the sexual aspects of their problems. An outcome appraisal for this program revealed a recidivism rate for the treated offenders (9.8%) that was substantially lower than that shown in the earlier program. These data suggest that adding the RP component improved outcome, but unfortunately such a comparison is confounded by the other changes in the program.

CONCLUSIONS

RP concepts have been adopted from the seminal work of Marlatt (Marlatt & Gordon, 1985) and adapted to the special needs and features of sex offenders. These adaptations include training the offenders in the application of RP concepts while they are completing comprehensive cognitive–behavioral treatment programs and then having the offenders supervised after discharge from treatment by someone skilled in RP procedures.

It is clear from both this chapter and our earlier evaluations of the treatment outcome literature (Marshall & Barbaree, 1990c; Marshall & Eccles, 1991; Marshall, Jones, et al., 1991; Marshall, Ward, Jones, Johnston, & Barbaree, 1991) that cognitive–behavioral treatment of sex offenders is generally effective. Although the evidence is limited and comparisons are difficult to make, it does seem that those programs that include RP components are generally more effective than those that do not. However, given the lack of adequate resources available to treat all those offenders who are in need, we need to know how simple we can make the treatment package and still retain effectiveness. Do we need to add both the internal and external management components to the full cognitive–behavioral program?

Indeed, it is always possible that simply extending the external management component could make formal treatment itself unnecessary. In fact, the nature of the external management required to reduce reoffending is not clear. Both Pithers and Marques not only have a supervisory component but also involve their clients in further treatment after discharge from prison. Clearly, we have only just begun the process of developing and evaluating RP approaches to dealing with sex offenders, and most of the research remains to be done. However, the observations to date are encouraging.

REFERENCES

Abel, G. G. (1987, May). *Surveillance groups*. A paper presented at the annual meeting of the Association for the Behavioral Treatment of Sexual Abusers, Newport, OR.

Abel, G. G., Levis, D. J., & Clancy, J. (1970). Aversion therapy applied to taped sequences of deviant behavior in exhibitionism and other sexual deviations: A preliminary report. *Journal of Behavior Therapy and Experimental Psychiatry, 1,* 59–66.

Abel, G. G., & Rouleau, J. L. (1990). The nature and extent of sexual assault. In W. L. Marshall, D. R. Laws, & H. E. Barbaree (Eds.), *Handbook of sexual assault: Issues, theories, and treatment of the offender* (pp. 9–21). New York: Plenum Press.

American Psychiatric Association. (1987). *Diagnostic and statistical manual of mental disorders* (3rd ed., rev.). Washington, DC: Author.

Annon, J. S., & Robinson, C. H. (1985). Sexual deviation. In M. Hersen & A. S. Bellack (Eds.), *Handbook of clinical behavior therapy with adults* (pp. 631–657). New York: Plenum Press.

Barbaree, H. E., & Marshall, W. L. (1986). Deviant sexual arousal, demographic and offense history variables as predictors of reoffense among child molesters and incest offenders. *Behavioral Sciences & the Law, 6,* 267–280.

Barbaree, H. E., & Marshall, W. L. (1989). *The Warkworth Sexual Behaviour Clinic.* Report to Correctional Services of Canada, Kingston, Ontario.

Barbaree, H. E., & Marshall, W. L. (in press). Treatment of the sexual offender. In R. M. Wettstein (Ed.), *Treatment of the mentally disordered offender.* New York: Guilford Press.

Baxter, D. J., Barbaree, H. E., & Marshall, W. L. (1986). Sexual responses to consenting and forced sex in a large sample of rapists and nonrapists. *Behaviour Research and Therapy, 24,* 513–520.

Bradford, J. M. W. (1990). The antiandrogen and hormonal treatment of sexual offenders. In W. L. Marshall, D. R. Laws, & H. E. Barbaree (Eds.), *Handbook of sexual assault: Issues, theories, and the treatment of the offender* (pp. 297–310). New York: Plenum Press.

Carnes, P. (1985). *Out of the shadows: Understanding sexual addiction.* Minneapolis, MN: Compcare Publishing.

Davidson, P. (1984, March). *Outcome data for a penitentiary-based program for sex offenders.* Paper presented at the conference on the Assessment and Treatment of the Sex Offender, Kingston, Ontario.

Finkelhor, D. (1984). *Child sexual abuse: New theory and research.* New York: Free Press.

Furby, L., Weinrott, M. R., & Blackshaw, L. (1989). Sex offender recidivism: A review. *Psychological Bulletin, 105,* 3–30.

Garlic, E. (1991). *Intimacy failure, loneliness and the attribution of blame in sexual offending.* Unpublished master's thesis, University of London.

Gordon, A. (1989). Research on sex offenders: Regional Psychiatric Centre (Prairies). *Forum on Corrections Research, 1,* 20–21.

Gordon, A., Weisman, R. G., & Marshall, W. L. (1980, November). *The effects of flooding with response freedom on social anxiety.* A paper presented at the 14th annual convention of the Association for the Advancement of Behavior Therapy, New York.

Hudson, S. M., Wales, D., Bakker, L. W., McLean, A., & Marshall, W. L. (1991). *Recognition of emotional expression by male prisoners.* Manuscript submitted for publication.

Hudson, S. M., Ward, T., & Marshall, W. L. (in press). The abstinence violation effect in sex offenders: A reformulation. *Behaviour Research and Therapy.*

Hunt, F. M. (1985). Contingent aromatic aversion. In A. S. Bellack & M. Hersen (Eds.), *Dictionary of behavior therapy techniques* (p. 78). New York: Pergamon Press.

Johnston, P., Hudson, S. M., & Marshall, W. L. (in press). The effects of masturbatory reconditioning with nonfamilial child molesters. *Behaviour Research and Therapy.*

Jones, R., Hudson, S. M., & Marshall, W. L. (1992). *Empathy in child molesters.* Manuscript submitted for publication.

Laws, D. R. (Ed.). (1989). *Relapse prevention with sex offenders.* New York: Guilford Press.

Laws, D. R., & Marshall, W. L. (1991). Masturbatory reconditioning with sexual deviates: An evaluative review. *Advances in Behaviour Research and Therapy, 13,* 13–25.

Leger, G. (1989). Research on sex offenders: Regional Treatment Centre (Ontario). *Forum on Corrections Research, 1,* 21.

Maletzky, B. M. (1990). *Treating the sexual offender.* Newbury Park, CA: Sage Publications.

Marlatt, G. A., & Gordon, J. R. (Eds.). (1985). *Relapse prevention: Maintenance strategies in the treatment of addictive behaviors.* New York: Guilford Press.

Marques, J. K. (1990, October). *Recent outcome data on the California Sex Offender Program.* A paper presented at the 9th Annual Clinical and Research Conference on the Assessment and Treatment of Sexual Abusers, Toronto.

Marques, J. K., Day, D. M., Nelson, C., & Miner, M. H. (1989). *The sex offender program and evaluation project: Third report to the legislative in response to PC 1365.* Sacramento: California State Department of Mental Health.

Marshall, W. L. (1973). The modification of sexual fantasies: A combined treatment approach to the reduction of deviant sexual behavior. *Behaviour Research and Therapy, 11,* 557–564.

Marshall, W. L. (1979). Satiation therapy: A procedure for reducing deviant sexual arousal. *Journal of Applied Behavioral Analysis, 12,* 10–22.

Marshall, W. L. (1984). L'avenir de la thérapie béhaviorale: Le béhaviorisme bio-social (illustré à partier d'une théorie sur la voil). *Revue de modification du comportement, 14,* 136–149.

Marshall, W. L. (in press). A revised approach to the treatment of men who sexually assault adult females. In G. C. Nagayama Hall & R. Hirschman (Eds.), *Sexual aggression: Issues in etiology and assessment, treatment and policy.* New York: Hemisphere/Harper & Row.

Marshall, W. L., & Barbaree, H. E. (1987). A manual for the treatment of child molesters. *Social and Behavioral Sciences Documents, 17,* 57.

Marshall, W. L., & Barbaree, H. E. (1988). The long-term evaluation of a behavioral treatment program for child molesters. *Behaviour Research and Therapy, 26,* 499–511.

Marshall, W. L., & Barbaree, H. E. (1990a). Sexual violence. In K. Howells & C. Hollin (Eds.), *Clinical approaches to aggression and violence* (pp. 205–246). New York: Wiley.

Marshall, W. L., & Barbaree, H. E. (1990b). An integrated theory of sexual offending. In W. L. Marshall, D. R. Laws, & H. E. Barbaree (Eds.), *Handbook of sexual assault: Issues, theories, and treatment of the offender* (pp. 209–229). New York: Plenum Press.

Marshall, W. L., & Barbaree, H. E. (1990c). Outcome of comprehensive cognitive–behavioral treatment programs. In W. L. Marshall, D. R. Laws, & H. E. Barbaree (Eds.), *Handbook of sexual assault: Issues, theories, and treatment of the offender* (pp. 363–385). New York: Plenum Press.

Marshall, W. L., Barbaree, H. E., & Butt, J. (1988). Sexual offenders against male children: Sexual preferences. *Behaviour Research and Therapy, 26,* 383–391.

Marshall, W. L., Barbaree, H. E., & Christophe, D. (1986). Sexual offenders against female children: Sexual preferences for age of victims and type of behaviour. *Canadian Journal of Behavioral Science, 18,* 424–439.

Marshall, W. L., Barbaree, H. E., Laws, D. R., & Baxter, D. J. (1986, September). *Rapists do not have deviant sexual preferences: Large-scale studies from Canada and California.* A paper presented at the 12th annual meeting of the International Academy of Sex Research, Amsterdam.

Marshall, W. L., & Barrett, S. (1990). *Criminal negligence: Why sex offenders go free.* Toronto: Doubleday.

Marshall, W. L., & Eccles, A. (1991). Issues in clinical practice with sex offenders. *Journal of Interpersonal Violence, 6,* 68–93.

Marshall, W. L., Eccles, A., & Barbaree, H. E. (1991). The treatment of exhibitionists: A focus on sexual deviance versus cognitive and relationship features. *Behaviour Research and Therapy, 29,* 129–135.

Marshall, W. L., Johnston, P., Ward, T., Jones, R., & Hudson, S. M. (1991). *Kia Marama: New Zealand's sex offender program.* Manuscript submitted for publication.

Marshall, W. L., Jones, R., Ward, T., Johnston, P., & Barbaree, H. E. (1991). Treatment outcome with sex offenders. *Clinical Psychology Review.*

Marshall, W. L., Laws, D. R., & Barbaree, H. E. (Eds.). (1990). *Handbook of sexual assault: Issues, theories, and treatment of the offender.* New York: Plenum Press.

Marshall, W. L., Payne, K., Barbaree, H. E., & Eccles, A. (1991). Exhibitionists: Sexual preferences for exposing. *Behaviour Research and Therapy, 29,* 37–40.

Marshall, W. L., & Seidman, B. (1991). [Intimacy and loneliness in sex offenders.] Unpublished data.

Marshall, W. L., Ward, T., Jones, R., Johnston, P., & Barbaree, H. E. (1991). An optimistic evaluation of treatment outcome with sex offenders. *Violence Update, March,* 1–9.

Pearson, H. J., Barbaree, H. E., Southmayd, S. E., & Marshall, W. L. (1991). *Treatment of exhibitionism and obscene telephoning with Buspirone: A case report.* Manuscript submitted for publication.

Pithers, W. D. (1990). Relapse prevention with sexual aggressors: A method for maintaining therapeutic gain and enhancing external supervision. In W. L. Marshall, D. R. Laws, & H. E. Barbaree (Eds.), *Handbook of sexual assault: Issues, theories, and treatment of the offender* (pp. 343–361). New York: Plenun Press.

Pithers, W. D., & Cumming, G. F. (1989). Can relapse be prevented? Initial outcome data from the Vermont Program for sexual aggressors. In D. R. Laws (Ed.), *Relapse prevention with sex offenders* (pp. 313–325). New York: Guilford Press.

Pithers, W. D., Marques, J. K., Gibat, C. C., & Marlatt, G. A. (1983). Relapse prevention with sexual aggressives: A self-control model of treatment and the maintenance of change. In J. G. Greer & I. R. Stuart (Eds.), *The sexual aggressor: Current perspectives on treatment* (pp. 214–239). New York: Van Nostrand Reinhold.

Pithers, W. D., Martin, G. R., & Cumming, G. F. (1989). Vermont Treatment Program for sexual aggressors. In D. R. Laws (Ed.), *Relapse prevention with sex offenders* (pp. 292–310). New York: Guilford Press.

Quinsey, V. L. (1990). *Strategy for the assessment, treatment and management of sex offenders*. A report to Correctional Service of Canada, Ottawa.

Quinsey, V. L., & Marshall, W. L. (1983). Procedures for reducing inappropriate sexual arousal: An evaluation review. In J. G. Greer & I. R. Stuart (Eds.), *The sexual aggressor: Current perspectives on treatment* (pp. 267–289). New York: Van Nostrand Reinhold.

Rice, M. E., Harris, G. T., & Quinsey, V. L. (1990). *Predicting sexual recidivism among treated and untreated extrafamilial child molesters released from a maximum security psychiatric institution*. Manuscript submitted for publication.

Riley, D. R., Hudson, S. M., & Anderson, G. A. (1991). *Demographic and social factors in the prediction of reoffending*. Manuscript submitted for publication.

Segal, Z. V., & Marshall, W. L. (1985). Self-report and behavioral assertion in two groups of sexual offenders. *Journal of Behavior Therapy and Experimental Psychiatry, 16*, 223–229.

Segal, Z. V., & Stermac, L. E. (1990). The role of cognition in sexual assault. In W. L. Marshall, D. R. Laws, & H. E. Barbaree (Eds.), *Handbook of sexual assault: Issues, theories, and treatment of the offender* (pp. 161–172). New York: Plenum Press.

Soothill, K. L., & Gibbens, T. C. N. (1978). Recidivism of sex offenders: A reappraisal. *British Journal of Criminology, 18*, 267–276.

Soothill, K. L., Jack, A., & Gibbens, T. C. N. (1976). Rape: A 22-year cohort study. *Medical Science and the Law, 16*, 62–69.

Stermac, L. E., Segal, Z. V., & Gillis, R. (1990). Social and cultural factors in sexual assault. In W. L. Marshall, D. R. Laws, & H. E. Barbaree (Eds.), *Handbook of sexual assault: Issues, theories, and treatment of the offender* (pp. 143–159). New York: Plenum Press.

CHAPTER 11

CHRONIC PAIN

Michael K. Nicholas
UNIVERSITY OF NEW SOUTH WALES

Chronic, nonmalignant pain is typically described as pain that is not due to malignancy and has persisted longer than the expected recovery period (Bonica, 1977). In most research contexts, an arbitrary period of 6 months is taken as a means of operationally defining pain as "chronic" (Black, 1975). Such pain may persist for many years with varying levels of severity and associated dysfunction or disability (Volinn, Lai, McKinney, & Loeser, 1988). It is often referred to as "intractable"; that is, it is refractory to treatment. Chronic pain has been associated with most areas of the body, but the most frequent sites are in the back, especially the lower back (e.g., Spanswick & Main, 1989; Sternbach, 1986).

Chronic pain associated with different sites may have different pathophysiological bases, and this may be so between individuals with chronic pain at the same site as well (e.g., low back pain). In many cases, no clear physical basis for the persisting pain can be found (Flor & Turk, 1984). But regardless of possible etiology, individuals with chronic pain are often seen as sharing common features, which has led investigators to consider chronic pain a syndrome rather than a symptom (Fordyce, Roberts, & Sternbach, 1985). In particular, individuals experiencing chronic pain, especially those presenting at hospital pain clinics, often report such features as general dysfunction in their daily activities (e.g., work, home, leisure, and social activities), mood and sleep disturbances, long-term use of various medications with associated side effects, and high levels of consumption of medical services. Many also display so-called pain behaviors (Fordyce, 1976), such as excessive resting, pain complaints, grimacing, and limping.

Evidence in support of chronic pain as a syndrome that is to some extent independent of the original cause of the pain comes from a range of sources. For example, a number of studies show that the level of dysfunction experienced by chronic pain patients is associated more with psychological variables, such as distress and maladaptive cognitions, than with pathophysiology (Keefe, 1989; Main, Wood, Hollis, & Spanswick, 1992). Fordyce (1976) and others (e.g., Keefe, Gil, & Rose, 1986; Sanders, 1979) have also argued that many of the problems experienced by chronic pain patients are due to the effects of learning, regardless of the original cause of pain. For example, if a patient finds that lying down results in easing of the pain, he/she may end up lying down for much of the time—resulting in a gradual withdrawal from normal activities, which, in turn, could increase the likelihood of depression (e.g., Lewinsohn & Libet, 1972) as well as the physical consequences of disuse, such as muscle wasting (Troup & Videman, 1989) from which many chronic pain patients suffer. Pain behaviors, such as resting, complaining about pain, and limping can also be reinforced by, for example, the solicitous attention of a concerned spouse or physician (Block & Boyer, 1984; Fordyce, 1976). Equally, attempts at engaging in more "well" behaviors, such as fitness exercises and return to work, can be discouraged through nonreinforcement or even punishment—in the form of either increased levels of pain or the response of significant others, such as employers who may refuse to accept the patient until he/she is declared 100% fit by his/her physician (which is unlikely) (Fordyce, 1976). The role of psychological variables in chronic pain has therefore been mainly concerned with the development and maintenance of the various features associated with chronic pain rather than the initial cause of the pain itself (Flor, Birbaumer, & Turk, 1990). Accordingly, the principal focus in cognitive and behavioral treatments for chronic pain is reduction in the disability, distress, and pain behaviors associated with the pain rather than resolution of the pain (Fordyce, Roberts, & Sternbach, 1985).

EPIDEMIOLOGY AND NATURAL HISTORY

Estimates of the prevalence of chronic pain indicate that approximately 10% of the population experience chronic pain conditions at any one time, although there are slight variations, due in part to differences in definition and measurement techniques. For example, a survey reported by Osterweis, Kleinman, and Mechanic (1987) indicated that about 10% of the U.S. population have pain conditions lasting more than 100 days a year. But a recent Swedish survey revealed that 15%–20% of a randomly selected sample reported continuous or nearly continuous pain for more than 6 months in the neck, shoulders, arms, lower back, and legs (Brattberg, Thorslund, & Wikman, 1989). Crook, Rideout, and Browne (1984) surveyed 372 randomly selected households on the roster of a family practice clinic in Canada and found that 11% of individuals interviewed had "persistent pain" (i.e., they were often troubled by pain, with 60% of this group having had pain for more than 3 years).

Evidence on the natural history of chronic pain problems is mainly derived from back pain studies that indicate that while most people (75%–80%) in industrialized countries experience episodes of low back pain (Horal, 1969; Steinberg, 1982), 80%–90% of these recover within 6 to 8 weeks (Waddell, 1987), but 5%–7% develop chronic, persistent back pain (Frymoyer, 1988; Spitzer, & Quebec Task Force on Spinal Disorders, 1987). In addition, Horal (1969) found that while acute back pain has a high spontaneous remission rate, it also has a high recurrence rate (90% of patients who were "sicklisted"). Horal and others (Dehlin, Hedenrud, & Horal, 1976; Hirsch, Jonsson, & Lewin, 1969) also found that repeat episodes lasted longer and were more severe than the initial occurrence. Relatively little is known about the long-term course of chronic pain and its associated problems, although if an individual is out of work for more than 1 year due to back pain, there is only a 25% chance of his/her returning to work, and after 2 years out of work the chances are almost nil (McGill, 1968). Even after rehabilitative treatments, only 35%–45% of chronic low back pain patients return to work (Linton, 1986). Advantageous results of surgery for chronic low back pain are also somewhat limited, though when performed on the small group of patients who have "appropriate signs and symptoms" of organic pathology, substantial pain relief and improved function are possible (Waddell, Bircher, Finlayson, & Main, 1984). Trief (1983), however, reported that while over 200,000 Americans undergo surgery each year to relieve back pain, after 5 years only 10% of these operations provided satisfactory relief. Furthermore, a study of workman's compensation patients who complained of persistent symptoms following initial surgery and subsequently had additional surgery revealed that most were worse after their third operation than they were before the first one (Waddell et al., 1979). Consistent with these rather gloomy outcomes is the finding that individuals with chronic pain problems consume health care services and compensation insurance funds at disproportionately high rates (Crook et al., 1984). For example, Frymoyer (1988) reported that the 5% of workers who have low back pain symptoms for more than 3 months account for 85% of the costs of compensation and loss of work.

Some studies have suggested that once developed in those patients with no clear signs and symptoms of a surgically treatable physical lesion, the condition does not improve within periods of 1 to 4 years (Main et al.,

1992). Others (Crook et al., 1984) have found that the frequency of pain episodes decreased (but not to zero) over a 2-year follow-up, with associated reductions in distress and use of health care services. There is also evidence that the prevalence of persistent pain varies with age. For example, a number of studies have found that the prevalence of pain problems is highest in the 45–64-year age group, with a gradual decrease in prevalence in subsequent years, apart from joint pain (Brattberg et al., 1989; Sternbach, 1986; Von Korf, Dworkin, Le Resche, & Kruger, 1988). In the case of back pain, the incidence rate appears highest in the 20–30-year age group with no clear sex bias (Flor & Turk, 1984). In sum, while there is evidence that the course of chronic pain and associated levels of dysfunction may fluctuate over the years, it seems that once pain has persisted for at least 1 year, even 3 months in some studies (Linton, Bradley, Jensen, Spangfort, & Sundell, 1989), return to prepain levels of functioning and a pain-free state is unlikely. This conclusion has obvious implications for considerations of relapse following treatment.

COGNITIVE–BEHAVIORAL TREATMENTS FOR CHRONIC PAIN

As mentioned earlier, the cognitive–behavioral treatments for chronic pain are rehabilitative in nature and are typically incorporated into multicomponent programs with each component being aimed at a different aspect of a patient's presenting problems. Most multicomponent pain management programs not only include sessions of cognitive–behavioral therapy, but also explicitly employ cognitive–behavioral principles in the application of all aspects of the program (Fordyce, 1976; Roberts, 1986). Thus, patients may be verbally reinforced by therapy staff for performing physiotherapy exercises. As they progress, the patients receive progressively less reinforcement from the staff, and at the same time the patients are encouraged to reinforce their own efforts. Ideally, the benefits of getting fitter will also help to reinforce the patients' efforts. Similarly, if cognitions such as fears that exercise might cause more damage are thought to be inhibiting a patient's progress, they are addressed by both educational means and training in ways of dealing with such unhelpful cognitions.

The components of most pain management programs usually consist of various exercise regimes to improve general or aerobic fitness and, in some cases, muscle strength (Fordyce, 1976; Lawrence, 1988; Turner, Clancy, McQuade, & Cardenas, 1990); relaxation techniques, along with biofeedback, to reduce muscle tension, facilitate sleep, and improve the management of stress (Gil, Ross, & Keefe, 1988; Linton, 1986); operant–

behavioral approaches to help patients increase their level of activity and reduce the frequency of pain behaviors through such methods as goal setting, planned gradual increments in activity and exercise levels, as well as reinforcement of achievements and nonreinforcement of pain behaviors by therapy staff (Fordyce, 1976; Keefe, 1982; Linton, 1986); cognitive–behavioral approaches to identify and modify maladaptive thinking processes and coping strategies (Philips, 1988; Turk, Meichenbaum, & Genest, 1983; Turner, 1982; Turner & Clancy, 1988); medication reduction regimes to gradually reduce the use of inappropriate medication; and education about chronic pain and its management (Gil et al., 1988; Philips, 1988).

Pain management programs are conducted in both inpatient and outpatient settings, usually in a group format with a range of health care disciplines involved (Fordyce, 1976; Keefe, 1982; Linton, 1986; Turk & Holzman, 1986). Inpatient programs tend to be 3 to 4 weeks in duration, while outpatient programs typically are conducted over 8 to 10 weeks with one session per week (Cinciripini & Floreen, 1982; Kerns, Turk, Holzman, & Rudy, 1986; McArthur, Cohen, Gottlieb, Naliboff, & Schandler, 1987; Philips, 1987; Turner & Clancy, 1988). In general, inpatient programs treat the more dysfunctional, distressed, and medication-dependent patients, relative to those attending outpatient programs (Gerber & Hanson, 1990; Kerns et al., 1986). Reviews of short-term outcome results from both inpatient and outpatient programs have revealed that improvements are usually obtained on measures of disability (e.g., return to work, increased uptime, increased exercise levels), mood (especially depression), medication use, cognitions about pain (especially on maladaptive, catastrophizing congnitions), use of health care resources (reduced), and pain severity (though often not to a clinically significant degree) (Linton, 1986; Keefe, Gil, & Rose, 1986; Turner & Romano, 1984). However, not all patients attending such programs improve on these dimensions, and many of those who do improve do not maintain their improvements at long-term follow-up (Turk & Rudy, 1991). The following section will review the evidence concerning the rate of relapse.

RELAPSE RATES FOLLOWING TREATMENT IN PAIN MANAGEMENT PROGRAMS

Relapse in Chronic Pain Patients

Before examining the rates of relapse following pain management programs, it would seem germane to consider the concept of "relapse" in such an intractable condition as chronic pain. It was established earlier that chronic pain is generally seen as a syndrome comprising a number of dimensions, including not only the experience of persisting pain but also pain behaviors, mood disturbance, dysfunction or disability in normal activities, and often maladaptive or unhelpful cognitions. Furthermore, chronic pain can persist for many years, although the severity, features, and associated problems often fluctuate over time. A recent paper by Tait, Chibnall, and Krause (1990), for example, revealed a relatively low ($r = .44$) correlation on a test–retest reliability assessment of a measure of disability administered 2 months apart using 46 chronic pain patients prior to treatment. The authors noted that, while significant, this correlation was lower than expected given that "disability status generally is viewed as a stable construct" (p. 177). Accordingly, determining relapse rates in such a condition is likely to be problematic. On an individual level, follow-up assessments after completion of treatment conducted at fixed points in time, such as 3, 6, or 12 months posttreatment, could well present a distorted picture. If the investigator happens to review the patient in a "good" period his/her results are likely to look considerably better than a review striking a "bad" period, such as during a temporary setback, which is not uncommon in chronic pain (Follick, Zitter, & Ahern, 1983). Although the aim of pain management programs is to help the patient both to prevent and to minimize setbacks, there is always the possibility of a setback's occurring for no apparent reason (given that the condition itself is imperfectly understood). Consequently, there is always the possibility that follow-up results in a given patient simply reflect the natural fluctuations in this chronic condition rather than the effects of treatment. Of course, when patients are assessed in groups it could be expected that the potential effects of individual variations would be minimized, although this approach risks overlooking the incidence of relapse.

Some reviewers (e.g., Turk & Rudy, 1991) have considered as evidence of relapse any decline from posttreatment levels of functioning during the follow-up period (e.g., in drug usage, exercise levels, or mood), with pretreatment levels on these variations as covariates. Others have used pretreatment levels of functioning as the baseline and relapse has been seen in terms of decline to baseline levels in the follow-up period (Cairns, Mooney, & Crane, 1982; Moore & Chaney, 1985). However, both approaches seem to make the assumption that the initial measures were stable. But rarely is any evidence presented in treatment outcome studies of baseline stability in the dependent measures employed, whether the baseline is pretreatment or posttreatment scores. Thus, the notion that decline following treatment represents a "return to baseline" in fact only refers to a baseline measured at one point in time and not a stable baseline. It could be the case that treatment has reduced the frequency, but not the amplitude, of natural fluctuations in the condition. If this were true, it could be argued that the treatment had had a lasting effect, albeit not quite what the investigators had intended. Thus, investigators could well overlook clinically significant improvements, such as generally reduced disruption in normal activities despite the occasional setback, due to limitations in their assessment methodology.

One obvious way around this problem is to employ a measure of performance that reflects improvement over an extended period, such as return to work or number of treatments received in the follow-up period versus those received in the pretreatment period. However, these sorts of measures also have methodological problems. For example, data on treatments received, especially in the pretreatment period, are often based on the recall of patients, which is known to be suspect (e.g., Linton, 1986). In addition, data on return to work or additional treatments are often subject to capricious influences well beyond the capacity of any treatment program to account for, such as the behavior of employers when selecting prospective employees or the treatment decisions of future medical caregivers (e.g., Follick et al., 1983). Nevertheless, some studies (Guck, Skultety, Meilman, & Dowd, 1985) have employed multi-criteria, presence–absence measures, such as Roberts and Reinhardt's (1980) operational definition of successful outcome, which reflects performance over a period of time and not just at one point, such as the last week (e.g., employed or, if not, unemployed or retired for reasons other than pain, a housewife by profession, doing volunteer work, or attending training; up and active at least 8 hours per day; receiving no compensation payments for pain; no pain-related hospitalizations since treatment and using no prescribed narcotic or psychotropic medications). Such an approach has the advantage of being clear-cut and not readily subject to week-to-week fluctuations, but it could result in a loss of potentially useful information that a measure reflecting degrees of disability due to pain could provide.

A complex construct like disability is unlikely to be adequately reflected in an all-or-nothing approach like that of Roberts and Reinhardt (1980). As an alternative, some investigators have employed inventories like the Sickness Impact Profile (SIP) (Bergner, Bobbitt, Carter, & Gibson, 1981) (e.g., Nicholas, Wilson, & Goyen, 1991; Peters & Large, 1990; Turner & Clancy, 1988). The SIP is a 136-item inventory that assesses dysfunction due to pain across a range of dimensions. Although the reference period for the SIP is stipulated as the current day, the author's personal experience with this measure suggests that when answering it patients are influenced by their perceptions of how they are functioning more generally. A similar but much shorter instrument than the SIP is the Pain Disability Index (PDI) (Tait, Pollard, Margolis, Duckro, &

Krause, 1987), which does not limit itself to the day of assessment as the reference period. Although not widely used as yet, it appears to have considerable promise (Tait et al., 1990). Similarly, the Multidimensional Pain Inventory (MPI) (Kerns, Turk, & Rudy, 1985) also addresses the degree to which pain is perceived by the patient to interfere with his/her daily activities over an unspecified period.

Considerations about appropriate measures of long-term outcome not only indicate the sorts of issues that need to be addressed in determining the content of a pain management program, they also demonstrate the limitations of attempts to evaluate these programs in isolation from the context in which they operate. In other words, some programs are primarily concerned with return-to-work outcomes (e.g., Hazard et al., 1989), while others, especially those dealing with older age groups, are more concerned with more general improvements in function (e.g., Nicholas et al., 1990). In each case, the meaning of "relapse" could be quite different. One needs to take into account each program's goals or purposes when evaluating outcomes and relapse rates.

Another way of dealing with the problem of the possible effects of natural fluctuations in chronic pain over time on the long-term evaluation of treatment programs is to employ a control group or an alternative treatment group that is also followed up. Unfortunately, most of the pain management outcome studies employing control groups have employed a wait-list control group, which typically covers the treatment period only (e.g., Philips, 1987; Turner, 1982), which means that only that period is controlled for. However, there is a steadily growing list of treatment comparison studies with long-term follow-ups (e.g., Kerns et al., 1986; Melin & Linton, 1988; Nicholas et al., 1991; Turner & Clancy, 1988; Turner et al., 1990).

In summary, the determination of relapse rates in chronic pain treatment studies is to some extent hampered by conceptual and methodological problems. It is with these issues in mind that the evidence on relapse rates is reviewed.

LONG-TERM OUTCOMES AND RELAPSE RATES

Reviews of long-term outcomes following pain management programs have indicated general maintenance of gains of 30%–70% over a period of 1 to 8 years (Keefe et al., 1986; Linton, 1986). However, as Turk and Rudy (1991) point out, this means that 30%–70% of patients treated relapse. Given some of the methodological problems mentioned above, as well as others such as high attrition rates in the follow-up period and a general reliance on questionable follow-up methods (e.g., mailed questionnaires, telephone contact), many findings should be treated with caution. This section examines outcomes on different variables, taking into account various methodological issues. Table 11.1 presents a summary of the findings from a broad selection of long-term outcome studies published from 1973 to 1991.

As can be seen in Table 11.1, determining the degree of maintenance of treatment gains is complicated by the different ways in which outcomes are presented and measured. Some studies report numbers of patients who meet various outcome criteria, while others report group mean scores for a number of domains. Furthermore, some follow-up methods, such as return to clinic for review, can be considered more reliable than others, such as mailed questionnaires, which are more open to influence by family members or ill-considered or incomplete responses. It can also be argued that those patients who return for review simply represent the motivated and successful cases, which could inflate the level of success achieved. An additional complication is the tendency for some studies to report variable follow-up periods, which are then averaged, such as 2 to 38 months with an average of 18.6 months (Corey, Etlin, & Miller, 1987). Given that relapse rates are likely to be higher with the passage of time and that follow-up response rates tend to decline with time, presenting follow-up data based on averaged periods not only makes it difficult to compare studies but also runs the risk of creating an inaccurate picture of relapse rates.

Quite apart from such methodological issues, a considerable amount of variation in response rates is evident between studies and over time, with longer-term follow-ups generally faring more poorly than shorter-term ones. There is, inevitably, some debate over how to treat nonresponders. One view is that they should be considered failures and hence be added to the relapse figures (e.g., Turk & Rudy, 1991). Another view is that providing no difference can be found between responders and nonresponders on pretreatment scores or on demographic or medical status variables, the nonresponders should be discarded (e.g., Hazard et al., 1989). As Turk and Rudy (1991) point out, the latter approach is based on the unproven assumption that such variables are predictive of outcome. At present, there seems to be no generally accepted approach, but the manner in which each study deals with the issue clearly needs to be borne in mind when comparing outcomes across studies.

An examination of those studies presented in Table 11.1 that report outcome in terms of numbers of patients rather than mean scores indicates that reduced disability was maintained by 37%–81% of patients who were followed up over a period of 1 month to 8 years. Reductions in medication use were maintained by 29%–100% of patients, depending on the drug. Improvements in mood were maintained by 94% of patients

TABLE 11.1. Summary of Long-Term Outcome Studies

Study	F/U period	F/U method	Return rate	Outcome
Fordyce et al. (1973)[a]	22 mos. mean	mail	31/36 (86%)	*Disability*: Reduced interference by pain in activities maintained from posttest gains; uptime greater at f/u than at pretest *Pain*: Estimates based on recall, but reduced pain levels at discharge (mean 6/10) maintained at f/u (mean 6.2/10)
Swanson et al. (1979)[a]	1 yr.	mail	not stated	*Disability*: 53% improved at postest, improved work status at f/u *Medication*: 29% maintained posttest levels *Pain*: No change
Gottlieb et al. (1977)[a]	6 mos.	mail	23/72 (32%)	*Disability*: 82% employed or in vocational training
Roberts & Reinhardt[a] (1980)	1–8 yr.	mail, ph.	26/34 (76%)	*Disability* and *medication*: 77% met all criteria for improvement
Malec et al. (1981)[a]	6 mos–2yr.	mail, ph.	32/40 (80%)	*Disability*: 28/40 (70%); at admission, 86% (of 28) unemployed cf. 25% at f/u; at f/u 14% had stopped all exercise, 46% kept up 50%–100% of exercises set *Medication*: (% at discharge vs. f/u): narcotics (0 vs. 23%), other analgesics (0 vs. 50%), relaxants (0 vs. 30%), antidepressants (3 vs. 3%) *Mood*: 70% rated better

Khatami & Rush[a] (1982)	1 yr.	mail	12/14 (completers)	*Mood:* mean BDI scores, 12.7 at admission; 3.6 at f/u *Medication:* (pills/day), at admission, mean 15.1; at f/u 7.2 *Pain:* mean ratings, at admission 53.9% at f/u 19.8%
Cinciripini & Floreen[a] (1982)	6 mos. 1 yr.	mail mail	70% 60%	*Disability:* disability payments reduced from 41% of total at admission to 16% at 6 mos. f/u, & 20% at 1 yr. f/u. 53% working at 6 mos., 50% at 1 yr *Medication:* none: 2.4% at admission, 92.2% at discharge, 64.7% at 6 m. f/u, 55% at 12m. f/u *Pain:* 4.6/10 at admission, 2.2 at discharge, 2.3 at 6 mos., 1.2 at 1 yr
Turner (1982)[bc]	1 mo. 1½–2 yr.	mail	34/34 (100%) 24/34 (71%)	*Disability:* mean SIP scores, for RT group at pretest (14.8), posttest (8.9), 1m. f/u (7.4). For CBT group (19.8), (10.4), (7.4); mean hours worked per week, for RT group pretest (23.8), posttest (23.8), 1 m. (25.3), 1.5 yr. (22.8); for CBT group pretest (18.4), posttest (18.9), 1 mo. (21.9), 1½ yr. (38) *Mood:* (BDI) mean scores for RT pre (12.4), posttest (8.7), 1 mo. (7.4); for CBT group at pretest (15.7), posttest (8.7), 1 mo. (5.6) *Pain:* (visual analogue scale) mean weekly pain for RT group at pretest (64.4), posttest (42.1), 1 mo. (55.6), 1½ yr. (25.8); for CBT at pretest (55.9), post (37.4), 1 mo. (33.8), 1½ yr. (20.6)
Lutz et al. (1983)[a]	23 mos. mean	mail	57 (74%)	*Disability, medication, pain:* 37%–59% improved from pretest to f/u on effects of pain on life-style, medication use, and pain levels

TABLE 11.1. (cont.)

Study	F/U period	F/U method	Return rate	Outcome
Guck et al. (1985)[a]	1–5 yr.	mail	random sample of 20 selected out of 77 (85% of total)	*Disability, medication:* 60% met all criteria *vs.* 0/20 untreated comparison group. *Pain, mood:* (BDI) treated group significantly better than untreated group
Kerns et al. (1985)[bc]	3 mos. 6 mos.	clinic attendance	15/20 (75%)	*Disability:* 65% relative to pretreatment, 16.3% for CBT group; change at 3 mos. f/u- 1.2% for BT group. At 6 mos., 11% for CBT, 11.5% for BT group. *Mood:* (BDI) change at 3 mos. f/u, 13.5% improvement for CBT, -6.7% for BT group; at 6 mos., 7.6% for CBT, 13.8% for BT group. *Pain:* change at 3 mos. f/u, 16.6% for CBT, 0.8% for BT; at 6 mos., 14.7% for CBT, 9.9% for BT group
Corey et al. (1987)[b]	18.6 mos. mean	mail phone	57/72 (79%)	*Disability:* all patients vocationally disabled at pretest; 71% working or equivalent at posttest, 69% at f/u. *Pain:* of those working or equivalent at f/u, mean posttest reductions in pain levels maintained. *Mood:* (coping ability): of those working or equivalent at f/u, mean gains at posttest maintained

Study	Follow-up	Method	Completion	Outcome
Philips (1987)[bc]	2 mos. 1 yr.	clinic attendance	22/25 (88%)	*Disability:* improvement on pretest mean score (44.9) to (40.2) posttest, (30.3) 2 mos. f/u, (27.6) at 1 yr. f/u *Mood:* (BDI) improvement across 4 occasions, from mean 15.9 to 11.4 to 12 to 9.4 at 1 yr. *Pain:* mean intensity (0–5), improvement across 4 occasions, from mean 2.4 to 1.7 to 1.7 to 1½ at 1 yr.
Melin & Linton[ac] (1988)	20 mos. mean	mail	26/28 (93%)	*Disability:* RT/BT: 19% mean improvement in activities of daily living pretreatment to f/u (3% improvement posttreatment to f/u), no improvement relative to wait-list and RT groups *Pain:* RT/BT group significant reduction relative to WL and RT groups *Mood:* (BDI) 48% improvement over pretest in RT/BT but no significant difference cf. WL and RT groups
Turner & Clancy[bc] (1988)	6 mos. 1 yr.	clinic attendance	43/53 (81%)	*Disability:* mean SIP scores, 92% held posttest gains; no difference between cognitive and operant groups at 1 yr. *Pain:* (McGill Pain Questionnaire) both groups continued to improve in f/u period *Pain behaviors* (observer-rated) pretest to posttest improvements in operant group maintained at f/u; cognitive group little change
Maruta et al, (1989)[a]	11 mos. mean	phone	100/100	*Mood:* (research diagnostic criteria) 54% identified as depressed at admission; at discharge, only 2/100 were depressed; at f/u, 8/100 were depressed

TABLE 11.1. (cont.)

Study	F/U period	F/U method	Return rate	Outcome
Hazard et al. (1989)[a]	12 wks. 1 yr.	mail, phone, clinic attendance	40/59 (68%)	*Disability:* return-to-work rate: 81% at 1 yr. f/u; mean Oswestry (disability) scores for those working at 1 yr. f/u: 39 at admission, 24 at discharge, 25 at 12 wks. f/u, 20 at 1-yr f/u *Mood:* (BDI) mean scores for those working at 1 yr. f/u: pretest (12.2), posttest (5.9), 12 wk f/u (8.3), 1 yr. (6.2) *Pain:* (Million Pain Analogue Scale) mean scores for those working at 1 yr. f/u: pretest (98), posttest (68), 12 wk f/u (66), 1 yr. (64)
Turner et al. (1990)[bc]	6 mos. 1 yr.	mail mail	45/57 (79%) 47/57 (82%)	*Disability:* compared to pretest, the 3 treatment groups maintained posttreatment improvements on SIP *Mood:* (CES-D Scale) the 3 groups generally maintained postest gains, none returned to baseline levels *Pain:* (McGill Pain Questionnaire) all 3 groups improved over pretest levels at both f/us
Skinner et al. (1990)[b]	1 mo.	clinic attendance	34/34 (100%)	*Disability:* mean Oswestry scores improved from 39.0 at 1 mo. baseline, to 37.6 at pretest, 32.2 at posttest, & 30.8 at f/u *Mood:* (Zung SDS) mean pre–post score improved from 28 to 23.6 and at 1 mo. f/u was 21.0

Study	Follow-up	Contact	N (%)	Outcomes
Cott et al (1990)[b]	2 mos.	contact with	176 (100%)	*Pain:* (VAS) mean pre-post scores improved from 61.2 to 51.3 & at 1 mo. f/u was 51.2 *Medication:* (mean number analgesics per week) 22.0 at pre, 10.4 at post, 6.3 at 1 mo. f/u
				Disability: of field-managed employer pain group, 82% and patients successful (resumed work, improved performance, job change, retraining, less disabled—if retired) vs. 6/17 (35%) office-treated pain group
Nicholas et al. (1991)[bc]	6 mos. 12 mos.	most by clinic attendance, some by mail	48/58 (83%) 39/58 (67%)	*Disability:* compared to pretreatment, posttest gains on mean SIP scores generally maintained in treatment conditions *Mood:* (BDI) pre–post gains in mean scores generally maintained in treatment groups *Pain:* mean weekly prepost gains in mean scores generally maintained at f/u

Note. BDI-Beck Depression Inventory; CES-D = Center for Epidemiological Studies Depression Scale; SIP = Sickness Impact Profile; VAS = Visual Analogue Scale; Zung SDS = Zung Self-rating Depression Scale; CBT = Cognitive–Behavioral Therapy; RT = Relaxation Training; BT = Behavioral Therapy.
[a]Inpatient treatment (in some cases [e.g., Hazard et al.] patients stay in nearby hotel and attend clinic most of each day for 3–4 weeks, which essentially is equivalent to inpatient treatment).
[b]Outpatient treatment (usually, patients attend clinic 3–4 hours on 1–2 days a week).
[c]Controlled trial (patients randomly assigned to treatment, alternative treatment, or wait-list conditions).

treated in Maruta, Vatterot, and McHardy's (1989) study, although the fact that the majority of studies reporting maintenance data on mood used mean figures rather than numbers of patients clearly restricts conclusions on this dimension.

When studies employing mean scores are examined, reduced disability posttreatment was maintained in most cases and even further reduced in the follow-up period in some cases (e.g., Hazard et al., 1989; Kerns et al., 1986; Philips, 1987; Skinner et al., 1990; Turner, 1982). Improved mood posttreatment was also maintained at follow-up in most studies and further improved in some (e.g., Kerns et al., 1985; Philips, 1987; Skinner et al., 1990; Turner, 1982). A similar picture emerges for average pain ratings, with most studies finding posttreatment improvements maintained, but fewer reporting further improvements than for disability or mood (e.g., Kerns et al., 1985; Turner, 1982; Turner & Clancy, 1988).

Considering both methods of reporting outcomes together, it seems that pre- to posttreatment improvements in the dependent variables are maintained in a substantial proportion of cases at long-term follow-ups. However, there is a considerable degree of variance in these figures, as reflected in the absolute-numbers approach to reporting outcome, as well as in the standard deviations reported with the mean scores. There is also quite a lot of variation in relapse rates between studies, which suggests that attention should be paid to other differences between the studies, such as patient sample, treatment contents, and follow-up methods. In this connection, it is interesting to compare the relative relapse rates of inpatient versus outpatient programs. It has been suggested by some that the mainly operant–behavioral inpatient programs may fare less well in relapse rates compared with the mainly cognitive–behavioral outpatient programs (Holzman, Turk, & Kerns, 1986). This view is based on the reasonable assumption that generalization of treatment effects is likely to be easier from outpatient programs as the patients are required to practice pain management strategies and exercises in the home environment throughout the treatment period and they do not face the task of attempting to transfer such skills only when the program is completed, as is the case in most inpatient programs. However, it should also be remembered that patients attending inpatient programs are generally more disabled than those attending outpatient programs, a factor that clearly makes straightforward comparisons difficult (e.g., Kerns et al., 1985; Hanson & Gerber, 1990). Furthermore, there are no long-term follow-up results available from studies comparing outcomes on patients randomly assigned to inpatient and outpatient programs, although at least two such studies are nearing completion (Nicholas et al., 1990; Peters & Large, 1991). Examinations of the studies presented in Table 11.1 indicates, somewhat curiously, that on the whole, inpatient and outpatient studies present their findings in ways that make "eyeball" comparisons difficult because most inpatient studies employ the number-of-patients approach while most outpatient studies employ the mean scores approach. As a result, all that can safely be said about the issue is that it is not proven.

In summary, while there is a large degree of variability in long-term outcomes between studies, some relapse in treatment gains is demonstrated by all of the studies examined. This suggests that there may be both general and specific factors that contribute to the variance in maintenance of treatment gains across studies. The following section examines these questions in an attempt to shed light on possible ways to reduce relapse rates.

FACTORS ASSOCIATED WITH RELAPSE

At least five main factors are frequently considered to contribute to posttreatment relapse. These include (1) the patient's home or work environment, (2) the behavior of the patient's medical caregivers, (3) the patient's beliefs about his/her pain and its treatment, (4) the patient's failure to employ the strategies and techniques taught during the treatment program, and (5) the content of the treatment program (Follick et al., 1983; Fordyce, 1976; Hanson & Gerber, 1990; Meichenbaum & Turk, 1987; Turk & Rudy, 1991).

Home Environment

Once the patient returns to the home environment, he/she is vulnerable to reinforcement of pain behaviors and nonreinforcement of well behaviors, particularly if this has been the pattern in the past (Fordyce, 1976). For example, Gil, Keefe, Crisson, and Van Delfsen (1987) reported that chronic pain patients who were satisfied with the level of social support they were receiving displayed higher levels of pain behavior than those patients who were less satisfied with the level of social support, irrespective of the availability of that support. Gil et al. (1987) interpreted this to mean that it is not the availability of social support that is important for the reinforcement of pain behavior but rather the perceived quality of that support. This finding was corroborated by Flor, Kerns, and Turk (1987), who found that patients with a solicitous spouse reported more pain, lower activity levels, and more satisfaction with their marriage compared to those with a less solicitous spouse. Interestingly, however, Flor et al. (1987) also found that it was the patients' perceptions of what their spouse did that was related to their pain and activity levels rather than what the spouse said he/she did. Thus, if there is no change in the perceived nature of social support, especially support that is contingent on pain behavior, following a patient's discharge from a pain management program, it is likely that pain behaviors will persist. This conclusion suggests that some family or spousal involvement in the treatment program could help to reduce relapse, either by changing the family's pain-contingent behavior or by changing the patient's perception of the support he/she is receiving. However, examination of those studies that have addressed this issue reveals little apparent effect associated with including spouses in the treatment program.

Moore and Chaney (1985), for example, randomly assigned chronic pain patients either to a cognitive–behavioral treatment that included spousal involvement or to one that did not. However, there were no differential maintenance effects at follow-up for either condition, although, interestingly, the level of marital satisfaction improved more in the group that did not include the spouses. A similar finding was reported by Turner and Clancy (1988), who compared a spouse-involved operant–behavioral group with a cognitive–behavioral group (with no spousal involvement). At 12 months follow-up, there were no significant differences between conditions, although the cognitive–behavioral group did improve more in the follow-up period than did the operant group. In a subsequent study by the same authors (Turner et al., 1990), comparing spouse-involved operant–behavioral treatment with an exercise-only condition (with no spousal involvement) also found no difference between conditions at 12 months follow-up—although, as the authors acknowledged, it could be argued that as both groups were only mildly disabled by pain pretreatment, major changes could not be expected.

All other studies that have included spouses in the treatment program have not controlled for this variable and thus can only be considered pre–posttreatment studies and their results therefore require replication in controlled trials. For example, Corey et al. (1987), in a quite innovative approach, conducted their treatment program in each patient's home and incorporated other family members in the program. Excellent long-term results were achieved, with 69.4% of patients assessed as successful an average of 18.6 months posttreatment. A similar approach was reported by Cott, Anchel, Goldberg, Fabich, and Parkinson (1990), who compared a large group of (mostly) chronic pain patients treated in their home by "field consultants" with a group of similar, but uninsured, patients who were given similar treatment in a clinical setting. Both conditions included family involvement, though the home-based condition was more comprehensive in its attention to environmental factors. Although the groups were not randomly assigned, the comparison between interventions does provide at least a guide to their relative efficacies. A

3-month follow-up revealed that the home-based group was significantly less disabled than the clinic-based group. Successful outcome, defined as either return to work or reduced limitations on work, exercise, or daily activities, was achieved by 84% of the home-based group versus 61% of the clinical group. In their inpatient program, Cinciripini and Floreen (1982) included family members, where possible in the last 3 days of the program, and they too reported good but declining maintenance effects at 1-year follow-up. Thus, while these studies all achieved impressive long-term outcomes, none actually established whether or not there had been changes, or perceived changes, in spousal behavior following treatment. It remains to be established that the inclusion of spouses in the treatment program aids relapse prevention (RP).

Work Environment

The contribution of the work environment to relapse has not been as systematically studied as the family role; however, there is evidence, both direct and indirect, that bears on the issue. Waddell, Morris, Di Paola, Bircher, and Finlayson (1986), for example, followed up some 185 back pain patients who had undergone various surgical procedures for their back conditions and found that the best predictors of return to work were length of time out of work and type of work. In other words, the longer the back patients studied were out of work, the less likely they were to return, and if the nature of their work made it difficult to perform, given their back conditions, return to work was also less likely. Thus, a bricklayer with back pain would probably have more trouble returning to his/her work than, say, a psychologist with back pain. Sandstrom (1985) also found that length of time out of work was a significant predictor of return to work in chronic low back pain patients, but only at older ages. More recently, Gallagher et al. (1989) also found that age and length of time out of work were significant predictors of return to work in low back pain patients, along with ease of ability to change occupations (with greater ability to change, the better the chances of return to work). Gallagher et al. (1989) interpreted their results to indicate that being out of work could result in a progressive loss of work-related skills and that treatment programs should therefore focus on overcoming such deficits, as espoused by the "work-hardening" programs (Tramposh, 1988). Certainly, this view is consistent with the high return-to-work rates achieved by treatment programs that included work simulation/hardening, such as those described by Hazard et al. (1989) and Mayer et al. (1987). Taking a different approach to this issue, Linton et al. (1989) demonstrated that when nurses with back pain were given a combined physical and behavioral therapy program, while still employed, follow-up review at 6 months posttreatment revealed that their absenteeism rates were significantly reduced compared to a wait-list control group. Taken together, these results indicate that not only is the practice of work-related skills important to improving return-to-work rates, but limiting the time out of work before treatment begins can also help.

The evidence that return to work may also be influenced by the worker's age and type of work suggests that the work environment itself plays an important role. Numerous anecdotal accounts indicate that workers with a history of accident or workman's compensation do find it difficult to obtain work, particularly when in competition with younger people with unblemished records and at times of economic recession (e.g., Mersky, 1988). A recent prospective study (Bigos et al., 1991) also found that report of back injury by workers in a large aircraft factory was most closely associated with the level of satisfaction workers derived from their jobs. Furthermore, solicitous behavior by the workers' superiors toward the workers during any out-of-work period due to acute back pain seemed to be an important factor in improving return-to-work rates in this study. It seems likely, therefore, that the achievement and maintenance of high return-to-work rates partly depends on early intervention (before too much time out of work has elapsed), adequate preparation for work during treatment, and the cooperative behavior of the future/ current employers.

Medical Management

It has been suggested that if the patient's medical caregivers continue to offer or provide further treatment following the patient's discharge from a pain management program, they effectively risk reinforcing persisting disability, passivity, and pain behaviors in the patient (Keefe, Gil, & Rose, 1986; Main & Parker, 1989; Turk & Rudy, 1991). Waddell et al. (1979), for example, found that patients with chronic low back pain who continued to complain about their symptoms following initial surgery and later underwent more surgery were mostly worse after the third operation than they were before the first. In an earlier study, Waddell, Main, Morris, Di Paola, and Gray (1984) reported that the amount of treatment received by 380 patients with backache of at least 3 months' duration was related more to their distress and illness behavior than to identified physical disease. Spanswick and Main (1989) reported similar findings in relation to the prescription and use of narcotic analgesics by chronic low back pain patients. These findings illustrate a point made by Keefe et al. (1986): that both the physician's and patient's behaviors need to be considered in these situations. Namely, if patients do not change what they say about their pain, despite improvements in function, they risk eliciting further interventions from their physicians and other caregivers. In this context, it is interesting to note that Pither and Nicholas (1991a) reported that a majority (65%) of 89 chronic pain patients assessed for a pain management program continued to strongly believe that doctors would ultimately cure their pain, despite a mean duration of pain of 9.7 years and numerous unsuccessful treatments. Such undiminished faith in surgical/medical treatments, despite contradictory experiences, provides an indication of the vulnerability of patients to continued offers of treatment. From this perspective, pain management programs need to focus on both the verbal pain behaviors of the patients and ways of improving coordination between a pain program and the patients' ongoing medical caregivers. Unfortunately, given the present state of "poorly integrated" (Pilowsky, 1988, p. 1) education about pain in medical schools, the problem of the physician's behavior may be expected to persist.

There is, however, some evidence that patients' verbal pain behaviors can be altered during pain management programs. Cinciripini and Floreen (1982), for example, reported significant reductions in observed pain talk by their patients as well as significant increases in pro-health talk. Unfortunately, as their follow-up data were based on mailed questionnaires, no information is available on the maintenance of these changes in the follow-up period, although 61% of the patients followed up did report no pain-related physician visits up to 12 months posttreatment. Interestingly, patients in this study also reported mean reductions in pain severity of 52% at discharge relative to baseline. Patients interviewed by Keefe et al. (1986) indicated that they would require reductions in pain severity of this magnitude to consider themselves improved. Examination of most of the studies presented in Table 11.1 reveals that few can match such reductions, despite reporting statistically significant reductions in pain severity. However, the importance of this issue is open to debate. It should be noted that the patients referred to by Keefe et al. (1986) were questioned about their required reductions in pain severity on entering their program. It is generally the intention of pain management programs to improve patients' capacities to cope with their persisting pain, such that a successful patient might be able to say something like: "Well, I've still got my pain, but it doesn't bother me as much as before." From this perspective, what patients say about their pain at the start of a pain management program is arguably less important than what they say at the end, bearing in mind that their earlier views have been shaped and reinforced by a health care system that mostly has focused on pain reduction as the primary goal of treatment. As they have to return to that general system upon discharge, it can also be argued that patients should be trained not only to talk about their pain in different ways, but also to be more assertive when dealing with their physicians so that they find it easier to decline offers of further treatment they do not want (e.g., Gerber & Hanson, 1990; Philips, 1988).

Patient Beliefs

A number of studies have demonstrated a close link between levels of distress and disability in pain patients and their beliefs and cognitions about pain (e.g., Crisson & Keefe, 1988; Dolce, 1987; Main & Spanswick, 1991; Rudy, Kerns, & Turk, 1988; Williams & Keefe, 1991; Williams & Thorn, 1989). Some treatment outcome studies have also found improvements on measures of unhelpful beliefs or cognitions about pain posttreatment, along with improvements on measures of disability and mood (e.g., Nicholas et al., 1991; Philips, 1987; Turner & Clancy, 1988). These studies have also reported maintenance of mean posttreatment gains in the follow-up period. Furthermore, beliefs that the pain was mysterious and that it would persist have been associated with poor compliance with physical and behavioral therapies for pain management by chronic pain patients (Williams & Thorn, 1989). More recently, Williams and Keefe (1991) found that patients who had completed a pain management program and held such beliefs in the enduring and mysterious nature of their pain were less likely to use cognitive coping strategies and more likely to catastrophize about their pain than patients who viewed their pain as understandable and unlikely to persist. In addition, the former group of patients was less likely to rate their coping strategies as effective in controlling and decreasing pain. This corroborates an earlier finding by Crisson and Keefe (1988), which indicated that chronic pain patients who viewed outcomes as controlled by chance also rated their abilities to control and decrease pain as poor and exhibited greater psychological distress. In sum, there is evidence that certain types of beliefs about pain are associated not only with greater distress and disability in chronic pain patients, but also with poor compliance with physical, behavioral, and cognitive pain management methods.

A number of investigators have also examined Bandura's (1977) concept of self-efficacy beliefs in relation to treatment outcome in chronic pain patients. Bandura's (1977) basic proposition is that a person's behavior is influenced, in part, by his/her belief in the ability to perform that behavior. Kores, Murphy, Rosenthal, Elias, and North (1990), for example, reported that the strength of patient's self-efficacy beliefs, as measured by a five-category rating scale, significantly improved following a pain management program. They also found that patients with high self-efficacy scores posttreatment rated themselves at follow-up (3 to 11 months later) as more improved, using less medication, and having substantially (although not significantly) less downtime than those with low posttreatment self-efficacy scores. Philips (1987) also found that an increase in self-efficacy ratings (defined as amount of perceived control over pain) was associated with improvements in avoidance behavior, mood, and affective reaction to pain following cognitive–behavioral treatment with a mixed group of chronic pain patients. More recently, Nicholas, Wilson, and Goyen (1992) reported that in a sample of chronic low back pain patients who had completed a cognitive–behavioral group treatment, increased ratings on a ten-item self-efficacy scale were associated with improvements in disability, as measured by SIP scores completed by both patients and their significant others, increased use of active coping strategies for dealing with pain, and reduced pain-related medication consumption.

Council, Ahern, Follick, and Kline (1988) reported that self-efficacy ratings for ten specific movements were predictive of both the performance of many of these movements (on a separate occasion) and questionnaire ratings of physical impairment in more general daily activities with a sample of chronic low back pain patients. Consistent with the Kores et al. (1990) study, Dolce, Crocker, and Doleys (1986a) found that increased self-efficacy expectancies posttreatment were predictive of increased exercise levels, work, and medication-free coping 6 to 12 months following a behavioral pain management program. Interestingly, Dolce, Crocker, Moletteire, and Doleys (1986b) reported an association between self-efficacy ratings and exercise levels in some of those patients whose exercise levels increased during treatment, but not in others. This finding was replicated by Dolce et al. (1986c). In reviewing these findings, Dolce (1988) proposed that those patients who improve during treatment but do not strengthen their self-efficacy beliefs may be more likely to relapse when treatment is completed. He suggested that such patients may not persist with the skills and strategies learned during treatment if they do not believe they can exercise them away from the treatment setting, especially if they attribute their improvement to external causes, such as the therapists on the program. To some extent, the results mentioned earlier by Kores et al. (1990) provide general support for this view, but Dolce's (1988) prediction of relapse in those patients who improve during treatment but do not strengthen their self-efficacy beliefs remains to be fully tested.

In summary, there is a considerable amount of evidence that a reduction in unhelpful beliefs and cognitions following cognitive–behavioral pain management treatment is associated with improvement on measures of disability and mood. Furthermore, there is some evidence that those patients who do not change unhelpful beliefs and cognitions following cognitive–behavioral pain management treatment have an increased risk of relapse. Unfortunately, as few treatment outcome studies seem to test for changes in unhelpful beliefs and cognitions posttreatment, the generality of these findings and the possibility of a causal role for cognitions remain to be established. It is also not clear how important a change in beliefs and cognitions is in RP, relative to such factors as the work or home environment and posttreatment medical management.

Compliance/Adherence with Treatment Strategies

Failure to practice or employ coping strategies, exercises, relaxation techniques, and other methods taught during treatment in the follow-up period has also been seen as contributing to relapse (Philips, 1988; Turk & Rudy, 1991; Meichenbaum & Turk, 1987). Lutz, Silbret, and Olshan (1983), for example, reported that of the 74% of patients who responded to a mail follow-up an average of 23 months after an inpatient pain management program, only 42% acknowledged the continued practice of individual therapeutic regimens. Furthermore, only 12.3% of respondents reported continued practice of the total package of therapeutic regimens, and continued practice of any one regimen was unrelated to the practice of others. Even so, Lutz et al. (1983) noted that 37%–59% of respondents reported improvements at follow-up, relative to pretreatment, on measures of pain, activity, and medication use. As Turk and Rudy (1991) pointed out, while such findings indicate a rather low continued practice rate, they also raise the question of the role of continued practice of pain management methods in the maintenance of treatment gains. It is conceivable, for example, that some patients may not need to continue their initial pain management regimen once they reach a certain level of functioning. From an operant point of view, it can be argued that while the treatment program may be necessary to get the patient up to "freeway speed," environmental sources of reinforcement (e.g., at work) can be expected to maintain the patient's improved functioning. In this view, continued practice of many pain management strategies is necessary only on an as-needed basis, whenever there is a flare-up in pain, for example. From the author's experience, anecdotal accounts from a number of discharged patients are consistent with this perspective. Certainly, there is presently no evidence that any particular rate of continued practice of exercises, relaxation, etc., is necessary for RP in chronic pain patients. That is, although there is evidence that maintaining a reasonable level of physical activity is important for chronic pain patients, it is not clear how often particular exercises should be performed (e.g., Troup, 1989). The few studies that have reported continued rates of practice of such techniques in the follow-up period generally found only modest practice frequencies, such as two to five times a week for many techniques or exercises, presuming such reports were reliable (e.g., Cinciripini & Floreen, 1982; Dolce et al., 1986a; Meilman, Skultety, Guck, & Sullivan, 1985; Nicholas et al., 1991; Philips, 1987; Turner, 1982). Interestingly, these studies also reported that many posttreatment improvements were generally maintained.

On the other hand, it could be argued that pre- to posttreatment improvements were not related to the practice of particular pain management techniques in the first place but to some other, unidentified factor associated with the treatment. Certainly, given the lack of dismantling studies in the pain management literature, where the contribution of different treatment components is examined, it is presently impossible to say with any confidence which components are necessary, for which problem, and for which patient. In this regard, the dismantling studies that have been conducted have reported somewhat inconclusive results, although there is a suggestion that different components have effects at different stages (e.g., Heinrich, Cohen, Naliboff, Collins, & Bonebakker, 1985; Kerns et al., 1985; Nicholas et al., 1991; Turner, 1982; Turner & Clancy, 1988; Turner et al., 1990).

Turk and Rudy (1991) also noted that continued practice of pain management strategies may not guarantee continued maintenance of initial treatment gains. It was mentioned earlier that in some patients, improvements on exercise measures were not matched with improvements in self-efficacy ratings (Dolce et al., 1986b) and that Kores et al. (1990) had found that those patients with low posttreatment self-efficacy ratings tended to have poorer outcomes at follow-up than those with high posttreatment self-efficacy ratings. Furthermore, Lutz et al. (1983) reported that the continued practice of one pain management technique in the follow-up period was unrelated to the performance of others. These findings suggest that individual behavioral measures, such as exercise levels, may not be reliable indicators of performance in other domains or on other occasions. Lutz et al.'s (1983) finding, for example, could suggest that while a patient with chronic low back pain continued to practice, say, exercises each day, if at the same time he/she was overdoing some other activities, a flare-up in pain intensity and possible relapse could be expected (e.g., Philips, 1988). Thus, in some circumstances it is conceivable that continued practice of selected treatment techniques may have little impact on RP.

In summary, the contribution of continued practice of pain management techniques and strategies to RP posttreatment remains unclear. It is particularly striking to note the apparent discrepancy between generally good maintenance of many treatment gains on the one hand and the relatively modest maintenance of treatment regimens on the other. However, it must be acknowledged that as few studies have reported data on this issue, any conclusions should be regarded as tentative. Clearly, though, greater attention ought to be paid to this issue in the treatment outcome literature; reporting the outcome only seldom tells us much about which factors may have been responsible.

STRATEGIES TO PREVENT RELAPSE

A number of studies, but by no means all, have reported particular strategies that have been employed, as part of the treatment program, to prevent relapse or to promote maintenance of treatment gains. These include preparation of each patient for discharge with plans for dealing with flare-ups in pain; setting specific posttreatment goals that are seen by the patient as relevant to his/her home or work environment; identifying activities and situations that should be avoided to reduce the risk of flare-ups; assertiveness training on ways of dealing with others in the home or work environment; and devising plans to deal with major setbacks, such as cut back on exercises or phone the pain clinic team or other former patients (e.g., Gil, Ross, & Keefe, 1988; Philips, 1988). Such predischarge preparations may also include the provision of written instructions or summaries of the treatment program for subsequent reference (e.g., Hanson & Gerber, 1990). Other strategies to enhance patients' learning and recall of information and techniques relevant to pain management have included the programmed repetition of key didactic sessions as well the exposure of patients in the program to successful former patients to emphasize the relevance of the program to the home/ work environment. Some programs have also employed short refresher courses or booster sessions for former patients in the follow-up period or even prearranged telephone calls from the pain team at set intervals (e.g., Cinciripini & Floreen, 1982; Hanson & Gerber, 1990; Ross et al., 1988).

When return to work is an important goal, a number of programs have arranged for discharged patients to attend "workstations" (e.g., Fordyce, 1976) where, for periods of up to several months, they are enabled to gradually build up their working hours in a real work environment, often under the supervision of a rehabilitation counselor associated with the pain program, until they are ready for a return to normal work. As mentioned earlier, some programs incorporate "work hardening" within the program itself (e.g., Hazard et al., 1989; Mayer et al., 1987). Typically, this involves engaging in activities such as lifting and carrying, which simulate the sorts of tasks patients are required to perform in their normal work settings. Of course, as with all exercises and activities in these programs, such activities are built up gradually throughout the program.

The inclusion of the patient's family in some aspects of the program is another common strategy. In some cases, this involves members of the family coming to the program a day or two before discharge (e.g., Cincir-ipini & Floreen, 1982). In others, the family may be involved throughout the program (e.g., Moore & Chaney, 1985; Corey et al., 1987; Cott et al., 1990). For the most part, the involvement of family members is confined to education about the approach to pain management employed in the program, and little attempt is made to address major or long-standing family/marital conflicts, which may best be dealt with by referral to appropriate agencies once the program is completed.

Quite apart from specific preparations for the follow-up period, the basic components of cognitive–behavioral pain management programs can also be seen as contributing to RP. These include training in self-control, which encompasses basic behavioral techniques such as self-monitoring and self-reinforcement for achieving set goals, as well as more cognitive techniques, such as identifying unhelpful cognitions, challeng-ing them, and substituting more adaptive cognitions (e.g., Hanson & Gerber, 1990; Philips, 1988; Turk et al., 1983). The cognitive techniques also include general problem-solving strategies, which may also be ap-plied by the patient to the normal vicissitudes of daily life stressors that may make their pain more difficult to cope with or, equally, that their pain may exacerbate (e.g., Turner, 1987). In this context, it is interesting to note Philips's (1987) finding that patients who had completed their cognitive–behavioral pain management program reported that their pain was less of a problem to them. Furthermore, there was an associated implication that the patients were better able to discriminate between their pain and other emotional problems. Thus, rather than attributing all or most of their problems to persisting pain, Philips's findings suggest that as a result of successful cognitive–behavioral treatment, chronic pain patients are better able to identify which problems are related to their pain and which are related to other factors. If this outcome were to be established, it would allow for more specific, and possibly more effective, targeting of problem areas so that, for example, pain-related problems could be dealt with in a pain management program and marital problems could be dealt with separately by appropriate agencies.

The major problem with all of these RP strategies is that apart from inclusion of the patients' spouses, none have been experimentally evalu-ated with chronic pain patients. Thus, it is difficult to know which strategy should be employed and which should not. Most programs appear to take a "scattergun" approach to this issue by including a range of methods, presumably in the hope that one or more may help a given patient, although one method may not suit all patients. Judging from the pub-lished studies, no method seems superior to another, although those studies with some of the lowest relapse rates appear to share some features. In particular, they either include the practice of exercises and work-related activities in the home/work environment during the program or many of the exercises and activities employed to simulate typical work tasks (e.g., Corey et al., 1987; Cott et al., 1990; Hazard et al., 1989; Linton et al., 1989; Mayer et al., 1987). However, it should also be noted that most of these studies, like others in this area, had various selection criteria for admission to their programs that could have resulted in unrepresentative samples with possible implications for the generalizability of the ensuing findings. For example, Hazard et al. (1989) rejected all patients who were denied financial payment for the program by their insurance carriers, while Cott et al. (1990) gave such patients a clinic-based program rather than the home-based one undertaken by patients with insurance coverage. Until there are controlled trials of these different strategies with randomly assigned patients, treatment programs will have to persist in employing as many as feasible of the RP strategies outlined here.

CLINICAL AND RESEARCH RECOMMENDATIONS

This chapter indicates that many of the gains achieved following cognitive–behavioral pain management programs are maintained at long-term follow-up by a substantial proportion of the patients treated. However, there is a degree of relapse evident in all studies and a great deal of variation in relapse rates between studies. A number of factors have been proposed to account for the relapse findings, but it is clear that considerably more research is required both to substantiate these proposals and to identify which interventions provide the most effective RP. Some of the shortcomings identified in the existing literature in this area include methodological issues, such as problematic and insufficient follow-up methods and imprecise follow-up periods, and a general lack of controlled trials with randomly assigned patients, especially studies comparing different RP strategies. Numerous questions remain unanswered: for example, the value of including spouses in the treatment program, the role of cognitive variables as predictors of long-term outcome, necessary rates of practice of physical exercise and relaxation techniques, and indeed their role, if any, in RP, and the relative merits of inpatient versus outpatient programs and for which patients. The value of follow-up booster sessions is also unclear.

It was suggested that many pain management programs appear to throw almost every conceivable RP measure at their patients in the hope that something will stick. While this may be seen as an inefficient way to proceed, it also highlights some important points about relapse and its prevention or minimization in chronic pain patients that this chapter has illustrated. Namely, relapse in chronic pain patients is related to many factors whose salience may not only vary over time but can also be only partially predicted or controllable. Thus, home and work environments, the behavior of future medical caregivers, and different exercises and techniques all appear to contribute to posttreatment relapse rates, but their relative impacts seem to vary, possibly according to such factors as the length of time the patients have been out of work (where work is a relevant issue), the patients' cognitions and beliefs about their pain and significant others, and the nature of the treatment program. Given all this complexity, and until a number of the questions about relapse mentioned above are resolved, it is not surprising that clinicians adopt as comprehensive an approach as possible to RP. Nevertheless, the chapter outlines the range of issues the clinican should consider when addressing the problem of RP in this difficult group of patients.

REFERENCES

Bandura, A. (1977). Self-efficacy: Toward a unifying theory of behavioral change. *Psychological Review, 84,* 191–215.

Bergner, M., Bobbitt, R. A., Carter, W. B., & Gibson, B. S. (1981). The Sickness Impact Profile: Development and revision of a health status measure. *Medical Care, 19,* 787–805.

Bigos, S. J., Battie, M. C., Spengler, D. M., Fisher, L. D., Fordyce, W. E., Hansson, T. H., Nachemson, A. F., & Wortley, M. D. (1991). A prospective study of work perceptions and psychosocial factors affecting the report of back injury. *Spine, 16,* 1–6.

Black, R. G. (1975). The chronic pain syndrome. *Surgical Clinics of North America, 55,* 999–1011.

Block, A. R., & Boyer, S. L. (1984). The spouse's adjustment to chronic pain: Cognitive and emotional factors. *Social Science and Medicine, 19,* 1313–1318.

Bonica, J. J. (1977). Neurophysiologic and pathophysiologic aspects of acute and chronic pain. *Archives of Surgery, 112,* 750–761.

Brattberg, G., Thorslund, M., & Wikman, A. (1989). The prevalence of pain in a general population. The results of a postal survey in a county of Sweden. *Pain, 37,* 223–228.

Cairns, D., Mooney, V., & Crane, P. (1982). Spinal pain rehabilitation: Inpatient and outpatient treatment results and development of predictors for outcome. *Spine, 9,* 91–95.

Cinciripini, P. M., & Floreen, A. (1982). An evaluation of a behavioral program for chronic pain. *Journal of Behavioral Medicine, 5,* 375–389.

Corey, D. T., Etlin, D., & Miller, P. C. (1987). A home-based management and rehabilitation program: An evaluation. *Pain, 29,* 219–230.

Cott, A., Anchel, H., Goldberg, W. M., Fabich, M., & Parkinson, W. (1990). Non-institutional treatment of chronic pain by field management: An outcome study with comparison group. *Pain, 40,* 183–194.

Council, J. R., Ahern, D. K., Follick, M. J., & Kline, C. L. (1988). Expectancies and functional impairment in chronic low back pain. *Pain, 33,* 323–332.

Crisson, J. E., & Keefe, F. J. (1988). The relationship of locus of control to pain coping strategies and psychological distress in chronic pain patients. *Pain, 35,* 147–154.

Crook, J., Rideout, E., & Browne, G. (1984). The prevalence of pain complaints in a general population. *Pain, 18,* 299–314.

Dehlin, O., Hedenrud, B., & Horal, J. (1976). Back symptoms in nursing aids in a geriatric hospital. *Scandinavian Journal of Rehabilitation Medicine, 8,* 47–53.

Dolce, J. J. (1987). Self-efficacy and disability beliefs in behavioral treatment of chronic pain. *Behaviour Research and Therapy, 25,* 289–299.

Dolce, J. J., Crocker, M. F., & Doleys, D. M. (1986a). Prediction of outcome among chronic pain patients. *Behaviour Research and Therapy, 24,* 313–319.

Dolce, J. J., Crocker, M. F., Moletteire, C., & Doleys, D. M. (1986b). Exercise quotas, anticipatory concern, and self-efficacy expectancies in chronic pain: A preliminary report. *Pain, 24,* 365–372.

Dolce, J. J., Doleys, D. M., Raczynski, J. M., Lossie, J., Poole, L., & Smith, M. (1986c). The role of self-efficacy expectancies in the prediction of pain tolerance. *Pain, 27,* 261–272.

Flor, H., Birbaumer, N., & Turk, D. C. (1990). The psychobiology of chronic pain. *Advances in Behaviour Research and Therapy, 12,* 47–84.

Flor, H., Kerns, R. D., & Turk, D. C. (1987). The role of spouse reinforcement, perceived pain, and activity levels of chronic pain patients. *Journal of Psychosomatic Research, 31,* 251–259.

Flor, H., & Turk, D. C. (1984). Etiological theories and treatments for chronic back pain: I. Somatic models and interventions. *Pain, 19,* 105–121.

Follick, M. J., Zitter, R. E., & Ahern, D. K. (1983). Failures in the operant treatment of chronic pain. In E. B. Foa & P. M. G. Emmelkamp (Eds.), *Failures in behavior therapy* (pp. 331–334). New York: Wiley.

Fordyce, W. E., Fowler, R. S., Lehmann, J. F., de Lateur, B. J., Sand, P. L., & Trieschmann, R. (1973). Operant conditioning in the treatment of disability due to chronic low back pain. *Archives of Physical Medicine and Rehabilitation, 54,* 399–408.

Fordyce, W. E., Roberts, A. H., & Sternbach, R. A. (1985). The behavioral management of chronic pain: A response to critics. *Pain, 22,* 113–125.

Frymoyer, J. W. (1988). Back pain and sciatica. *New England Journal of Medicine, 318,* 291–300.

Gallagher, R. M., Rauh, V., Haugh, L. D., Milhous, R., Callas, P. W., Langelier, R., McClallen, J. M., & Frymoyer, J. (1989). Determinants of return-to-work among low back pain patients. *Pain, 39,* 55–68.

Gil, K. M., Keefe, F. J., Crisson, J. E., & Van Delfsen, P. J. (1987). Social support and pain behavior. *Pain, 29,* 209–218.

Gil, K. M., Ross, S. L., & Keefe, F. J. (1988). Behavioral management of chronic pain: Four pain management protocols. In R. D. France & K. R. R. Krishnan (Eds.), *Chronic pain* (pp. 376–413). Washington, DC: American Psychiatric Press.

Gottlieb, H., Streit, L. C., Koller, Maderasky, Z., Hockersmith, V., Kellman, M., & Wagner, J. (1977). Comprehensive rehabilitation of patients having chronic low back pain. *Archives of Physical Medicine and Rehabilitation, 58*, 101–108.

Guck, T. P., Skultety, F. M., Meilman, P. W., & Dowd, E. T. (1985). Multidisciplinary pain centre follow-up study: Evaluation with a no-treatment control group. *Pain, 21,* 295–306.

Hanson, K. E., & Gerber, K. E. (1990). *Coping with chronic pain: A guide to patient self-management.* New York: Guilford Press.

Hazard, R. G., Fenwick, J. W., Kalisch, S. M., Redmond, J., Reeves, V., Reid, R., & Frymoyer, J. W. (1989). Functional restoration with behavioral support: A one-year prospective study of patients with chronic low-back pain. *Spine, 14,* 157–161.

Heinrich, R. L., Cohen, M. J., Naliboff, B. D., Collins, G. A., & Bonebakker, A. D. (1985). Comparing physical and behavior therapy for chronic low back pain on physical abilities, psychological distress, and patients perceptions. *Journal of Behavioral Medicine, 8,* 61–78.

Hirsch, C., Jonsson, B., & Lewin, T. (1969). Low-back symptoms in a Swedish female population. *Clinical Orthopaedics, 63,* 171–176.

Holzman, A. D., Turk, D. C., & Kerns, R. D. (1986). The cognitive–behavioral approach to the management of chronic pain. In A. D. Holzman & D. C. Turk (Eds.), *Pain management: A handbook of psychological treatment approaches* (pp. 31–50). New York: Pergamon Press.

Horal, J. (1969). The clinical appearance of low back disorders in the City of Gothenberg, Sweden. *Acta Orthopaedica Scandinavia, 118,* (Suppl.) 8–73.

Keefe, F. J. (1982). Behavioral assessment and treatment of chronic pain: Current status and future directions. *Journal of Consulting and Clinical Psychology, 50,* 896–911.

Keefe, F. J. (1989). Behavioral assessment methods for chronic pain. In R. D. France & K. R. R. Krishnan (Eds.), *Chronic pain* (pp. 298–321). Washington, DC: American Psychiatric Press.

Keefe, F. J., Gil, K. M., & Rose, S. C. (1986). Behavioral approaches in the multidisciplinary management of chronic pain: Programs and issues. *Clinical Psychology Review, 6,* 87–113.

Kerns, R. D., Turk, D. C., Holzman, A. D., & Rudy, T. E. (1986). Comparison of cognitive–behavioral approaches to the outpatient treatment of chronic pain. *The Clinical Journal of Pain, 1,* 195–203.

Kerns, R. D., Turk, D. C., & Rudy, T. E. (1985). The West Haven–Yale Multidimensional Pain Inventory (WHYMPI). *Pain, 23,* 345–356.

Khatami, M., & Rush, A. J. (1982). A one-year follow-up of the multimodal treatment for chronic pain. *Pain, 14,* 45–52.

Kores, R., Murphy, W. D., Rosenthal, T., Elias, D., & North, W. C. (1990). Predicting outcome of chronic pain treatment via a modified self-efficacy scale. *Behaviour Research and Therapy, 28,* 165–169.

Lawrence, L. M. (1988). Physiotherapy in chronic pain. In R. D. France & K. R. R. Krishnan (Eds.), *Chronic pain* (pp. 452–483). Washington, DC: American Psychiatric Press.

Lewinsohn, P. M., & Libet, J. (1972). Pleasant events, activity schedules, and depression. *Journal of Abnormal Psychology, 79,* 291–295.

Linton, S. J. (1986). Behavioral remediation of chronic pain: A status report. *Pain, 24,* 125–141.

Linton, S. J., Bradley, L. A., Jensen, I., Spangfort, E., & Sundell, L. (1989). The secondary prevention of low-back pain: A controlled study with follow-up. *Pain, 36,* 197–208.

Lutz, R. L., Silbret, M., & Olshan, N. (1983). Treatment outcome and compliance with therapeutic regimens: Long-term follow-up in a multidisciplinary pain program. *Pain, 17,* 301–308.

Main, C. J., & Parker, H. (1989). The evaluation and outcome of pain management programmes for chronic low back pain. In M. Roland & J. Jenner (Eds.), *Back pain: New approaches to education and rehabilitation* (pp. 129–155). Manchester: Manchester University Press.

Main, C. J., Wood, P. L. R., Hollis, S., & Spanswick, C. C. (1992). The distress and risk assessment method (D.R.A.M.): A simple patient classification to identify distress and evaluate the risk of poor outcome. *Spine, 17,* 42–52.

Main, C. J., & Spanswick, C. C. (1991). A comparison of cognitive measures in low back pain: Statistical structure and clinical validity at initial assessment. *Pain, 46,* 287–298.

Malec, J., Cayner, J. J., Harvey, R. F., & Timming, R. C. (1981). Pain management: Long-term follow-up of an inpatient program. *Archives of Physical Medicine and Rehabilitation, 62,* 369–372.

Maruta, T., Vatterot, M. K., & McHardy, M. J. (1989). Pain management and an antidepressant: Long-term resolution of pain-associated depression. *Pain, 36,* 335–38.

Mayer, T. G., Gatchel, R. J., Mayer, H., Kishino, N., Keeley, J., & Mooney, V. (1987). A prospective 2-year study of functional restoration in industrial low back injury. An objective assessment procedure. *Journal of the American Medical Association, 258,* 1763–1767.

McArthur, D. L., Cohen, M. J., Gottlieb, H. J., Naliboff, B. D., & Schandler, S. L. (1987). Treating chronic low back pain. I. Admissions to initial follow-up. *Pain, 29,* 1–22.

McGill, C. M. (1968). Industrial back problems, a control program. *Journal of Occupational Medicine, 10,* 174–178.

Meichenbaum, D., & Turk, D. C. (1987). *Facilitating treatment adherence: A practitioner's guidebook.* New York: Plenum Press.

Meilman, P. W., Skultety, F. M., Guck, E. T., & Sullivan, P. (1985). Benign chronic pain: 18-month to 10-year follow-up of a multidisciplinary pain unit treatment program. *Clinical Journal of Pain, 1,* 131–137.

Melin, L., & Linton, S. J. (1988). A follow-up study of a comprehensive behavioural treatment programme for chronic pain patients. *Behavioural Psychotherapy, 16,* 313–322.

Mersky, H. (1988). Back pain and disability. Letter to the editor. *Pain, 34*, 213.

Moore, J. E., & Chaney, E. F. (1985). Outpatient group treatment of chronic pain: Effects of spouse involvement. *Journal of Consulting and Clinical Psychology, 53*, 326–334.

Nicholas, M. K., Williams, A. C. deC., Richardson, P. H., Pither, C. E., Justins, D. M., Chamberlain, J. H., Harding, V. R., Shannon, E. M., Ralphs, J. A., & Fraser, M. (1990, April). *The establishment of a programme for the controlled evaluation of inpatient behavioural pain management*. Paper presented at the 6th World Congress on Pain, Adelaide, Australia.

Nicholas, M. K., Wilson, P. H., & Goyen, J. (1991). An evaluation of cognitive and behavioral treatments for chronic low back pain, with and without relaxation training. *Behaviour Research and Therapy, 29*, 225–238.

Nicholas, M. K., Wilson, P. H., & Goyen, J. (1992). Comparison of cognitive–behavioral group treatment and an alternative, nonpsychological treatment for chronic low back pain. *Pain, 48*, 339–347.

Osterweis, W., Kleinman, A., & Mechanic, D. (Eds.). (1987). *Pain and disability: Clinical, behavioral, and public policy perspectives*. Washington, DC: National Academy Press.

Peters, J. L., & Large, R. G. (1990). A randomized controlled trial evaluating in and out-patient pain management programs. *Pain, 41*, 283–294.

Philips, H. C. (1987). The effects of behavioural treatment on chronic pain. *Behaviour Research and Therapy, 25*, 365–377.

Philips, H. C. (1988). *The psychological management of chronic pain*. New York: Springer.

Pilowsky, I. (1988). An outline curriculum on pain for medical schools. *Pain, 33*, 1–2.

Pither, C. E., & Nicholas, M. K. (1991a). The identification of iatrogenic factors in the development of chronic pain syndromes: Abnormal treatment behaviour? In M. R. Bond, J. E. Charlton, & C. J. Woolf (Eds.), *Proceedings of the VIth World Congress on Pain* (429–434). Amsterdam: Elsevier.

Pither, C. E., & Nicholas, M. K. (1991b). Psychological approaches in chronic pain management. *British Medical Bulletin, 47*, 743–761.

Roberts, A. H. (1986). The operant approach to the management of pain and excess disability. In A. D. Holzman & D. C. Turk (Eds.), *Pain management: A handbook of psychological treatment approaches* (pp. 10–30). New York: Pergamon Press.

Roberts, A. H., & Reinhardt, L. (1980). The behavioral management of chronic pain: Long-term follow-up with comparison groups. *Pain, 25*, 337–343.

Rudy, T. E., Kerns, R. D., & Turk, D. C. (1988). Chronic pain and depression: Toward a cognitive–behavioral mediation model. *Pain, 35*, 129–140.

Sanders, S. H. (1979). Behavioral assessment and treatment of clinical pain: Appraisal and status. In M. Hersen, M. Eisler, & P. Miller (Eds.), *Progress in behavior modification* (p. 8). New York: Academic Press.

Sandstrom, J. (1985). Clinical and social factors in rehabilitation of patients with chronic low back pain. *Scandinavian Journal of Rehabilitation Medicine, 18*, 35–43.

Spanswick, C. C., & Main, C. J. (1989). The role of the anaesthestist in the management of chronic low back pain. In M. Roland & J. Jenner (Eds.), *Back pain: New approaches to education and rehabilitation* (pp. 108–126). Manchester: Manchester University Press.

Spitzer, W. O., & Quebec Task Force on Spinal Disorders. (1987). Scientific approach to the assessment and management of activity-related spinal disorders: A monograph for clinicians. *Spine, 12* (Suppl. S1–S59).

Steinberg, G. G. (1982). Epidemiology of low back pain. In M. Stanton-Hicks & R. A. Boas (Eds.), *Chronic low back pain* (pp. 1–14). New York: Raven Press.

Sternbach, R. A. (1986). Survey of pain in the United States: The Nuprin pain report. *The Clinical Journal of Pain, 2,* 49–53.

Swanson, D. W., Maruta, T., & Swensen, W. M. (1979). Results of behavior modification in the treatment of chronic pain. *Psychosomatic Medicine, 41,* 55–61.

Tait, R. C., Chibnall, J. T., & Krause, S. (1990). The Pain Disability Index: Psychometric properties. *Pain, 40,* 171–182.

Tait, R. C., Pollard, C. A., Margolis, R. B., Duckro, P. N., & Krause, S. (1987). The Pain Disability Index: Psychometric and validity data. *Archives of Physical Medicine and Rehabilitation, 68,* 438–441.

Tramposh, A. K. (1988). Work-related therapy for the injured reduces return-to-work barriers. *Occupational Health and Safety,* April, 55–82.

Trief, P. M. (1983). Chronic back pain: A tripartite model of outcome. *Archives of Physical Medicine and Rehabilitation, 64,* 53–56.

Troup, J. D. G., & Videman, T. (1989). Inactivity and the aetiopathogenesis of musculoskeletal disorders. *Clinical Biomechanics, 4,* 173–178.

Turk, D. C., & Holzman, A. D. (1986). Commonalities among psychological approaches in the treatment of chronic pain: Specifying the meta-constructs. In A. D. Holzman & D. C. Turk (Eds.), *Pain management: A handbook of psychological treatment approaches* (pp. 257–268). New York: Pergamon Press.

Turk, D. C., Meichenbaum, D. H., & Genest, M. (1983). *Pain and behavioral medicine: A cognitive–behavioral perspective.* New York: Guilford Press.

Turk, D. C., & Rudy, T. E. (1991). Neglected topics in the treatment of chronic pain patients—relapse, noncompliance, and adherence enhancement. *Pain, 44,* 5–28.

Turner, J. A. (1982). Comparison of group progressive-relaxation training and cognitive–behavioral group therapy for chronic low back pain. *Pain, 50,* 757–765.

Turner, J. A., & Clancy, S. (1988). Comparison of operant–behavioral and cognitive–behavioral group treatment for chronic low back pain. *Journal of Consulting and Clinical Psychology, 56,* 261–266.

Turner, J. A., Clancy, S., McQuade, K. J., & Cardenas, D. D. (1990). Effectiveness of behavioral therapy for chronic low back pain: A component analysis. *Journal of Consulting and Clinical Psychology, 58,* 573–579.

Turner, J. A., & Romano, J. M. (1984). Evaluating psychologic interventions for chronic pain: Issues and recent developments. In C. Benedetti, C. R. Chapman, & G. Moricca (Eds.), *Advances in pain research and therapy* (p. 7). New York: Raven Press.

Volinn, E., Lai, D., McKinney, S., & Loeser, J. D. (1988). When back pain becomes disabling: A regional analysis. *Pain, 33,* 33–40.

Von Korff, A., Dworkin, S. F., Le Resche, L., & Kruger, A. (1988). An epidemiologic comparison of pain complaints. *Pain, 32,* 173–183.

Waddell, G. (1987). A new clinical model for the treatment of low back pain. *Spine, 12,* 632–644.

Waddell, G., Bircher, M., Finlayson, D., & Main, C. J. (1984). Symptoms and signs: Physical illness or illness behaviour? *British Medical Journal, 289,* 739–741.

Waddell, G., Kummel, E., Lotto, W. N., Graham, J. D., Hall, H., & McCulloch, J. A. (1979). Failed lumbar disc surgery and repeat surgery following industrial injuries. *Journal of Bone and Joint Surgery, 61A,* 201–207.

Waddell, G., Main, C. J., Morris, E. W., Di Paola, M., & Gray, I. C. M. (1984). Chronic low back pain, psychological distress and illness behaviour. *Spine, 9,* 209–213.

Waddell, G., Morris, E. W., Di Paola, M., Bircher, M., & Finlayson, D. (1986). A concept of illness as an improved basis for surgical decisions in low back disorders. *Spine, 11,* 712–719.

Williams, D. A., & Keefe, F. J. (1991). Pain beliefs and the use of cognitive–behavioral coping strategies. *Pain, 46,* 185–194.

Williams, D. A., & Thorn, B. E. (1989). An empirical assessment of pain beliefs. *Pain, 36,* 351–358.

CHAPTER 12

MARITAL DISTRESS

Paula Truax
Neil Jacobson
UNIVERSITY OF WASHINGTON

It is no secret that divorce rates have skyrocketed over the past several decades. Marital distress rates for intact marriages are also remarkably high, with 50% of married couples reporting significant distress (Mace & Mace, 1980). It would be difficult to imagine that the institution of marriage could have survived unscathed through the myriad technological, life-style, and value changes over the past century. Thus, the current state of nuclear family is in crisis. Both divorce and marital distress take a significant toll on spouses, children, and society at large (cf. Emery, 1982).

Along with the increased potential for marital dissolution and significant levels of marital distress has been the development of marital therapy. Since the '60s, the practice and study of marital therapy have exploded in an attempt to meet the ever-increasing demand for marital repair and enhancement. Nearly every theoretical perspective and therapeutic technique has been applied to help couples improve their marital satisfaction (Gurman, Kniskern, & Pinsof, 1986). Despite the wide practice of marital therapy and accompanying anecdotal writings, there is a relative dearth of controlled clinical trials evaluating its effectiveness. Even fewer studies have assessed marital therapy's long-term efficacy. The extent to which couples maintain their therapeutic gains is unknown.

An important exception to this rule has been behavioral marital therapy (BMT), which, since its origin in the late '60s, has been at the leading edge of scientific inquiry into marital therapy (see Baucom & Hoffman, 1986; Beach & O'Leary, 1985; Gurman et al., 1986; Hahlweg &

Markman, 1988; Jacobson, Follette, & Elwood, 1984). BMT's consistently supported efficacy in relieving marital distress has won it the status of the "state-of-the-art technology" or "gold standard" against which newcomers to marital therapy research compare their therapies (cf. Johnson & Greenberg, 1985; Snyder & Wills, 1989). Parallel to BMT's position at the hub of marital therapy research, this paper focuses primarily on BMT and secondarily on other researched marital therapy approaches as they compare to BMT. The first section follows BMT's development from its conception to its form at present.

BMT'S HISTORICAL DEVELOPMENT

Behavioral marital therapy has undergone a number of changes since its birth in the late '60s. Consistent with the traditional behavioral commitment to empirical observation, BMT interventions have been refined and improved in cadence with new experimental findings. This reciprocal relationship between empirical study and technological development has resulted in omitting, revising, and adding to the original interventions that have characterized BMT.

BMT in the '60s and '70s

Along with behavioral therapy's *zeitgeist* in the late '60s, many of the earliest attempts to apply behavioral techniques to married couples were extrapolations from behavioral interventions for institutionalized populations and children (Jacobson, 1991a). These early interventions included contingency contracting, quid pro quo agreements (cf. Jacobson & Margolin, 1979; Stuart, 1969), and token economies (cf. Stuart, 1969). With contingency contracting and quid pro quo agreements, written statements are used to specify how each spouse's behavioral change will be contingent upon the other spouse's corresponding changes. If a wife wants her husband to talk to her more and the husband wants to watch football on TV without being nagged, the husband may agree to 1 hour of conversation in exchange for 1 hour of nag-free TV watching. In token economies, one spouse is in charge of awarding tokens for a desired behavioral change while the receiving spouse "cashes in" the tokens for another desired behavior. Thus, the wife may give the husband a token for each hour of conversation that he exchanges for TV time.

As the following sections indicate, these interventions were moderately helpful in the short term, although no long-term follow-ups are available. These less-than-impressive initial results combined with contractual/token interventions' unknown durability pointed to a need for change. Indeed, by the time these outcome studies reached fruition, most behavioral marital therapists had dropped contractual interventions from their repertoire. The more recent behavioral marital therapy literature corroborates this observation and consistently declares these interventions obsolete (Jacobson, 1983).

This behavioral revolution opened marital therapy to much needed empirical scrutiny. At the same time, there were significant limitations to directly transposing interventions from grossly impaired and skill-deficient populations to married couples. These contractual interventions were believed to efficiently teach couples behavioral reciprocity while addressing the target complaints. In effect, however, the behavioral patterns that led to marital distress may have been inadvertently reinforced. Distressed couples are frequently caught in an aversive control cycle in which their relationship-improvement behaviors are contingent upon their partner's efforts to improve the relationship. Marital therapists hear all too frequently, "I won't change until he does," and "I'm not about to make the first move." Distressed couples are typically expert at "keeping score." The very process of making their behavior mutually contingent upon the other may entrench them even more deeply in their dysfunctional patterns. Thus, even though these contractual/token interventions were temporarily effective in relieving distress over instrumental concerns, durable improvement was unlikely.

BMT in the '80s

In an effort to circumvent this problem, the next generation of BMT was based primarily on behavioral observations of married couples (Jacobson & Margolin, 1979). Such observations suggested that couples' cognitions about their own and their partner's behavior were related to whether behavioral changes occurred and whether such changes contributed to improved marital satisfaction. Thus, cognitive interventions were added to the BMT package within the social learning perspective. Behavioral change remained the primary goal, although cognitive techniques were used to facilitate behavioral change. Cognitive changes were perceived as a potential means to an end rather than an end in themselves.

During this era, BMT became characterized by a time-limited series of procedures (approximately 20 sessions) including careful assessment, setting a collaborative context for the couple's behavioral change, behavioral exchange, communication training, problem-solving skills, and generalization. The explicit behavioral interventions included didactics (verbal and written), role playing, and therapist modeling, as well as providing and encouraging reinforcement for new target behaviors. The facilitative cognitive interventions were primarily to increase positive expectancies about therapeutic success.

Since behavioral treatment of any kind hinges on accurate behavioral analysis of existing strengths and problems, assessment is taken very seriously. Assessment typically involves at least the initial two sessions. Usually, the couple is interviewed together in the first session and individually in the second session. Both sessions' focus is on behavior-specific information about the presenting problem as well as on past and current strengths in the relationship. The goals for the couple are to help them begin thinking about their relationship in behavioral/learning model terms and to "set the stage for therapeutic change by building positive expectancies and trust in the couple, and by actually providing them with some benefits" (Jacobson & Margolin, 1979, p. 51). The therapist's goal is to get a better understanding of the functional relationship between the spouses' behaviors.

In the third session, the therapist presents a formulation of the couple's strengths and weakness, proposes a plan for change, and introduces a new context in which change will be more likely. Consistent with the goal of developing positive expectancies, strengths are emphasized first, followed by a behavioral description of the presenting problems. To educate the couple on behavioral reciprocity and to help them move away from a position of blame, marital problems are framed as the inadvertent mutual reinforcement of dysfunctional behaviors stemming from skill deficits. The therapeutic plan typically involves increasing the number of positive behavioral exchanges and skills training in communication and problem solving. Therapist statements of optimism and research findings supporting BMT's efficacy are presented to increase positive change expectancies. The couple is also asked to adopt a collaborative relationship view in which problems are mutually maintained. The defeating circular logic of "I won't change until he or she does" is challenged. Couples are encouraged to improve their marriage by focusing on each member's behavior, without waiting for the other to change. Before the conclusion of the third session, the therapist requests a commitment from each spouse to follow through with weekly therapy sessions and homework and at least to attempt a collaborative relationship view.

Characteristically, the subsequent three sessions are devoted to increasing the couple's positive behavioral exchanges. Spouses are instructed to increase their partner's marital satisfaction by engaging in behaviors they believe will be pleasing for their spouse. The goals of this intervention include (1) trying out their new collaborative focus; (2) illustrating behavioral reciprocity; (3) inadvertently reducing the frequency of negative behaviors, because of time spent engaging in positive behaviors; and (4) increasing each spouse's reinforcement potential. Because spouses are encouraged simply to increase the frequency of previously mastered behaviors rather than to attempt new or complex behaviors, successful implementation is more likely. Positive expectancies and relationship efficacy are increased, while therapy becomes a discriminative stimulus for the reinforcement of relationship-changing behavior.

Training in basic communication skills, including nonverbals (e.g., posture, eye contact) and paraphrasing, usually follows behavioral exchange. Because couples vary widely in their basic communication skills, this, like the other modules, is implemented differently depending on the couple's need. For couples genuinely deficient in basic communication skills, the interventions would be skills training and practice on important nonverbal and verbal skills. Although most couples have mastered basic communication skills and use them consistently in other contexts (e.g., with friends, at work), they may not be using them in marital interactions. In this case, the goal is to have the couple practice the skills in the presence of one another, so they may experience reinforcing results and thus increase the likelihood that the behavior will be emitted in the same context in the future.

After behavioral exchange has helped the couple to get in touch with positive marital rewards and communication training has set the stage for skills training, therapy's primary focus shifts to problem-solving training. Except for approximately the last three sessions, the remainder of therapy is devoted to teaching problem-solving skills and applying them to increasingly complex and emotionally charged issues. The goal is to collaboratively discuss salient problems and come to an agreement on mutual behavioral change. Couples are trained to follow a specific format and adhere to some basic rules. The format involves (1) careful, behavior-specific problem definition; (2) acceptance of mutual responsibility; (3) mutual verbal commitment to work on solving the problem; (4) brainstorming solutions; (5) evaluating the pros and cons of each proposal; and (6) developing a mutual change agreement. The basic rules are to avoid overgeneralizations (e.g., "never," "always") and derogatory adjectives (e.g., "lazy," "inconsiderate"); to be neutral rather than negative; to talk only about observable behaviors; to paraphrase; to focus on solutions; and to be willing to compromise. All of the general behavioral techniques discussed above are used throughout this module. The couple learns in an interactive didactic format with the skills modeled by the therapist. The couple is coached in how to improve the reinforcement value of their behavior and attend to the reinforcing aspects of the interaction (e.g., feeling heard and understood) rather than to the negative aspects (e.g., change agreement is not immediately reached). The eventual goal for the couple to experience the natural reinforcements in the process as well as in the outcome.

Although the primary goal of the final three sessions is relapse prevention (RP), it is viewed more as a consolidation of the generalization and maintenance foundations embedded in the first 17 sessions. Throughout therapy, generalization from therapy to daily life is facilitated through weekly homework assignments and phasing out therapist reinforcement by increasingly drawing attention to natural reinforcers within the marriage. Maintenance is also inherent with the skills-training rationale, since the goal is mastery of a relationship-building toolbox for application to future as well as current problems.

Unique to the final sessions, with their RP, focus on the following: "state of the relationship meetings," personalization of the problem-solving format, anticipation of future problems, and the extension of intervals between sessions. Couples are encouraged to have weekly state-of-the-relationship meetings after therapy termination so that problem solving will continue and improvements will be reinforced. To increase the likelihood that couples will continue active problem solving, they are aided in finding a format that meets problem-solving goals but incorporates the couple's natural problem-solving style. For example, couples are initially taught to save problems for predetermined problem-solving sessions rather than attempting to discuss them in the heat of the moment. Some couples may find it extremely uncomfortable to wait, however, and may be able to solve problems on the spot as long as they adhere to the problem-solving rules. Others may solve problems best without any kind of rigid format except to wait until a circumscribed time. Future problems and plans for circumventing undue distress are also anticipated (e.g., retirement, birth of a child). In an effort to simulate life after therapy termination, the between-session intervals are increased so that skills can be implemented with a minimum of therapist intervention. The goal is to elicit positive expectancies about maintenance of in-therapy gains while troubleshooting any potential problems.

As the data presented in the following section indicate, the immediate effects of this version of BMT are substantial, with approximately 71% of the marriages significantly improved. The long-term benefits are less clear, however. By 2-year follow-up, at least 25% had relapsed (Jacobson, Schmaling, & Holtzworth-Munroe, 1987). As Baucom and Hoffman (1986) noted in their review of BMT outcome, "many couples still experience some notable distress following short-term BMT" (p. 605).

A metareview of the inter- and intramodal BMT comparisons suggests that some therapy factors are related to enhanced durability. When several factors differentiate compared therapies, isolating salient factors in RP is difficult. Nevertheless, at least one factor stands out as prominent in the more durable therapies: the extent to which therapists are allowed to make careful functional analyses of all behavioral facets (i.e., overt behaviors, thinking, feeling) and tailor the treatments accordingly. Although BMT of the '80s was a vast improvement over the fare of the '60s and '70s this generation's interventions were based on general observations of the typical distressed couple, rather than on individualized behavioral analyses and interventions (Baucom, 1984).

BMT in the '90s

The newest generation of BMT has made a gradual, natural migration back to its theoretical roots in behavioral empiricism. This growth has proceeded in two steps. The first began with a more flexible application of the BMT interventions to easily observable and definable behaviors through identifying interactional themes and troubleshooting. The second expanded to address all behavioral aspects, including the more challenging operationalized external manifestations of thinking and feeling through emotional-acceptance interventions.

Initially, the identification of interactional themes and troubleshooting arose in response to the frequent therapeutic need for a strategy to handle between- and within-session arguments, particularly when these conflicts interfered with problem-solving training. Thus, when a couple arrives at therapy with a recent unresolved argument, the therapist has each spouse describe the conflict in his or her own words. Those data are then used to illustrate how each spouse inadvertently reinforces the destructive behavioral pattern. After several enactions of a similar behavioral pattern, an interactional theme is identified that characterizes a key aspect of the couple's conflict. The couple is then encouraged to identify and debrief its occurrence at home. The couple or therapist may also attempt to identify the behaviors necessary to "rechoreograph their dance."

Because of the recency of these interventions, no systematic outcome studies have evaluated their relative efficacy or long-term effectiveness. Clinically, however, these interventions have grown beyond auxiliary facilitators of standard problem-solving training. Frequently, more therapeutic energy has been devoted to the troubleshooting and interactional theme interventions than to the more regimented prefab strategies. While data needed to confirm this shift, the preliminary anecdotal reports are promising.

Another issue that has emerged through these interventions is that changing the discussed behaviors may not always be possible or ultimately desirable. Although couples frequently focus on instrumental concerns (e.g., housework, child care) when describing their unhappiness, they usually use terms like intimacy, understanding, sharing, and togetherness to describe their ideal relationship (Pineo, 1961). This is what sets apart intimate relationships from other types of relationships. Functional compatibility can be achieved with any variety of dyads. If functional compatibility were the primary goal, a new partner could fill that role each week. Instead, it seems that knowing and being known are fundamental reinforcers. Although a focus on instrumental concerns has been consistently found to reduce immediate marital distress, these changes often do not last.

We know that traditional BMT is more effective at reducing negative behaviors than at increasing positive behaviors (cf. Baucom & Hoffman, 1986; Hahlweg, Schindler, Revenstorf, & Brengelmann, 1984). Indeed, even in a BMT therapy directly aimed at increasing positive instrumental behaviors, these behaviors were not substantially increased (Turner, 1972). The most consistently supported difference between distressed and nondistressed couples is that distressed couples engage in more negative behaviors while nondistressed couples emit a higher proportion of positive behaviors (Revenstorf, Hahlweg, Schindler, & Vogel, 1984). These findings are not surprising; they suggest that the simple reduction of negative behaviors without a simultaneous rise in positive behaviors may not be sufficient to help distressed couples genuinely become happy. As Jacobson himself frequently remarks of traditional BMT: It does a good job of helping couples to be better friends but often doesn't make them better lovers. Baucom and Hoffman (1984) remark in their discussion upon the consistent failure to increase positive behaviors:

> The communication skills taught are generally aimed at problem solving. Thus, a number of destructive communications that interfere with the process often tend to be emphasized. . . . In order to have meaning, many positive communications must be spontaneous, emerging from the person's internal thoughts and feelings about the partner or the topic. (p. 600)

Thus, one important key in improving long-term BMT durability may be identification and intervention of the behaviors associated with positive intimate experiences.

Consequently, the most recent BMT innovations have focused on broadening the target behavioral scope to include intimacy behaviors. This constellation of interventions is called "emotional acceptance." The goal is to have couples use the problem interaction to become more intimate rather than to solve the problem themselves, particularly when the problems are not reasonably solvable.

The operational definition of intimacy is difficult, however. While it is generally agreed that intimacy is related to the simultaneous feelings of knowing and being known by another, there is no universally accepted group of overt intimacy behaviors. Thus, the challenge is twofold: (1) to identify salient behavioral sequences likely to promote the feeling of knowing and being known, and (2) to effectively intervene to bring about these behavioral changes.

Skinner (1976) proposes that the extent to which someone is known is synonymous with the extent to which his or her behavior can be predicted. Predictability requires an acute knowledge of both public and private behaviors (p. 190). Similarly, being known is the feeling that one's behavior can be accurately predicted. Public behaviors can be observed by anyone, but private behaviors must be conveyed by the experiencer. Thus, the better spouses are at mutually expressing internal experiences and reinforcing such expression, the greater are the chances that they will feel intimate. Consistent with this conceptualization, the primary goal of emotional-acceptance interventions is to help spouses create a context with which they will be likely to get in contact with the reinforcing feelings of mutual knowledge of one another. The behavioral goals are to increase the expression of pertinent internal experiences and to reinforce this expression.

Interactions around central relationship problems are usually chosen as a focal intervention point because they have the unqiue advantage of simultaneously involving salient private experiences as well as the most negative feelings about not knowing or being known. Typically, such arguments involve each spouse attending to and reporting certain aspects of his or her private experience, such as anger and hostility, while ignoring others. Because the complaining spouse's causal explanation of his or her distress usually involves faults in the listening spouse, the listening spouse is likely to experience these expressions as punishing and to respond with his or her own anger and blame. The result is that each person focuses on how the other is responsible for his or her negative internal experiences, rather than on gaining new information about one another's internal experiences.

The therapeutic goal is to facilitate intimacy-building interactions around major relationship issues through mutual behavioral change. To this end, the complainer is helped to identify and express internal experiences that do not involve blaming, such as desperation or vulnerability. The listening spouse is simultaneously encouraged to attend to and express his or her internal experiences when hearing the new information. Since the listening spouse is less likely to experience feelings of blame and more likely to feel compassion or "softening", the overt response will likely be more reinforcing, thereby increasing the future likelihood of other such expressions. The primary intervention is aimed at creating a context that maximizes the likelihood that such intimacy behaviors will be emitted and reinforced. Specific interventions include (1) providing directives about how to behave more intimately; (2) making suggestions about how to express internal experiences that may have never been aired; (3) reminding the couple of the positive feelings derived from their behavioral differences; (4) emphasizing behavioral sequences that exemplify how the relationship benefits from their differences; (5) pointing out that behavioral differences are a result of different learning histories rather than something each does to the other; (6) educating the couple on how expressing and listening to one another's internal experiences will be mutually reinforcing; and (7) helping the couple understand that interactions that promote intimacy may have more reinforcement potential than actually solving the problem.

Emotional-acceptance interventions may be used with intimacy development as the primary goal, and also either either before or after problem solving. Before problem solving, emotional acceptance is aimed at facilitating problem-solving collaboration. Afterwards, emotional acceptance may help the couple improve their marital satisfaction even if the problem itself has not been resolved.

Like interactional themes and troubleshooting, emotional acceptance is very new. Although plans to investigate it empirically are under way, no systematic data have been collected to date.

These recent dramatic shifts in the face of BMT have evoked criticisms of atheoretical eclecticism (Baucom & Epstein, 1991; Gurman, 1991; Johnson & Greenberg, 1991; Snyder & Wills, 1991). Yet BMT's current focus on careful functional analysis including emotion and cognition is far more consistent with behavioral empiricism than was any of the BMT that came before it. As many BMT researchers have recently noted, its early exclusive focus on instrumental behaviors was to a large extent misguided (Jacobson, 1991a). Although the techniques paralleled the behavioral therapy *zeitgeists*, the transposition of "canned" interventions from relationships with clear power differentials, or populations with clear skill deficits, sidestepped careful behavioral analyses of salient reinforcers for couples. As B. F. Skinner (1976), the behaviorism originator, so aptly wrote:

> A small part of the universe is contained within the skin of each of us. There is no reason why it should have any special status because it lies within this boundary, and eventually we should have a complete account of it from anatomy and physiology. No very good account is now available, however, and it therefore seems all the more important that we should be in touch with it in other ways. We feel it and in some sense observe it, and it would seem foolish to neglect this source of information just because no more than one person can make contact with one inner world. *Nevertheless, our behavior in making that contact needs to be examined* (emphasis added). (p. 24)

As may be legitimately asked, then: "What separates BMT from other approaches such as emotion-focused marital therapy?" Indeed, the comprehensive behaviorism that characterizes "new-wave BMT" neither mandates nor excludes any particular interventions. Instead, behavioral empiricism can be considered more a philosophy to guide intervention choices than a specified set of therapeutic interventions. Perhaps the three most important components of this philosophical perspective are that (1) all public and private experiences are inherently behavior; (2) all behavior is operantly shaped; and (3) while behaviors may be functionally related, they are not causally linked. Behaviorism treats all behavior as essentially the same. Cognitive and emotional experiences are not unique in how they are either developed or modified. Neither do they have special causal properties. Just as sitting in a chair by the computer does not cause typing behavior, neither does thinking "I should get going on this paper" cause typing behavior. Instead, all behaviors (including thinking and feeling) are operantly related to the current external content. The complicating factor, however, is that our only access to internal experiences is through external manifestations. Thus, the goal of emotional-acceptance interventions is to help create a context in which behaving "acceptingly" will be reinforced rather than to change the internal experience of "acceptance." Even though the internal experience may change concurrently, it is also under environmental control and is not believed to be causal.

The application of behavioral empiricism is new to psychotherapy in general and even newer to marital therapy. Considerable refinement and research are needed to accurately identify salient functional relationships and develop interventions that will facilitate durable changes in marital satisfaction reports.

MARITAL THERAPY AND RELAPSE RATES

Despite a plethora of BMT outcome studies, the research designs and assessment methods have typically been most finely tuned to evaluate immediate outcome rather than long-term maintenance. The following two subsections address assessment issues relevant to relapse prediction and outcome studies pertinent to BMT's development in attempting to increase maintenance.

Assessment

As with any outcome evaluation, the target goal must be defined. This is essential to accurately evaluate within-study changes, to make meaningful between-study comparisons, and to predict relapse. With marital therapy research this is a multifaceted task. Since two clients are involved, both individual well-being and marital satisfaction are pertinent. Because the marital therapy focus is relationship enhancement, most outcome studies use marital satisfation reports to evaluate therapeutic success (Whisman, Jacobson, Fruzzetti, & Waltz, 1989). Despite the obvious logic of this choice, there are potential limitations. Individual well-being and marital satisfaction are related (Whisman, Schmaling, & Jacobson, 1988) but not synonymous. Clients who do not experience a positive relationship between individual and marital satisfaction may contribute to either under- or overestimating therapeutic success. A decision to end a relationship because of unresolvable, entrenched marital unhappiness may result in increased feelings of personal well-being. Thus, marital therapy's success is underestimated. Conversely, therapeutic success may be overestimated when marital satisfaction is increased at the expense of uncomfortable individual compromises that result in decreased individual well-being. Not only does this highlight potential ethical issues of exchanging individual well-being for a more harmonious marriage, it also points to a potential relapse predictor. If marital success is based on huge individual compromises, relapse may be more likely. A focus on marital satisfaction to the exclusion of individual well-being may also obscure potentially important differences between treatments.

Even with the general agreement among marital therapy researchers that marital happiness is the most salient variable, the ideal measurement strategy is unclear. There is some dispute over whether self-reports or behavioral observation provides more accurate data (Jacobson, Follette, & Elwood, 1984). In general, self-report instruments are more concise and considerably easier to implement. The most frequently used measures include the Dyadic Adjustment Scale (DAS) (Spanier, 1976), the Marital Satisfaction Inventory (MSI) (Snyder, 1979), and the Locke–Wallace Marital Adjustment Scale (Locke & Wallace, 1959). Their primary goal is to evaluate each spouse's subjective marital satisfaction. The goal in behavioral observation is to identify salient behaviors or contingencies that are outside of the subject's awareness or are impacted by the subject's individual context. Each method has somewhat different goals (e.g., Coding System for Interpersonal Conflict [Rausch, Barry, Hertel, & Swain, 1974]; Marital and Family Interaction Coding System [Olson & Ryder, 1975]; Marital Interaction Coding System [Hops, Wills, Patterson, & Weiss, 1972]; Couples Interaction Scoring System [Gottman, 1979]; Kategoriensystem fur Interpersonelle Kommunikation [Schindler, 1981], but most focus on passing behaviors into positive and negative verbal and nonverbal behaviors (Jacobson, Elwood, & Dallas, 1981). The positivity or negativity is determined by whether the behavior is thought to contribute to improved communication or increased marital happiness. The rationale for behavioral observation's additional time, expense, and energy is that its objectivity adds accuracy (Gottman, 1985; Weiss & Frohman, 1985).

The frequently documented lack of correspondence between behavioral observation and self-report data (e.g., Birchler, Clopton, & Admas, 1984; Floyd, 1988; Gottman, 1979; Margolin, Hatten, John, & Yost, 1985) make this seem unlikely, however. Unless targeted behavioral changes are also accompanied by subjective improvement, it makes little sense to deem observational reports more accurate. The relationship between the observed behaviors and the internal state of marital satisfaction is oinly inferred. Because marital therapy's primary goal is to change an internal experience (i.e., marital satisfaction), external observations can only identify "signs" of this change. Actual behavioral "samples" of the therapeutic goal can only be observed if the goal itself is observable (e.g., smoking behavior) (Jacobson, Follette, & Elwood, 1984). Because each couple brings a different cumulative history to the assessment session, it cannot be assumed that behaviors that appear as signs of marital happiness to observers are being evaluated positively by couples.

The above discrepancy is perplexing, however. Possibly, the coding systems are focused on the wrong behaviors, or we are making the wrong conclusions based on the observed behaviors. It is also possible that although behavioral observations tend not to manifest the predicted relationships immediately following therapy, they may provide important predictive information. Behavioral observation measures may help to differentiate the relapse potential of couples reporting similar posttest marital satsifaction. This is supported by a (Gottman, 1979) study finding that despite positive correlations between positive behaviors and marital satisfaction at posttest, the frequency of posttest positive behaviors was correlated with a greater likelihood of separation at 6-month follow-up (Baucom & Mehlman, 1984). Although there are few studies using behavioral observation data to predict future marital satisfaction or status, the data available suggest that a uniform abandonment of behavioral observation methodology would ignore potentially important RP information.

In addition to reconciling the differences between behavioral observation and self-report measures, decisions must be made about how to treat two spousal accounts of the same relationship. Because each spouse has an opinion about his or her own marital happiness, both of their opinions should be considered in an assessment of therapeutic success. The most common solution is to sum or average data from each partner into a single combined score (Whisman et al., 1989). What this method gains in parsimony, however, it loses in sensitivity to between-spouse differences. One might expect that couples wth large discrepancies between their marital satisfaction ratings would be quite different from couples with similar scores even if both couples had the same averages. A couple's ability to maintain therapeutic gains may well be impacted by the discrepancy between their marital satisfaction levels. Baucom (1984) addressed this issue by investigating whether alternative models of handling dual scores were differentially predictive of marital status 6 months after therapy. The models were (1) summative (adding both spouses' scores); (2) difference (subtracting one spouse's score from the other's; (3) wife- and husband-gender (using each spouse's score independently); and (4) weak-link (using the lowest of the two scores). The weak-link, wife-gender, and summative models were the more powerful in predicting marital status than were the difference or husband-gender models. These findings suggest that the method used to handle dual scores has potential relevance to these scores' helpfulness in predicting therapeutic maintenance.

An additional issue impacting on outcome and follow-up data interpretation is the definition of study eligibility, recovery, and relapse. In contrast to other psychological disorders that rely on the standardized DSM-III-R (American Psychiatric Association [APA], 1987) criteria to establish clinically significant syndromes, no such criteria exist for marital distress. Although a V code specifies that a "marital problem" can be established when "the focus of attention or treatment is a marital problem that is apparently not due to a mental disorder," this is of little help. Distinct distressed and nondistressed groups are difficult to define. The logic quickly becomes circular. Criterion averages for each group are typically extrapolated from means of groups defining themselves as distressed or nondistressed by their therapy-seeking behavior (MSI) (Snyder, 1979) or marital status (DAS) (Spanier, 1976). Although marital satisfaction level is likely to impact on whether couples seek therapy or get divorced, other factors such as socioeconomic status, religion, and children are also involved. Thus, some proportion of unhappy couples do not seek therapy or get divorced. Similarly, some nondistressed couples seek enhancement therapy or come to an amicable dissolution of their marriage. Although better alternatives are not immediately clear, these limitatons should be acknowledged.

This difficulty in separating clinical distress from marital bliss compounds the evaluation of therapeutic success. Until recently, marital therapy success was declared when differences between pre- and posttest group means were statistically significant. Whether a treatment effect exists in the statistical sense has little to do with the clinical significance of the effect, however (Jacobson, 1988; Jacobson, Follette, & Revenstorf, 1984; Jacobson, Follette, Revenstorf, Baucom, Hahlweg, & Margolin, 1984; Jacobson & Truax, 1991). For a treatment to be clinically significant, it must make a durable and significant life difference. If the therapeutic goal is to reduce physically abusive fighting and the number of fights per year is reduced from 50 to 45 across all subjects, the change will likely be statistically significant, but recovery or normalcy could hardly be declared. Response variability is also ignored when simple statistical comparisons are used. Jacobson and colleagues (1988) propose that couple scores be evaluated individually for clinically significant and statistically reliable change. Clinically significant change is established when a couple moves from a clinically distressed group (as defined by criterion measure) to a nonclinically distressed group (as defined by a posttest criterion measure score that is (1) at least 2 standard deviations above mean for distressed group; (2) within 2 standard deviations of the normal population; or (3) closer to the normal mean than to the distressed mean). Statistically reliable change is established when the result of dividing the difference between the pre- and posttest scores by the standard error of the difference score is greater than 1.96 (see Jacobson et al., 1988, for equations). Recovery requires that both criteria are met. Relapse occurs when the couple moves from the recovered to the distressed group. Although it is also reasonable that change should be maintained for a reasonable period of time to be considered clinically significant, no such measures are available in the current clinical significance statistics.

Outcome Studies

As noted previously, the primary goal of BMT research has been to produce immediate results. Perhaps because of rapid changes in the field or because of the difficulty in assessing marital therapy success, most follow-ups have been short. Many follow-ups have spanned only a few months, and although one recent study has followed its subjects for 4 years (Snyder & Wills, 1989), no other comparative marital therapy outcome study has extended its follow-up period beyond 2 years.

There are many controlled BMT outcome studies and generally uniform conclusions to be found across a number of thorough, complete reviews (cf. Gurman, Kniskern, & Pinsof, 1986). Thus, the following discussion reviews a select sample of BMT outcome studies, specifically those that influenced BMT's development in the direction of improving maintenance. Special attention is given to findings that provide information beyond other reviews' frequent conclusions that (1) BMT is better than no treatment; (2) BMT is basically the same as other marital therapies; and (3) none of BMT's component parts are more effective than any others, alone or in combination. In an effort to be sensitive to the methodological concerns raised above, the following information is presented when available: (1) behavioral and self-report measures; (2) the

method for combining both spouses' scores; (3) marital satisfaction
eligibility requirements; and (4) clinical significance statistics.
The first important developmental step in BMT was a shift from
contingency contracting and token economy interventions to communication and problem-solving approaches. Although several studies established contracting and token economies' effectiveness against waiting-list
control groups with typically small samples or case studies, the interventions were often contaminated by unstandardized communication
or problem-solving training, and comparisons were not generally made
with other potentially effective treatments (cf. Azrin, Naster, & Jones,
1973; Emmelkamp, Van der Helm, Macgillavry, & Van Zanten, 1984;
Ewart, 1978; Margolin, Christensen, & Weiss, 1975; Rappaport & Harrell, 1972; Stuart, 1969; Turner, 1972). The first controlled comparative
outcome study to parse out contingency contracting from communication
and problem-solving training was conducted by Baucom (1982, 1984).
Fifty-four couples reporting marital distress as the primary problem
(average group score was in the distressed range) participated in one of
four 10-week experimental groups: (1) problem-solving/communication
training plus contingency contracting; (2) problem-solving/communica-
tion training only; (3) contingency contracting only; and (4) waiting-list
control. Direct comparison of averaged marital satisfaction ratings at
posttest showed all active treatment conditions to be similarly superior to
the control group. At 3-month follow-up the therapeutic gains and lack of
marital satisfaction differences between treatments were maintained with
between 57% and 77% improved and between 8% and 14% deteriorated.
Although no differences emerged between the treatment groups on
marital satisfaction alone, the combined treatment condition was the only
one to show significant, lasting improvement on self-report (marital satisfaction) and behavioral observation (communication)-dependent measures. In contrast, contingency contracting alone did not show significant
improvement on either of the two behavioral observation (communication) measures. Although the differences between the treatments were
not as dramatic as might have been expected given the intuitive appeal
and theoretical support for communication and problem-solving training,
the fact that the behavioral observations were unaffected by the contingency contracting intervention is potentially important. As discussed
above, behavioral observation methods may reveal more predictive information about treatment maintenance than is immediately apparent. A
longer follow-up may have uncovered more differences between the
treatment conditions. Although only partially warranted by the controlled
outcome data, contingency contracting as a primary BMT intervention
was largely abandoned after these findings.
Simultaneously, the social learning perspective was gaining popular-

ity among behavioral researchers. In an effort to create a more effective and durable therapy, marital therapy researchers shifted their focus to include more cognitive interventions, in order to facilitate behavioral change (Jacobson & Margolin, 1979). As a result, contingency contracting was replaced with behavioral exchange. To avoid the aversive control component inherent when explicity contracting behavioral reciprocity, behavioral exchange required each spouse to commit to collaborative stance in which behavioral changes would be enacted to increase their partner's marital satisfaction without waiting for their partner to do so. Behavioral exchange was added to the communication/problem-solving component.

The research goal was then to establish whether behavioral exchange could stand alone or whether it was most effective in combination with communication/problem-solving training. In a component analysis of BMT (Jacobson, 1984), 36 couples seeking therapy with marital distress as their primary concern were randomly assigned to one of four conditions: (1) communication/problem-solving training plus behavioral exchange (BMT); (2) communication/problem-solving training only; (3) behavioral exchange only; and (4) waiting-list control. At posttest, all three active conditions improved relative to the control group, although no significant overall summed marital satisfaction differences were found between the active conditions. Overall, 72.1% of couples improved, and 58% recovered. A notable difference, however, was that despite effective reduction of negative exchanges in all three active conditions, only the behavioral exchange condition led to increases in self-reported positive behaviors. This advantage was not maintained at the 6-month follow-up, however. The behavioral exchange condition showed strong trends toward deterioration, whereas treatment gains in the other two conditions were generally maintained. Although the behavioral measure was 2 weeks of daily self-tracking before and after therapy rather than objective behavioral observation, the results are a striking parallel to Baucom and Mehlman's (1984) finding that positive behaviors at posttest predicted relapse. [Possibly, increasing positive behaviors without addressing relationship problems acts as a "Band-aid" or increases a couple's expectations to an unrealistic, unmaintainable level. Nevertheless, these findings suggested that while behavioral exchange was effective at doing what it was designed to do—immediately change behavior—administered alone, it was not as durable as therapies involving vehicles for problem resolution. At 2-year follow-up the differences between the conditions were diminished, although couples in the combined treatment were most likely to be happily married and least likely to be separated or divorced. Thus, further BMT development has included both behavioral exchange and communication/problem-solving training.

The second prominent question that emerged in this second BMT generation was: What are the effects of cognitive interventions in inducing and maintaining change? Since these interventions were new to BMT, it was unclear, whether they added effectiveness and if so, whether cognitive changes operated as facilitators for behavioral changes or were legitimate goals in their own right. Baucom and Lester (1986) investigated this question with 24 maritally distressed couples randomly assigned to participate in one of three 12-week groups: (1) behavioral marital therapy alone (6 weeks of communication/problem-solving training and 6 weeks of quid pro quo contracting [to avoid the cognitive interventions in behavioral exchange]); (2) behavioral marital therapy plus cognitive behavioral therapy (6 weeks of BMT and 6 weeks of cognitive interventions on marital attributions and partner and relationship expectations); or (3) waiting-list control. Similar to previously reviewed studies at posttest, the active conditions were found to be significantly better in improving marital satisfaction (spouse's scores analyzed individually) than the control group, but no statistically significant differences between the active conditions emerged. While more consistent cognitive changes were noted in the combined condition, the group differences were not significant. Behavioral changes were also similar in both active conditions. Fifty percent of the males in both conditions entered the nondistressed range. In contrast, 75% of the women in the combined condition recovered, while only 50% in the BMT-only condition entered the nondistressed range. Although treatment gains were generally maintained at 6-month follow-up, the trend toward a greater percentage of females responding to the combined treatment was eliminated. Although the follow-up was short, no evidence supported the inclusion of cognitive interventions in BMT. The fact that the intended cognitive changes were produced but had no apparent impact on immediate or follow-up marital satisfaction further supports this conclusion.

In Baucom and Lester's (1986) discussion, they addressed an issue that has troubled many researchers of standardized treatment approaches. Because subjects are randomly assigned to treatment conditions, there is no room to modify the therapy to best meet the needs of the individual client. This is an important factor, which reduces the generalizability of controlled outcome studies to actual clinical practice. While it is frequently argued that research's random assignment does simulate the rather random process by which couples seek a therapist (e.g., the *Yellow Pages*), even the most limited clinicians are probably more flexible in individualizing their therapy than are most controlled outcome studies. In response to this observed flexibility need, Jacobson et al. (1989) conducted an outcome study comparing the structured research-based version of BMT (i.e., 20 sessions, circumscribed session order) with a clinically flexible version of the same treatment (i.e., no specific number of sessions, individually based intervention order and length). Thirty distressed (DAS scores averaged 80 for husbands and 83 for wives) married couples were randomly assigned to one of the two treatments. At posttest, both treatments elicited significant marital satisfaction improvement, but like previous studies, no between-condition differences were found. At 6-month follow-up, however, the structured-format couples were more likely to have deteriorated while the flexibly treated couples were more likely to have maintained their treatment gains. The 2-year follow-up is in progress, hence though no data are currently available. These findings suggest that the therapist's ability to tailor treatments to client needs may be integral to maintaining therapeutic gains.

Until recently, the vast majority of controlled marital therapy outcome studies have been involved comparisons between BMT variations and its components. Other therapeutic approaches in common clinical practice have been significantly underrepresented in research. Within the last few years, some newcomers to marital therapy research have compared alternative therapies to BMT (Johnson & Greenberg, 1985, 1987; Snyder & Wills, 1989, 1991). As we show below, these studies supported the need for therapist flexibility in individualizing treatments and expansion of the target behavior range beyond simple instrumental behaviors.

Johnson and Greenberg (1985) compared emotion-focused therapy and a version of BMT. Emotion-focused therapy involved identifying negative interactional patterns (i.e., pursue–distance or attach–withdraw) and guided spouses in expressing unacknowledged underlying feelings such as fear, vulnerability, or resentment. Spouses were aided in learning how to respond effectively to the newly expressed needs of their partner. The goal was to create new emotional experiences and interactional patterns. The version of BMT evidence in this study used contingency contracting combined with teaching, modeling, and rehearsing effective communication. Forty couples with at least one spouse in the distressed range (DAS score of 100 or below) were randomly assigned to one of two 8-session treatment conditions or a waiting-list control group. Both treatment groups made significant gains over untreated controls, although the emotion-focused treatment was superior to BMT at therapy's conclusion and a 2-month telephone follow-up.

Another study by Snyder and Wills (1989) compared BMT with insight-oriented therapy. Insight-oriented therapy focuses on developmental issues, collusive interactions, incongruent contractual expectations, irrational role assignments, and maladaptive relationship rules to help resolve conflictual emotions within the individual or couple.

Specific interventions include probes, clarification, and interpretation. BMT involved the four major components in Jacobson and Margolin's (1979) original BMT guide: communication skills, problem-solving skills, relationship enhancement, and contingency contracting. These goals were facilitated through shaping, homework, instruction, modeling, rehearsal, and feedback. Fifty-nine couples reporting marital distress as the primary presenting problem (although the sample mean of husband and wifes self-report MSI score was within the distressed range, no criterion measure was used for selection) were randomly assigned to 25 sessions of insight-oriented marital therapy, BMT, or a waiting-list control group. Both groups made significant gains at posttest and 6-month follow-up. No between-treatment group differences were found. At 4-year follow-up, however, quite a different picture emerged (Snyder, 1990). BMT couples were much more likely to be divorced than were the insight-oriented marital therapy couples (38% compared to 3%).

In a marital therapy research world that has been repeatedly inbred by researchers from one theoretical perspective, these newcomers provide a much-needed fresh perspective (cf. Baucom, 1984; Jacobson, 1991a). As empiricists, we have much to learn from these studies. Snyder's (1990) maintenance over the 4-year follow-up is particularly impressive. Before drawing conclusions from these comparative studies, however, some important methodological concerns should be addressed. The primary problem in both studies (Johnson & Greenberg, 1985; Snyder & Wills, 1989, 1991) was BMT's implementation (Jacobson, 1991b). The most obvious problem was that both implemented only a portion of the full BMT package and focused almost exclusively on instrumental concerns. In both cases, the BMT manuals focused on behavioral modification technology to the virtual exclusion of the clinical skills integral to its implementation. The alternative treatments included many clinical skill guidelines consistent with BMT. These oversights exemplify how frequently and profoundly behavioral therapy is misunderstood. Perhaps this misunderstanting can be attributed to an even more serious methodological problem that blurs the interpretation of these findings: The supervision for the BMT conditions was provided by experts in the alternative therapies rather than experts in BMT. Whereas the former problem may be at least partially attributable to BMT's many changes over the last few years, the latter truly makes it difficult to know whether the BMT conditions accurately reflected any current or former version of BMT.

Despite these questions about the accuracy of BMT's representation, both emotion-focused and insight-oriented marital therapy are effective treatments that deserve further attention. Of particular interest is the apparent similarity between these two perspectives' investment in helping the couple behave more intimately with each other by coming in contact with and mutually sharing novel personal information. In contrast, the BMT that performed inferiorly focused on communicative changes to facilitate the negotiation of instrumental changes. Although this focus on instrumental concerns produced positive marital satisfation changes, the changes were not as significant as those resulting from emotion-focused therapy (Johnson & Greenberg, 1985) and less durable than those from insight-oriented therapy (Snyder, 1990). Possibly, couples in the BMT conditions were making changes that led to immediate relief but could not be maintained (Jacobson, 1991b). This result may have been exacerbated by primarily focusing on decreasing negative behaviors rather than on developing a base for positive behaviors. In contrast, the alterative therapies focused on helping the couple have more intimate and satisfying interactions about their reported problems.

RELAPSE PREVENTION

As has been frequently noted throughout this chapter, marital therapy research has focused primarily on immediate outcome, with follow-up as a secondary goal. Identification of the RP properties in treatments is typically post hoc, rather than part of a priori predictions. The additional time and expense of recommencing therapy at a basic level after 1 or 2 years, coupled with the potentially serious consequences of a temporary marital distress reprieve for important joint decisions (i.e., childbearing or financial decisions), point to the need for increased attention to assessing and enhancing long-term outcomes. This need is substantiated by findings that between-therapy differences have consistently emerged during follow-ups.

The goals in this section are twofold: (1) to review the marital therapy research aimed specifically at RP and (2) to highlight the data-based and theoretical components in enhancing RP.

Research

We were only able to locate two marital therapy studies directly aimed at enhancing RP. Both focused on ways to help couples generalize from the therapeutic environment to the couple's environment. One compared standard weekly therapy sessions with a modified time format (Bogner & Zielenbach-Coensen, 1984), while the other evaluated the effects of booster sessions (Whisman, 1991).

Bogner and Zielenbach-Coenen (1984) challenged the basic psychotherapy weekly-session format by comparing standard weekly sessions of BMT with a modified time format in which sessions were phased out at the end of therapy. The predictions were that couples could more rapidly tackle problems in the beginning and gain confidence in their newly learned skills so that sessions could be phased out at the end. Twenty-four couples with relationship distress as the primary complaint were randomly assigned to one of three conditions: (1) weekly-session BMT (nine weekly sessions); (2) modified-time-format BMT (nine sessions with 2 weeks separating sessions 7 and 8 and 3 weeks between sessions 8 and 9); (3) waiting-list control group. In both BMT conditions, the problem-solving and communication training was presented in sessions 4 through 6 during 1½-hour long sessions. Session 7 involved intensive training in crisis management (3½ hours). At posttest, both treatment groups were significantly improved (based on averaged marital satisfaction scores), but the modified-time-format couple improved significantly more. As predicted, the modified-time-format couples were also more likely to maintain their gains at 8-month follow-up, with the average modified-time-format couple scoring in the normal range and the average weekly-format couple scoring in the unhappy range. Thus, it appears that increasing the intervals between the final therapy sessions does indeed facilitate the couple's ability to benefit from marital therapy initially and in the long term.

Another strategy that has long been advocated for generalizing from the therapeutic environment to the couple's daily life is "booster" sessions (Hall & Hall, 1980). In contrast to other theoretical perspectives that purport that psychotherapy produces permanent changes within its participants, behavioral philosophy points to the importance of the environment for change and maintenance. Although the therapeutic goal is to help couples create a reciprocally reinforcing environment within their relationship through mutual behavioral change, the therapeutic environment provides an important reinforcement source for the initial changes. The maintenance of change is dependent on reinforcement availability. If the reinforcement quality of either spouse's behavioral changes is not great enough or flexible enough to endure new stresses, relapse is likely. Thus, booster sessions may help the couple fine-tune their relationship-maintaining behaviors to be more flexible or more mutually reinforcing.

Whisman (1991) investigated the effectiveness of booster sessions in RP with 27 maritally distressed couples (averaged DAS scores 98 or below) randomly assigned to either a standard BMT condition or a standard BMT condition plus booster sessions. Couples in both conditions participated in 20 therapy sessions conducted by graduate student therapists. Booster couples had two mandatory booster sessions at 3 and 6 months after therapy and three optional sessions during the same 6-month period. As expected, couples in both treatments exhibited significant marital satisfaction improvement immediately after therapy, with 77% of the booster couples and 50% of the nonbooster couples significantly improved. Fully recovery was experienced by 46% of the booster couples and 36% of the nonbooster couples. by the 12-month follow-up, 69% of the booster couples had maintained their gains, while only 36% of the nonbooster couples had not deteriorated. Although these clinically significant statistics seem to support the efficacy of booster sessions, the between-treatment differences were not statistically significant. While a larger sample may have increased statistical power, the fact that nearly a third of the booster couples reentered the distressed range by the 1-year follow-up suggests that booster sessions—as implemented in this study—were not sufficient to prevent relapse. These findings suggest that booster sessions deserve further attention and refinement, but they do not unequivocally support booster sessions' efficacy. Whisman (1991) outlined several ways the efficacy of booster sessions could have improved, including using experienced therapists; improving the booster session content; scheduling additional booster sessions during the first 3 posttherapy months; and extending the length of the maintenance component.

RP CONCLUSIONS AND GUIDELINES

Although research aimed directly at parsing out treatment differences responsible for enhanced maintenance is rare, some characteristics emerge as unique to the more durable therapies: (1) flexibility in treatment content; (2) flexibility in treatment format; (3) identifying and modifying salient behaviors (i.e., overt, emotional, cognitive); (4) focusing on reasonably changeable behaviors; and (5) effectively generalizing from therapy to the clients' world.

Despite some common themes across distressed couples, each couple presents idiosyncratically. Thus, while it is important to keep in mind overriding principles about what is helpful to couples, the priority and emphasis on the various components should be calibrated according to the couple's needs. As Jacobson et al. (1989) found in their comparison of a structured versus a flexible application of BMT, therapeutic gains were more effectively maintained in the flexibility treated group. This need for flexibility is consistent with the behavioral philosophy. Each person enters his or her relationship with vastly different behavioral repertoires acquired through myriad prior experiences. Upon entering the reationship, each of these behaviors is then strengthened or weakened by the reinforcing properties of the other spouse's behaviors, and vice versa. Each couple creates its own environment, which supports some behaviors in some contexts and reinforces others in other contexts. The possibilities for marital distress behavioral patterns quickly grow. It is no wonder that the early one-size-fits-all marital therapies were not as durable as those that could directly address each couple's salient behaviors. This highlights the importance of conscientious and careful assessment of the presenting concerns. Another possibility that has been frequently proposed (cf. Jacobson, 1991b), although not empirically tested, is matching clients to treatments according to how they conceptualize their distress. Some couples may have numerous cognitive distortions and may thus benefit from a cognitively oriented therapy. Other couples may have primarily instrumental concerns and thus can be more effectively helped with a traditional BMT focus.

Another factor that appears to be important in how durably couples learn new behaviors is the format of the treatment sessions. The standard weekly 1-hour therapy sessions may not provide the optimal environment for acquiring new skills (Bogner & Zielenbach-Coenen, 1984). Allowing enough time for each new set of skills to be learned and adequately practiced in one session may help couples to genuinely incorporate the new behaviors into this repertoire. If, for example, the skill to be learned is listening and reflecting, a 1-hour session may provide only enough time to present the concept and have one spouse practice it. Homework possibilities are then limited and the spouse who did not get listened to may become frustrated. Because the couple couldn't practice the skill at home, a portion of the subsequent session would involve relearning some of material from the previous week and possibly dealing with negative feelings from the inequality of the previous week. If instead the sessions were designed so that concepts could realistically be presented, practiced, and examined couples may be able to more effectively practice at home and experience less frustration from learning partial skills. Thus, marital therpists may benefit from structuring the length and spacing of sessions according to the interventions and point of view of the therapy.

Perhaps the most fertile ground for enhancing marital therapy outcome and maintenance lies in the accurate identification of the behaviors salient to the couple's distress. As discussed earlier in this chapter, the early BMT focus on resolving instrumental complaints (e.g., who does the dishes; whether to move or not) may not have included a broad enough range of target behaviors. The findings that traditional BMT is good at reducing negative behaviors but largely ineffective at increasing positive behaviors supports this view (cf. Snyder & Wills, 1989). Possibly, the behaviors salient to helping distressed couples become more like nondistressed, non-therapy-seeking couples were being overlooked. This is supported by Snyder's (1990) finding that insight-oriented marital therapy was superior to bare-bones BMT at a 4-year follow-up. Although no behavioral observation data were collected at the 4-year follow-up, the posttest behavioral assessment suggested that nonverbal positiveness was significantly increased for the insight-oriented group but not for the BMT group. We do not know whether this positive behavior increase was maintained after 4 years or whether it was integral to preventing relapse, but this was one posttest difference that emerged despite similar marital satisfaction ratings. Because there were numerous intervention differences, the specific constellation of interventions responsible for the outcome differences is difficult to pinpoint. Yet, from a behavioral perspective, the primary differences between the two conditions was that the insight-oriented therapy included interventions to help spouses more effectively share internal cognitive and emotional experiences. Through gaining new information about their learning histories (i.e., insight) while learning skills for listening and expressing these internal experiences, spouses learned to share more intimate experiences. Although more data are clearly needed to substantiate the RP potential of this more comprehensive behavioral focus, this projection is theoretically sound and consistent with the available research.

A related factor is that RP may require focusing attention on reasonably maintainable behavioral changes. Although huge behavioral changes may improve marital satisfaction in the short run, it is unlikely that the available reinforcement will be sufficient to maintain them. In Jacobson's (1984) component analysis of BMT, he found that a simple focus on having spouses attempt to improve their patner's marital satisfaction by increasing their positive behaviors was as effective as the other BMT components at posttest, but the changes were not maintained over time. Possibly, the therapeutic environment provides reinforcers to maintain behaviors that do not exist in the relationship (e.g., encouragement that this will improve the marriage; praise for attempting all items on their list). If, with the therapist's encouragement, a husband attempts to improve his wife's satisfaction by buying her flowers, washing her car, fixing dinner, and taking care of the kids while the wife buys special food, gives nightly back rubs, and asks questions about his day, both may feel more satisfied overall although there is no natural reinforcement for each of the behavioral changes. Behaviors that are naturally reinforcing within the relationship are far more likely to be maintained. If, instead, the couple has an interaction that leads to increased understanding and ends in a spontaneous embrace, the interactive behaviors are more likely to be repeated outside of the therapeutic context. Similarly, this also applies to problems that are apparently insoluble such as a disagreement about whether to have children. Attempting to resolve the conflict itself may more deeply entrench couples in their hopelessness or lead to an unworkable solution. Instead, helping the couple better understand one another's internal experiences without rushing to a conclusion may increase intimate feelings and eventually facilitate a satisfactory agreement. Thus, therapists should pay special attention to behaviors that are naturally reinforcing in and out of the sessions.

Perhaps the greatest challenge in promoting RP involves designing interventions that facilitate generalization from therapeutic environment to the couple's daily life. Unless each partner becomes self-sufficient in providing reinforcement for the other, even the most immediately effective therapy will fail once therapist reinforcement is phased out. Several steps have been recommended to improve generalization: (1) maximizing the couples natural reinforcement potential; (2) assigning homework throughout therapy; (3) increasing intervals between final sessions; (4) including booster sessions; and (5) predicting stressful life events.

Whenever possible, spouses should be encouraged to express naturally occurring positive reinforcement for one another (Jacobson & Margolin, 1979). Therapist praise statements should be oriented toward modeling possible responses rather than being the primary reinforcement source. Not only will overuse of therapist reinforcement lead to a dependence on therapy for change to be maintained, but the therapist may be reinforcing behaviors that are not inherently reinforcing for the listening spouse. Careful assessment of each aspect of both spouse's internal experiences when various behaviors are omitted will help to determine which changes will genuinely lead to maintainable marital satisfaction improvement. The therapist can then help spouses attend to and express salient positive experiences.

Homework assignments have long been advocated as a way to encourage couples to transfer skills from therapy to real life. Although research has not directly evaluated the role of homework assignments in maintaining marital therapy gains, homework compliance has been associated with treatment maintenance in other behavioral therapies (e.g., assertion problems) (Kazdin & Mascitelli, 1982). Intuitively, it seems obvious that the target behaviors occur outside the therapy session, so that the natural reinforcement can be experienced and any problems can be problem-solved in the session. In early sessions, homework assignments may need to be explicitly spelled out by the therapist. As therapy progresses, generalization will be improved if the couple plays a more active role in designing between-session tasks. The extent to which the between-therapy work can ultimately be incorporated into the couple's daily life may also determine its durability. Not surprisingly, the only skills couples report using 2 years after BMT were those they could incorporate into their day-to-day discussions (e.g., prefacing complaints with expression of appreciation; stating problems in behaviorally specific terms; and expressing feelings). Other skills such as problem-solving sessions or state-of-the-relationship meetings typically did not occur because they were too time-consuming or stilted (Jacobson et al., 1987).

Increasing the intervals between the final therapy sessions has been found to increase couples' ability to maintain their gains (Bogner & Zielenbach-Coenen, 1984). As couples near the end of therapy, the increased intervals may help them to practice and experiment with workable skill variations outside of therapy while relying on the natural reinforcers in their environment to maintain them. The less frequent the sessions, the less salient therapy becomes as a primary reinforcement source. At the same time, couples know that they can discuss any concerns that arise in the upcoming session. A variation on increasing the intervals between the final sessions is booster sessions, which have also been found to prevent relapse (Whisman, 1991). The primary difference between increasing between-session intervals and increasing booster sessions occurs when intensive therapy is conceptualized as ending. With increased intervals, the final sessions are seen as integral to the therapy process. For booster sessions, they typically ocur after intensive therapy is "over" and serve the purpose of augmenting what was already learned. Although no research is available comparing these two formats, there are apparent advantages to each. Increased-intervals couples are likely to continue to perceive themselves "in therapy" and thus to continue more intensive change efforts. Booster-session couples may see therapy as over and forget about maintaining therapeutic changes. In contrast, increased-intervals couples may become dependent on being "in therapy" and feel unable to solve their disputes without therapeutic intervention, while booster-sessions couples see themselves as "on their own" and become more effective at independent resolution. Clearly, more knowledge is needed before one approach can be recommended over another.

Of all the variables that have been investigated in predicting relapse, the occurrence of stressful life events has been consistently related to whether or not gains are maintained. Jacobson et al. (1987) found that stressful events were better predictors of relapse 2 years after BMT than were therapist attributes or maintenance of treatment-derived relationship skills. Predicting stressors and aiding couples in independently handling crises that arise during therapy may help a couple's marriage to suffer less when subsequent stresses arise. Booster sessions or increased between-session intervals may also help to deal with unexpected problems. However, since no amount of foresight can predict every problem, couples need to learn joint problem solving by using problem discussions to become more intimate.

FUTURE DIRECTIONS

Further investigation of RP in marital therapy can proceed in many directions. Movement from a focus on immediate outcome to one on long-term maintenance is essential for evaluating the success of marital therapy.

Recommendations for research into marital therapy's long-term effectiveness are as follows.

1. *Longer and more rigorous follow-ups.* All but one study, which followed its subjects for 4 years, have followed their subjects for a maximum of 2 years. Even these relatively short-term follow-ups are plagued with poor subject retention and truncated assessment methods. Future researchers are behooved to treat the follow-up phase with the same attention and rigor as the treatment phase. Subjects may be given incentives to encourage continued participation, and assessment methods at each phase should be comprehensive.

2. *Identifying therapy factors related to long-term maintenance.* Several new therapies show promise in helping couples maintain their therapeutic gains. Yet, little research has been done to confirm their effectiveness. The existing research has focused on comparisons of different therapy packages rather than on the actual therapeutic differences responsible for outcome differences. With numerous factors separating the various therapies, it is difficult to determine exactly why one therapy is more effective than another. Thus, it is difficult to truly improve therapy based on these findings. In fact, such an approach is antithetical to the scientific method which requires exact knowledge of how studied substances are different. Instead a focus on the actual process differences between compared approaches may shed light on the factors that would genuinely fine-tune marital therapy.

REFERENCES

American Psychiatric Association. (1987). *Diagnostic and statistical manual of mental disorders* (3rd ed., rev.). Washington, DC: Author.

Azrin, N. H., Naster, B. J., & Jones, R. (1973). Reciprocity counseling: A rapid learning-based procedure for marital counseling. *Behavior Research & Therapy, 11,* 365–382.

Baucom, D. H. (1982). A comparison of behavioral contracting and problem-solving/communications training in behavioral marital therapy. *Behavior Therapy, 13,* 162–174.

Baucom, D. H. (1984). The active ingredients of behavioral marital therapy: The effectiveness of problem-solving/communication training, contingency contracting and their combination. In K. Hahlweg & N. S. Jacobson (Eds.), *Marital interaction: Analysis and modification* (pp. 73–88). New York: Guilford Press.

Baucom, D. H., & Epstein, N. (1991). Will the real cognitive–behavior marital therapy please stand up? *Journal of Family Psychology, 4,* 394–401.

Baucom, D. H., & Hoffman, J. A. (1986). The effectiveness of marital therapy: Current status and application to the clinical setting. In N. S. Jacobson & A. S. Gurman (Eds.), *Clinical handbook of marital therapy* (pp. 597–620). New York: Guilford Press.

Baucom, D. H., & Lester, G. W. (1986). The usefulness of cognitive restructuring as an adjunct to behavioral marital therapy. *Behavior therapy, 17,* 385–403.

Baucom, D. H., & Mehlman, S. K. (1984). Predicting marital status following behavioral marital therapy: A comparison of models of marital relationships. In K. Hahlweg & N. S. Jacobson (Eds.), *Marital interaction: Analysis and modification* (pp. 89–104). New York: Guilford Press.

Beach, R. H., & O'Leary, K. D. (1985). Current status of outcome research in marital therapy. In L. L'Abate (Ed.), *Handbook of family psychology and therapy* Vol. 2). Homewood, IL: Dorsey Press.

Birchler, G. R., Clopton, P. L., & Adams, N. L. (1984). Marital conflict resolutions: Factors influencing concordance between partners and trained coders. *American Journal of Family Therapy, 12,* 15–28.

Bögner, I., & Zielenbach-Coenen, H. (1984). On maintaining change in behavioral marital therapy. In K. Hahlweg & N. S. Jacobson (Eds.), *Marital interaction: Analysis and modification* (pp. 27–35). Guilford Press.

Emery, R. R. (1982). Interparental conflict and the children of discord and divorce. *Psychological Bulletin, 92,* 310–330.

Emmelkamp, P., van der Helm, M., MacGillavry, D., & van Zanten, B. (1984). Marital therapy with clinically distressed couples: A comparative evaluation of system-theoretic, contingency contracting and communication skills approaches. In K. Hahlweg & N. S. Jacobson (Eds.), *Marital interaction: Analysis and modification* (pp. 36–52). New York: Guilford Press.

Ewart, C. K. (1978, August 31). *Behavior contracts in couple therapy: An experimental evaluation of quid pro quo and good faith models.* Paper presented at the American Psychological Association Meeting Toronto, Canada.

Floyd, R. J. (1988). Couples' cognitive/affective reactions to communication behaviors. *Journal of Marriage and the Family, 50,* 523–532.

Gottman, J. M. (1979). *Marital interaction: Experimental investigations.* New York: Academic Press.

Gottman, J. M. (1985). Observational measures: A reply to Jacobson. *Behavioral Assessment, 7,* 317–321.

Gurman, A. S. (1991). Back to the future, ahead to the past: Is marital therapy going in circles? *Journal of Family Psychology, 4,* 402–406.

Gurman, A. S., Kniskern, D. P., & Pinsof, W. M. (1986). Research on marital and family therapies. In S. L. Garfield & A. E. Bergin (Eds.), *Handbook of psychotherapy and behavior change.* New York: Wiley.

Hahlweg, K., Reisner, L., Kohli, G., Volmer, M., Schindler, L., & Revenstorf,

D. (1984). Development and validity of a new system to analyze inter-personal communication: Kategoriensystem für partnerschaftliche interaktion. In K. Hahlweg & N. S. Jacobson (Eds.), *Marital interaction: Analysis and modification*. (pp. 182–198). New York: Guilford Press

Hahlweg, K., Schindler, L., Revenstorf, D., & Brengelmann, T. C. (1984). The Munich marital therapy study. In K. Hahlweg & N. S. Jacobson (Eds.), *Marital interaction: Analysis and modification* (pp. 3–26). New York: Guilford Press.

Hahlweg, K., & Markman, H. J. (1988). Effectiveness of behavior marital therapy: Empirical status of behavioral techniques in preventing and alleviating marital distress. *Journal of Consulting and Clinical Psychology, 56,* 440–447.

Hall, S. M., & Hall, R. G. (1980). Maintaining change. In J. M. Ferguson & C. B. Taylor (Eds.), *The comprehensive handbook of behavioral medicine* (Vol. 3). New York: SP Medical and Scientific Books.

Hops, H., Wills, T. A., Patterson, G. R., & Weiss, R. L. (1972). *Marital interaction coding system.* University of Oregon and Oregon Research Institute, Eugene (Available from ASIS/NAPS, c/o Microfiche Publication, 305 E. 46th St, New York, New York, 10017).

Jacobson, N. S. (1978). A review of the research on the effectiveness of marital therapy. In I. Paolino & B. McCrady (Eds.), *Marriage and marital therapy,* New York: Brunner/Mazel.

Jacobson, N. S. (1983). Clinical innovations in behavioral marital therapy. In K. Craig (Ed.), *Clinical behavior therapy.* New York: Brunner/Mazel.

Jacobson, N. S. (1984). A component analysis of behavioral marital therapy: The relative effectiveness of behavior exchange and communication/problem-solving training. *Journal of Consulting and Clinical Psychology, 52,* 295–305.

Jacobson, N. S. (1985). The role of observational measures in behavior therapy outcome research. *Behavioral Assessment, 7,* 297–308.

Jacobson, N. S. (1988). Defining clinically significant change: An introduction. *Behavioral Assessment, 10,* 131–132.

Jacobson, N. S. (1991a). To be or not to behavioral when working with couples: What does it mean? *Journal of Family Psychology, 4,* 436–445.

Jacobson, N. S. (1991b). Toward enhancing the efficacy of marital therapy and marital therapy research. *Journal of Family Psychology, 4,* 373–393.

Jacobson, N. S., Elwood, R., & Dallas, M. (1981). Assessment of marital dysfunction. In D. H. Barlow (Ed.), *Behavioral assessment of adult disorders* (pp. 439–479). New York: Guilford Press.

Jacobson, N.S., Follette, W. C., & Elwood, R., (1984). Outcome research in behavioral marital therapy: Methodological conceptual reappraisal. In K. Hahlweg & N. S. Jacobson (Eds.), *Marital interaction: Analysis and modification* (pp. 113–129). New York: Guilford Press.

Jacobson, N. S., Follette, W. C., & Revenstorf, D. (1984). Psychotherapy outcome research: Methods for reporting variability and evaluating clinical significance. *Behavior Therapy, 15,* 336–352.

Jacobson, N. S., Follette, W. C., Revenstorf, D., Baucom, D. H., Hahlweg, K., & Margolin, G. (1984). Variability in outcome and clinical significance of behavior marital therapy: A reanalysis of outcome data. *Journal of Consulting and Clinical Psychology, 52,* 497–504.

Jacobson, N. S., Follette, W. C., & Revenstorf, D. (1986). Toward a standard definition of clinically significant change. *Behavior Therapy, 17,* 308–311.

Jacobson, N. S., & Margolin, G. (1979). *Marital therapy: Strategies based on social learning and behavior exchange principles.* New York: Brunner/Mazel.

Jacobson, N.S., & Revenstorf, D. (1988). Statistics for assessing the clinical significance of psychotherapy techniques: Issues, problems and new developments. *Behavioral Assessment, 10,* 133–145.

Jacobson, N. S., Schmaling, K. B., & Holtzworth-Munroe, A. (1987). Component analysis of behavioral marital therapy; 2-year follow-up and prediction of relapse. *Journal of Marital and Family Therapy, 13,* 187–195.

Jacobson, N. S., Schmaling, K. B., Holtzworth-Munroe, A., Katt, J. L., Wood, L. F., & Follette, V. M. (1989). Research-structured vs. clinically flexible versions of social learning-based marital therapy. *Behavioral Research Therapy, 27,* 173–180.

Jacobson, N. S., & Truax, P. (1991). Clinical significance: A statistical approach to defining meaningful change in psychotherapy research. *Journal of Consulting and Clinical Psychology, 59,* 12–19.

Johnson, S. M., & Greenberg, L. S. (1985). Differential effects of experiential and problem-solving interventions in resolving marital conflict. *Journal of Consulting and Clinical Psychology, 53,* 175–184.

Johnson, S. M., & Greenberg, L. S. (1987). Emotionally focused couples therapy: An outcome study. *Journal of Marital and Family Therapy, 11,* 313–317.

Johnson, S. M., & Greenberg, L. S. (1991). There are more things in heaven and earth than are dreamed of in BMT? A response to Jacobson. *Journal of Family Psychology, 4,* 407–415.

Kazdin, A. E., & Mascitelli, S. (1982). Behavioral rehearsal, self-instructions, and homework practiced in developing assertiveness. *Behavior Therapy, 13,* 346–360.

Locke, H. J., & Wallace, K. M. (1959). Short-term marital adjustment and prediction tests: Their reliability and validity. *Journal of Marriage and Family Living, 21,* 251–255.

Mace, D., & Mace, V. (1980). Enriching marriages: The foundation stone of family strength. In N. Stinnett, B. Chesser, J. DeFrain, & P. Knaub (Eds.), *Family strengths: Positive models for family life.* Lincoln, NE: University of Nebraska Press.

Margolin, G., Christensen, A., & Weiss, R. L. (1975). Contracts, cognition and change: A behavioral approach to marriage therapy. *The Counseling Psychologist, 5,* 15–25.

Margolin, G., Hatten, D., John, R. S., & Yost, K. (1985). Perceptual agreement between spouses and outside observers when coding themselves and a stranger dyad. *Behavioral Assessment, 7,* 235–247.

Olson, D. H., & Ryder, R. G. (1975). *Marital and Family interaction Coding System (MFICS).* Unpublished manuscript, University of Minnesota, Minneapolis.

Pineo, C. (1961). Disenchantment in the later years of marriage. *Marriage and Family Living, 23,* 3–11.

Rappaport, A. F., & Harrell, J. E. (1972). A Behavioral-exchange model for marital counseling. *Family Coordinator, 21,* 203–213.

Rausch, H. L., Barry, W. A., Hertel, R. K., & Swain, M. A. (1974). *Communication, conflict and marriage.* San Francisco: Jossey-Bass.

Revenstorf, D., Hahlweg, K., Schindler, L., & Vogel, B., (1984). Interaction analysis of marital conflict. In K. Hahlweg & N. S. Jacobson (Eds.), *Marital interaction: Analysis and modification* (pp. 159–181). New York: Guilford Press.

Schindler, L. (1981). *Empirische Analyse partner schatlicher Kommunikation.* Unpublished doctoral dissertation, Universitat Tubingen, Tubingen, Germany.

Schindler, L., Hahlweg, K., & Revenstorf, D. (1983). Short- and long-term effectiveness of two communication training modalities with distressed couples. *The American Journal of Family Therapy, 11,* 54–64.

Skinner, B. F. (1976). *About behaviorism.* New York: Vintage Books.

Snyder, D. K. (1979). Multidimensional assessment of marital satisfaction. *Journal of Marriage and the Family, 41,* 813–823.

Snyder, D. K. (1990). *Long-term effectiveness of behavioral versus insight-oriented marital therapy: A four-year follow-up study.* Unpublished manuscript.

Snyder, D. K., & Wills, R. M. (1989). Behavioral versus insight-oriented marital therapy: Effects on individual and interspousal functioning. *Journal of Consulting and Clinical Psychology, 57,* 39–46.

Snyder, D. K., & Wills, R. M. (1991). Facilitating change in marital therapy and research. *Journal of Family Psychology, 4,* 426–435.

Spanier, G. B. (1976). Measuring dyadic adjustment: New scales for assessing the quality of marriage and similar dyads. *Journal of Marriage and the Family, 38,* 15–28.

Stuart, R. B. (1969). Operant interpersonal treatment for marital discord. *Journal of Consulting and Clinical Psychology, 33,* 13–29.

Turner, A. J. (1972, October). *Couple and group treatment of marital discord: An experiment.* Paper presented at the meeting of the Association for the Advancement of Behavior Therapy, October 1972, New York, New York.

Weiss, R. L., & Frohman, P. E. (1985). Behavioral observation as outcome measures: Not through a glass darkly. *Behavioral Assessment, 7,* 309–315.

Whisman, M. A. (1991). *The use of booster maintenance sessions in behavioral marital therapy.* Unpublished doctoral dissertation, University of Washington, Seattle.

Whisman, M. A., Jacobson, N. S., Fruzzetti, A. E., & Waltz, J. A. (1989). Methodological issues in marital therapy. *Advances in Behavioral Research and Therapy, 11,* 175–189.

Whisman, M. A., Schmaling, K. B., & Jacobson, N. S. (1988). Treatment of relationship dysfunction: An empirical evaluation of group and conjoint behavioral marital therapy. *Journal of Consulting and Clinical Psychology, 56,* 929–931.

CHAPTER 13

SOCIAL COMPETENCE: INTERVENTIONS WITH CHILDREN AND PARENTS

Sandra T. Azar
CLARK UNIVERSITY

Elizabeth S. Ferguson
CLARK UNIVERSITY

Craig T. Twentyman
UNIVERSITY OF HAWAII AT MANOA

Writing a chapter on relapse prevention (RP) in social skills training presents both a unique opportunity and a perilous task. On the one hand, the concept of "relapse" in this area has not yet received much attention and a discussion focusing on central issues would be useful. However, because the definition of "socially competent behavior" continues to be open to question (McFall, 1982), "relapse" in such interventions may be less clearly defined than in the other areas in this volume. Thus, much of what constitutes the very core of this chapter is still being debated. Nevertheless, the issue of how to achieve socially competent behavior and maintain it over time is a fundamental clinical task.

In an effort to make the task within the "competence" level of the authors, some ground rules were established. First, a decision was made to focus on only two domains of "social competence," children's peer relationships and parenting, both of which entail developmental issues that introduce unique difficulties in producing treatment maintenance. Second, while other approaches have been explored within these domains (e.g., client-centered and educational), this chapter is restricted to behavioral and cognitive–behavioral approaches since these are by far the best researched. Finally, because RP in social competence interventions is an emerging area, emphasis will be placed on basic issues facing the field in hopes of guiding future empirical work.

PROBLEMS IN "DIAGNOSING" SOCIAL COMPETENCE

Despite the fact that no less than 17 DSM-III-R diagnoses include some mention of social competence disturbance (Dodge, 1989), the definition of this construct has been subject to much debate. Recent reviews have made a distinction between two important terms: "social competence" and "social skill." The first term, "social competence," which appears in the title of this chapter, has been used broadly in the intervention literature. Indeed, McFall (1982) has argued that it has been used too widely, encompassing everything from treatment of sexual dysfunction to depression. The second term, "social skill," has at times been used synonymously with social competence, but it appears to have a narrower meaning and, therefore, may have greater utility in discussing the issue of relapse. Even this term, however, is not without problems. At times it is used to imply a trait exhibited consistently across situations, an assumption that has not received empirical support. Consequently, a more manageable, domain specific view of the term "social skill" has come to be used. In the words of Combs and Slaby (1977):

> Social skills are the ability to interact with others in a given social context in specific ways that are societally acceptable or valued and at the same time personally beneficial, mutually beneficial, or beneficial primarily to others. (p. 162)

Even this definition poses problems, especially when RP is discussed. First, words like "societally valued" pose ethical dilemmas and definitional problems in culturally diverse settings. Discrepancies between trained skills (e.g., restricting parental use of physical punishment) and the values of the cultural context in which they ultimately are to be used may impact on the occurrence of relapse and the nature of efforts to prevent it. Second, the requirement that behaviors be "beneficial" to multiple constituencies raises problems for defining when relapse occurs. The subjective evaluations of social agents (e.g., teachers, peers, and social workers) have typically been utilized to "diagnose" social incompetency. These different sources have not necessarily agreed (Giovannoni & Becerra, 1970; Gresham, 1981). When no consensus exists, who should take precedence in determining the occurrence of relapse? Even if a single source is utilized, the literature has not set standards for when "disorder" is present. For instance, peer sociometric ratings have been utilized to select socially incompetent children, resulting anywhere from 16% to 50% of normal populations being selected for intervention (Hops, 1983). Such discrepancies and the lack of definitional clarity they represent make an examination of the effectiveness of RP efforts more difficult. Finally, identifying crucial contexts may also pose problems for identifying relapse (e.g., in how many or in which types of contexts, would poor social skills be exhibited before "relapse" can be said to occur?).

Despite these problems, this general approach to defining social competency has gained wide acceptance. It assumes that there are specific identifiable cognitive and behavioral skills that form the basis of socially competent behavior. A variety of approaches to delineating the relevant skills exist, with some investigators taking a molar view (e.g., assertiveness, child management skills) and others choosing a more molecular one (e.g., eye contact). Skill selections have also reflected either component or process views (Beck & Forehand, 1984). The former focuses on the behaviors associated with socially competent performance and the latter on cognitive and perceptual processes (e.g., perspective taking, monitoring contextual cues). Other dimensions to consider in arriving at definitions have begun to emerge (e.g., gender) (Waldrop & Halverson, 1975). "Relapse" for each of the above would look different.

Adding further confusion are suggestions that "meta-skills," which are even further removed from social behavior, be considered. These skills are not social per se but may be essential to successful social interaction (Hops, 1983). For example, poor motor ability hinders a child's social interaction on the playground and may decrease developmentally crucial contacts with peers.

This debate has led to increased efforts to define "social skill" with greater specificity. Although this basic research may ultimately improve treatment maintenance by leading to greater clarity in selecting affected individuals and relevant target skills, current interventions appear not to have attended to such findings. Hughes (1986), in a review of 32 recent intervention studies with children, found 56% reported no empirical evidence justifying the skills targeted and 66% did not even make an attempt to verify that trainees were deficient in them prior to treatment. Such lack of connection between basic research and interventions will hinder the development of RP efforts.

We chose to focus on two "contexts" of social skill problems: peer relationships in childhood and parenting. Difficulties with peers in childhood have long been indicated as boding poorly for later adjustment (Asher, Oden, & Gottman, 1977; Kohlberg, LaCrosse, & Ricks, 1972;

Parker & Asher, 1987), and the interpersonal skills required of parents are believed to be the cornerstone of socialization and crucial determinants of developmental outcomes in children (Sameroff & Chandler, 1975; Sears, Maccoby, & Levin, 1957). Thus, both are important domains for intervention attempts and for an examination of relapse issues. The skills involved in both of these areas, however, may be "moving targets," varying with children's development (Azar & Siegel, 1990; Foster, De-Lawyer, & Guevremont, 1985). For example, Coie, Dodge, and Coppotelli (1982) found that over the course of childhood, some social behaviors (e.g., supportiveness) were consistently tied to peer status, but others (e.g., disruptive behavior) varied in importance across developmental eras. Similarly, the communications skills required of parents to produce smooth interpersonal interaction and foster development in an infant (e.g., tactile stimulation) are very different from those required of parents of a teenager (e.g., negotiation skills) (Azar & Siegel, 1990). RP in both these domains consequently may be complex and may provide the most stringent test of such interventions. These shifting "targets" must be anticipated and evaluations may require both short- and long-term follow-up periods to determine effectiveness, evaluating important skills in one developmental period and looking for impact on skills in another.

COURSE OF THE "DISORDER" AND RELAPSE

In creating and evaluating RP strategies, a detailed knowledge of the course of any given disorder is required. Available information is quite limited in the areas of peer relationship problems and parenting disorders. The prevalence of social skill problems in childhood is highly dependent upon definitions of the deficiency chosen and the person rating the child's deficiency. Between 2% and 50% of the "normal" population have been termed socially incompetent, that is, isolated, rejected, withdrawn (Hops, 1983). Using peer ratings, 6% to 11% of third through sixth graders have been identified as having no friends in their classroom (Gronlund, 1959; Hymel & Asher, 1977). If figures based on rates of social interaction are considered, however, higher numbers are found (e.g., one third) (O'Connor, 1969). While contradictory evidence exists (Kupersmidt, 1983; West & Farrington, 1973), there appears to be some stability and predictive validity to childhood peer problems as measured in a *global* manner. Sociometric status, for example, has been shown to be relatively stable after the preschool years (Howes, 1987; Li, 1985; Rubin & Daniels-Bierness, 1983).

The continuity of *specific* types of skills deficits, however, may vary. Coie and Dodge (1983), for example, reported continuity of active peer rejection of fifth graders over a 5-year period, whereas social isolation did not show continuity. Rejected children display disruptive and aggressive behavior, which may be more firmly ingrained in a child's repertoire.

Figures regarding the continuity of parenting problems are harder to come by and as in the child literature, those available vary with measurement method. When extreme parenting difficulties are considered, such as physical abuse, prevalence figures range from a low of 4.9 per 1,000 children for reports by professionals (Burgdorf, 1988) to a high of 19 per 1,000 in general population surveys (Straus & Gelles, 1986). Reincidence figures indicate a high rate of relapse (e.g., between 20% and 70% depending on the type of abuse and whether agency records or research criteria are used) (Williams, 1983). Since the samples in many of these studies technically cannot be considered untreated (i.e., at the very least they received some form of case management) and the methodologies used are also problematic (e.g., reporting biases and short follow-up periods), actual relapse figures may be much higher. Not much is known about predictors of relapse. One small-scale study found that income source, marital status, and parental abuse history were all associated with reabuse (Ferlinger, Glenwick, Gaines, & Green, 1988). Even if abuse itself does not reoccur, it has been our clinical observation that excessive punishment and emotional abuse may continue to be present.

Even less is known about the continuity of more subtle parenting disturbances associated with poor child outcome (e.g., noncontingent responsivity, understimulation, overcontrol, low verbal interaction, and warmth) (Belsky, 1983). Since poor child outcome appears to be due to the presence of continuous negative transactions with caregivers (Sameroff & Chandler, 1975), there may be stability here as well.

Our knowledge regarding the natural course of social skills problems clearly requires improvement. Long-term follow-ups of children and parents are needed to assess the natural course of interpersonal skills deficits, identifying those problems that spontaneously "remit" and those that remain problematic. RP efforts cannot be examined except against such a background of empirical data. In addition, since some skills deficits as extreme as child abuse may have high stability over time and others may not (e.g., childhood shyness) (Parker & Asher, 1987), determining those factors that predict better outcomes may provide clues for developing RP efforts as well as tell us the most important "targets" for intervention.

INTERVENTION STRATEGIES

Social competence interventions with both children and parents include many common strategies. (For detailed reviews, the reader is referred to

Gresham & Lemanek [1983], Hops [1983], and Dodge [1989] in the child area and Gordon & Davidson [1981] and Azar & Wolfe [1989] in the parenting area.) Techniques are typically grouped under three general headings: operant, social learning theory, and cognitive approaches.

The first, *operant conditioning,* involves the identification of observable and well-defined behavioral deficits in the client's repertoire, as well as interfering negative behavior. Through the methods of contingent reinforcement and punishment, more positive social behaviors are developed. Such techniques have been recommended when the behavior in question is nonverbal, does not require problem solving, or when the focus is on a few observationally "discrete" behaviors. In these approaches, modeling is not employed and tangible reinforcers are utilized, not self-reinforcement.

Operant techniques have been used most commonly to train very young children and developmentally delayed older ones (e.g., sharing, initiating play). Parents, peers, and teachers have been used as reinforcement agents using either social approval or token reinforcers. In one of the earliest efforts of this type, Hart, Reynolds, Baer, Brawley, and Harris (1968) attempted to increase the cooperative play of a socially isolated 5-year-old girl by having her teacher prompt social initiations by other children and verbally reinforce her for responding. The teacher then shaped the target child's responses to include only those deemed positive. Other studies have utilized peers. Kohler and Fowler (1985) attempted to increase the prosocial behavior of three girls (ages 5, 6, and 7). While teachers monitored their social behavior, the other children in the classrooms were used as training "assistants." Each day, three children were chosen and trained to invite the target child to play during a free-play period. Behaviors targeted for reinforcement included play invitations, use of social niceties (e.g., "I'm sorry," "Thank you"), and rejection of the target child's demands to others. The target child and her "assistants" received stickers on days they met training criteria.

Operant approaches have been used less frequently with parents. When they have been employed with parents, the samples have typically been intellectually low functioning. For example, two case studies with low-functioning abusive and neglectful mothers employed a bug-in-the-ear transmitter to prompt and verbally reinforce more positive parental behavior (Crimmins, Bradlyn, St. Lawrence, & Kelly, 1984; Wolfe et al., 1982). In another effort, Fantuzzo, Wray, Hall, Goins, and Azar (1986) trained mentally retarded mothers identified as maltreating using a board game. Mothers generated verbal responses to hypothetical parenting and social situations, with more elaborate responses gradually socially reinforced and shaped by a nonprofessional trainer. The therapist's contingent reinforcement has also been combined with desensitization to increase an abusive father's tolerance for his son's crying (Sanders, 1978).

More common than operant approaches have been ones based in social learning theory. At the core of such interventions are modeling and behavioral rehearsal. The client practices new modeled responses to increase or refine his/her already existing repertoire of skills. Skills can be presented in a variety of formats (e.g., therapist and peer modeling, written scripts, films, didactic instruction, and training manuals like Patterson's [1971] *Families*). In most cases, feedback on the target behavior is then provided and refinements are made through coaching. Technology has been used to facilitate the impact of this feedback (e.g., video feedback and coaching through headphones). Correct responses are reinforced by therapists or clients themselves.

In the child literature, symbolic modeling (e.g., film modeling) has been used more often with preschoolers, while coaching (i.e., verbal presentation of rules and standards for behavior, rehearsal, response feedback, and discussion) is more commonly employed with the peer problems of older children (Gresham & Lemanek, 1983). Oden and Asher (1977) used coaching successfully to increase children's social participation, cooperation, communication, and validation of support. Using a symbolic modeling film, O'Connor (1969, 1972) conducted a series of studies examining the impact on preschoolers' low rates of interaction.

Such approaches have also been very common in the general parent training literature (Patterson, 1971; Forehand & McMahon, 1981) and with abusive parents (Azar & Wolfe, 1989). Barth, Blythe, Schinke, Stevens, and Schilling (1983) utilized role plays with maltreating parents using scripts of parenting interactions that provided both behavioral and cognitive responses. Sandler and his colleagues (Denicola & Sandler, 1980; Wolfe & Sandler, 1981) have conducted a series of studies with abusive parents demonstrating the efficacy of child management skills training that relied on role modeling, rehearsal, and feedback to communicate parenting strategies.

More recently, *cognitive techniques* have also been utilized in social competence interventions. In these approaches, clients are trained in "process-oriented" skills said to underlie socially competent behavior: interpersonal problem solving, perspective taking, imagery techniques, and cognitive restructuring to decrease inappropriate expectancies and negative self-statements. Such training has also been used to decrease behaviors interfering with competent responses (e.g., anger).

Using cognitive methods, Billings and Wasik (1985) implemented a self-instructional training program with preschoolers to decrease academic, off-task, disruptive behavior. The children modeled the presented task and repeated the trainer's instructions in a progressively quieter voice until they performed the task with silent internal instructions. Shure, Spivack, and Jaeger (1971) taught preschool children alternative, causal, and consequential thinking for classroom interpersonal situations. Rickel, Eshelman, and Loigman (1983) have suggested that a stable relationship exists between the learning of these problem-solving skills and observed behavior utilizing such training.

Cognitive approaches have only recently been employed with parents. Azar (1989) described a cognitive–behavioral group treatment package for use with maltreating parents. Social learning theory-based strategies (e.g., child management skills training—use of reinforcement, appropriate discipline techniques, parent–child communication skills) were combined with (1) cognitive restructuring to decrease unrealistic expectations and mis-attributions regarding children's behavior; (2) problem-solving techniques to increase ability to deal with childrearing problems; and (3) cognitive anger control and stress management training (Novaco, 1975). Problem solving and anger control training have also been successfully used alone (Dawson, deArmas, McGrath, & Kelly, 1986; MacMillan, Guevremont, & Hansen, 1988; Nomellini & Katz, 1983).

All of these approaches have been utilized with both professional and nonprofessional trainers and used in both individual consultations and groups. Training has been done in homes, clinicians' offices, classrooms, and specially constructed settings (e.g., rooms with one-way mirrors and constructed home settings). Each has received some empirical support. To date, the most effective in terms of immediate impact have been those combining several different therapeutic methodologies (e.g., modeling with instruction, rehearsal, feedback, and role playing). Presumably, integrative approaches address all of the primary objectives of social skills training (Dodge, 1989): that is, enhancing knowledge of the required behaviors, assisting the individual to translate that knowledge into active responses, and helping him/her maintain and generalize the behavior.

Effectiveness, however, has not been demonstrated for all pop-ulations. While parent training (social learning theory-based) has general-ly been shown to be effective in changing parental behavior in middle- and upper-middle-class families (Gordon & Davidson, 1981; Johnson & Katz, 1973), its effectiveness with lower socioeconomic status parents has been questioned (Patterson, 1974; Patterson, Cobb, & Ray, 1973). Char-acteristics such as high emotional and financial stress have been cited as reasons for this (Dumas, 1984; Dumas & Wahler, 1983; Wahler, 1980). Some studies, however, have not shown differences related to socioeco-nomic status (Mira, 1970; Rogers, Forehand, Griest, Wells, & McMahon, 1981; Strain, Young, & Horowitz, 1981). Those studies showing dif-ferences appear to use more discussion and verbal teaching of learning principles rather than engaging clients in "action-oriented" modeling, role play, and coaching (Knapp & Deluty, 1989).

Marital distress has also been implicated as interfering with the effectiveness of parent training, although as with socioeconomic status, there are contradictory findings (Brody & Forehand, 1985; Oltmanns, Broderick, & O'Leary, 1977; Reisinger, Frangia, & Hoffman, 1976). The impact seems stronger on long-term outcome (McMahon & Wells, 1989).

Less is known regarding individual differences in the effectiveness of social skills training with children. While it has met with success in a variety of groups (e.g., learning disabled, inpatient, handicapped, rejected, and socially isolated children), lower effectiveness has been found with aggressive children. Adaptations may be required with this group (e.g., instituting environmental management to suppress anger before beginning training [Sallis, 1983]).

Ethnic and socioeconomic differences in outcome have been found in studies employing film modeling with children (Gottman, 1977). This has been attributed to film role models being different than the target children in race and social class.

More information is needed to determine which clients will not succeed in such approaches. With such knowledge, improvements can be made in both the mode in which material is presented and the components employed. Ultimately, this may strengthen maintenance of treatment effects as well.

RELAPSE AND FACTORS ASSOCIATED WITH ITS OCCURRENCE

Dropouts in Treatment—Early "Relapse"

Dropping out of an intervention might be construed as the earliest form of "relapse." Little is known about dropout rates in child social skill interventions, while some limited information is available on parenting interventions (mainly social learning theory-based). Forehand, Middlebrook, Rogers, and Steffe (1983) found a 28% dropout rate across the 45 parenting studies they reviewed, which they suggested compares favorably with the general psychotherapy literature. It may be, however, that only studies with low dropout rates reported figures, and thus the actual rates may be higher. Attrition appeared to be higher during assessment than treatment, which may reflect the extensive assessment that occurs in behavioral treatments. Data from one recent prevention study with parents, however, found that parents who were not assessed prior to treatment showed higher attrition rates than did a group that was (38% vs. 13%) (Dush & Stacy, 1987).

Depressed parents (McMahon, Forehand, Griest, & Wells, 1981) and ones lower in socioeconomic status (McMahon et al., 1981; Worland, Carney, Weinberg, & Milich, 1982) appear to be at greater risk for dropping out. Process variables (e.g., parental expectancies and client–therapist interactions) and therapist characteristics may also play a role (Chamberlain, Patterson, Reid, Kavanagh, & Forgatch, 1984; Patterson & Forgatch, 1985). Because of the involuntary nature of most treatment in the child abuse area, the issue of attrition may be of particular concern. Indeed, data with maltreating parents suggest high dropout rates (e.g., 45%) (Reid, 1985). Wolfe, Aragona, Kaufman, and Sandler (1980) found that parents court ordered into treatment were more likely to complete parent training than those who were not court ordered (32% vs. 87%). Another study that involved a more comprehensive service approach (including day care, group sessions for the parents, and home treatment), however, did not find differential effects for court-involved families (Irueste-Montes & Montes, 1988). It has been suggested that incentives be provided to reduce attrition (e.g., movie tickets, monetary incentives, the provision of transportation, lunch and baby sitting, and contracting), but their effectiveness has not been examined yet.

Because the reoccurrence of child abuse is so dangerous, relapse during treatment is a major problem for clinicians. Cohn (1979), in reviewing traditional interventions with abusive and neglectful parents in 11 federally funded demonstration projects, found a 30% relapse rate during treatment. Similar figures for behaviorally oriented treatments are not available. While initiating therapeutic contracts for reducing the use of physical punishment during treatment may be helpful (Azar & Wolfe, 1989), empirical support for their use is not available as yet.

Maintenance of Treatment Effects without Programming

In both the parenting and child intervention literature, some data exist on maintenance of treatment effects without specific programming. For the most part, however, follow-up periods have been relatively short.

Because studies on parent training typically have focused on children with behavioral problems, an examination of maintenance of parental changes has been of less interest. In reviewing 47 studies, Moreland, Schwebel, Beck, and Wells (1982) found only 6 that examined such maintenance. Behavioral training has generally been shown to be effective in changing parental behavior up to periods of 18 months (Patterson & Fleischman, 1979; Webster-Stratton, 1982, 1984). Social learning theory parental training also appears to do better than no treatment or other common approaches used with child behavioral problems (e.g., child guidance, juvenile court services, and client-centered) when follow-up ranged from 6 to 18 months (Gordon & Davidson, 1981).

Follow-up data in programs designed to change abusive parents' behavior have been considerably more limited. Single case studies have indicated maintenance of selected parental behaviors (e.g., decreased negative behavior) at follow-up periods from 2 to 8 months (Azar, 1989). Few of these, however, examined recidivism for abuse itself. One exception is a study by Wolfe, Kaufman, Aragona, and Sandler (1981), which employed a group treatment package that included child management skills training and anger control and stress management training and found no recidivism at 1 year follow-up in eight abusive parents. Another is a study by Azar and Twentyman (1984), which also demonstrated no recidivism at 1 year follow-up with a package that included cognitive strategies (Azar, 1989).

In social skills training with children, similarly short follow-ups have been the rule. Schloss, Schloss, Wood, and Kiehl (1986) reviewed follow-up data from 25 studies done between 1980 and 1985. Only 15 studies collected such data, with the follow-up periods ranging from 2 weeks to 1 year (the modal period was 2 to 3 weeks). Twelve studies showed continued effectiveness at the time of maintenance assessment.

A number of factors appear to be associated with poor maintenance in parent training programs: socioeconomic distress, marital discord, multiple life stressors, and social isolation (Dadds, Sanders, Behrens, & James, 1987; Dadds, Schwartz, & Sanders, 1987; Dumas & Wahler, 1983; Griest & Forehand, 1982; McMahon et al., 1981; Wahler, 1980). These factors may ultimately play a causal role in the relapse process and may need to be addressed in RP programming. Studies that have shown better maintenance (e.g., over periods from 1 to 4½ years) (Baum & Forehand, 1981) provided treatment for less socioeconomically distressed parents.

Negative findings for the impact of stress have also appeared in the child maltreatment area. Szykula and Fleischman (1985) found that parent training was successful in reducing the need for out-of-home placement of children in families when stress levels were low and the treatment occurred early in the course of problems (i.e., families without multiple incidents of maltreatment). These findings suggest that high-stress families may be particularly vulnerable to relapse and thus require added preventive efforts (e.g., management of external stressors and early intervention). These factors also argue for extensive assessment of the ecological context of parenting as crucial in understanding potential obstacles to maintenance (Sanders, Dadds, & Bor, 1989).

Parameters of treatment may also be involved in the relapse process. Approaches that were time limited (e.g., maximum of 12 weeks) and used graduate student therapists have not fared as well as those that employed open-ended treatment and experienced trainers (McMahon & Wells, 1989).

ATTEMPTS TO INFLUENCE MAINTENANCE

Programming for maintenance is rare in social skills interventions with both children and parents. For example, in Sanders and James's (1983) review of the general parent training intervention literature, only four such studies were identified. Our review of the literature in these two domains provided similarly poor results. A few examples of applications of methods commonly considered in the domain of RP (Stokes & Baer, 1977) do exist, but only limited data on their effectiveness in extending treatment effects over time are available. This work has mostly involved single case studies or ones with no control condition, limiting generalization.

Booster Session/Fading of Treatment

"Fading" has been used to increase temporal generality in behavioral interventions. A few examples of this strategy exist in the peer competency literature. VanHasselt, Griest, Kazdin, Esveldt-Dawson, and Vries (1984) used fading in a social skills training study with an inpatient 7-year-old boy who was aggressive and had poor social interactions. The fading involved reducing the frequency of token rewards (a small car or a toy soldier) from three times to once a day, discontinuing prompts, and delaying reinforcement (from immediate to only at the end of the day). Improvements in behaviors targeted for treatment (decreasing aggression and increasing prosocial peer interactions) were still evident at 1 month and 1 year follow-ups. This fading took place in a controlled environment (inpatient unit), and it is unclear whether it would have been as successful with naturally occurring "risk" factors present.

In another example, Greenwood, Walker, and Hops (1977) gradually removed the behavioral components of a social skills program (e.g., rules and progress charts) with a classroom of children and found the addition of fading to be more effective than a training-only condition. Rhode, Morgan, and Young (1983) examined the impact of reinforcement thinning and self-evaluation of appropriate classroom behavior within a special education classroom, using fading of self-evaluation from every 15 minutes in a resource room to every 30 minutes. Once training was transferred to the regular classroom, evaluations were further faded to every other day to finally only private nonverbal self-evaluations. Over a 12-session follow-up period, appropriate behavior maintained at 54% higher than at baseline.

At least one effort in the parenting area has included fading. Herbert and Baer (1972) trained a mother in self-recording using a wrist recorder to monitor instances of her attention to her child, at first on a daily basis and then intermittently, gradually decreasing the frequency. Follow-up indicated maintenance of parental behavioral changes.

Booster sessions in the posttreatment period have also been employed. In a large prevention effort with second to fourth graders, for example, Weissberg et al. (1981) provided weekly encore sessions after the training of social problem-solving skills (42-lesson curriculum) was complete where children reviewed and applied skills to recent problems experienced. These children showed greater gains than control children on cognitive and behavioral social problem-solving skills and expressed greater confidence in their ability to deal effectively with interpersonal problems. They also did better on teacher ratings of shy-anxious behavior and global ratings of likability and school adjustment. Weissberg and Allen (1986) suggest that social problem-solving programs that end after the skills are trained in the classroom do not allow time to practice the newly acquired skills in multiple real-life situations. Such encore sessions, however, may be indistinguishable from actual treatment sessions, especially in cost, and, therefore, may not technically constitute a RP effort.

Other efforts of this sort have occurred in the parenting area. Patterson (1974) collected home data over a 12-month period, providing retraining at signs of deterioration. Wahler (1975) successfully employed a refresher course during the posttreatment period. Unfortunately, no control groups were utilized in either of these efforts. Other studies have not shown a positive impact of continued contact/booster work (e.g., with low SES mothers) (Wahler, 1980).

Other procedures have been suggested but have not been evaluated as yet. For example, switching to a leaner schedule of therapist social reinforcement or specifying to the parents contingencies for returning to the clinic (e.g., a predetermined maintenance plan) might be tried. The latter would increase client sense of control and self-efficacy, both of which are important to RP (Marlatt & Gordon, 1985).

Multiple Exemplars

Another technique to promote maintenance involves training in multiple settings or exemplars (Stokes & Baer, 1977). Here, the idea is to prepare the client for the multitude of settings in which his/her newly learned behavior will be utilized. RP efforts utilizing this strategy have focused on high-risk situations. Wolfe et al. (1981) combined standard child management training with anger control and relaxation training to help parents deal with the inevitable stressful situations they would encounter both during and posttreatment. No recidivism was found at 1 year follow-up. Unfortunately, because no condition without these components was included, it is unclear what was responsible for the maintenance found.

Azar and Twentyman (1984), using the 10-week cognitive–behavioral package described earlier, conducted a comparative outcome study that provides better information regarding RP. This study compared this package in two forms (group treatment with and without weekly home visits to increase generalization) to an insight-oriented group and a wait-list control group. While all treated groups fared better at posttest and at a 2-month follow-up than no-treatment controls, only the cognitive–behavioral plus home training condition showed no recidivism at 1 year follow-up. The adjunct home training allowed for many exemplars of difficult situations to occur in the trainers' presence, permitting *in vivo* coaching and feedback as well as individualization of the program.

In probably the most specific effort of this type, Sanders and Dadds (1982) employed a planned activities procedure whereby parents were taught to engage children in activities in "high-risk" target community settings. The procedure involved the selection and arrangement of appropriate activities and discussions with the child regarding the rules for the situation and the consequences operating for appropriate and inappropriate behavior. Following the situation, a review of the child's behavior and delivery of any relevant consequences occurred. This procedure followed standard child management training, and levels of positive changes in parental behavior either maintained or improved further. In a later report, efforts were directed successfully at high-risk situations in the home (e.g., bedtime and school exit) as well, but with no differences found when compared with a child-management-training-alone condition (Sanders & Christensen, 1985).

Training in multiple settings has not been a common therapeutic practice with children. Wiig and Bray (1983), in teaching prosocial communication to young children, used the classroom teacher as the main or initial trainer who then sent home activity sheets. These sheets enabled parents to reinforce the skills from school and to facilitate the generalization from one environment to another. It has also been suggested that arranging the training setting to be similar to natural environments may help in both generalization and maintenance. For example, Walker and Buckley (1974) rearranged the special classroom used in training to resemble the regular classroom. Maintenance of appropriate behavior at 77% of treatment levels was found at a 15-day follow-up. This approach of "equating stimulus conditions" to encourage transfer through the "rule of identical elements" may prove to be important.

Reducing Risk Factors and Social Ecological Work

The context in which social interactions occur and the social network of the individual have been suggested as playing a role in relapse. McCrady

(1989), for example, has presented a convincing argument regarding the role that social networks play in the relapse process in addictions and suggests specific programming that might be done to improve spousal support during the maintenance period. Similarly, the mood state of the parents and the nature of their interactions with other adults (e.g., aversive interactions with others) have been implicated as impacting on long-term outcome in parent training (Panaccione & Wahler, 1986).

Some efforts to improve maintenance by intervening with social networks have been attempted with parents. Dadds, Schwartz, and Sanders (1987), for example, showed that maritally distressed families who received only child management training, but not an adjunctive marital intervention, failed to maintain short-term improvements in maternal behavior at 6-month follow-up. Similar programs have also been tried with abusive parents. Gilbert (1976) utilized a spouse to reinforce an abusive mother's newly acquired responses. Ecobehavioral attempts by Lutzker and his colleagues addressed contextual issues including leisure activities, health issues, and marital discord, all of which may detract from parents' motivation to maintain gains (Campbell, O'Brien, Bickett, & Lutzker, 1983; Lutzker & Rice, 1984). These approaches have shown lower rates of multiple incidents of reabuse or reneglect over a 5-year period. Other case studies have focused on intra-individual factors that may increase risk for "relapse" (e.g., depression [Conger, Lahey, & Smith, 1981]). Research employing larger samples and group designs are needed to assess the long-term impact of such interventions.

Other suggestions for utilizing social networks during the posttreatment phase have been made. Nay (1979) suggested that families meet with nonprofessional volunteers for ongoing support and reinforcement for intervention efforts. Groups like Parents Anonymous could also be used for ongoing support with abusive parents during the maintenance phase. Another alternative might be to pair already trained parents with parents new to parent training to provide ongoing monitoring, feedback, and support for behavioral changes (Sanders & James, 1983).

While many child social skills training studies have employed significant others to prompt and reinforce children's behavior during treatment, systematic attempts to influence the skill level of the child's social network postintervention have not yet been attempted. Such attempts would likely facilitate coping and maintenance of treatment gains. It is also possible that some spillover to posttreatment might occur with peers and teachers who have acted as prompters and who now have had positive experiences with target children, but no empirical evidence is currently available to support this hypothesis.

Self-Management Training

Marlatt and Gordon's (1985) work in RP strongly argues the need for coping skills in the relapse period (e.g., self-control skills to maintain the newly trained behaviors in high-risk situations). Efforts in this direction have appeared in both the child and parenting competency training literature.

In the child literature, there are a few examples of self-management-based RP efforts in the form of correspondence training, self-evaluation, and self-monitoring. In correspondence training, for example, elementary school children have compared their own behavioral ratings with those of their teacher (Robertson, Simon, Rachmann, & Drabman, 1979). Rewards were given for ratings that matched the teacher's. Teacher matching was eliminated when it was deemed that students were capable of accurate assessments. Bolstad and Johnson (1972) designed a similar study using self-evaluation with disruptive elementary schoolchildren. In this case, self-evaluation cards were awarded points for accurate self-observations in comparison to ratings of independent observers. Sixty-nine percent maintained at or below one half of baseline disruptive behavior for the seven-session extinction period.

In the parenting area, Wells, Griest, and Forehand (1980) employed self-control training in conjunction with standard behavioral parent training with parents of noncompliant children. They found the addition of such training did not affect parental behavior at 2 months follow-up but did improve child behavior. They explained their lack of differential parental maintenance effects by suggesting that parents in both standard parental training and enhanced treatment could modify their behavior during a follow-up observation, but only those who had actually been using techniques in the posttreatment period would be able to influence their children's behavior.

In summary, it is striking that so few efforts have been directed at RP in these two domains. Most of the studies reported here were carried out a number of years ago and have not been replicated. It appears that many of the early researchers in this area abandoned treatment outcome work. Instead, they moved toward more basic research examining phenomena associated with parenting and child social skills problems. Perhaps in the next decade, with this information now in hand, more efforts regarding intervention will occur.

A RESEARCH AGENDA

Based on the present review, five global directions for enhancing RP efforts are recommended. First, efforts aimed at identifying the defining qualities of socially competent peer and parenting responses need to continue, as well as the development of ways to optimally measure them. These efforts should be aimed at uncovering those problems that have continuity in children's and parents' lives and those that shift across developmental eras. Particular efforts need to be directed at understanding gender, socioeconomic and cultural differences, so that interventions might be attuned to the defining qualities of social competence based on these dimensions and any obstacles to maintenance such differences may present. In particular, information regarding fathers' interactions with children has been noticeably thin (Horton, 1984). Problems with the reliability and validity of current measurement methods have been delineated (Connolly, 1983; Elliott, Sheridan, & Gresham, 1989). The use of multiple methods has been suggested, as well as refinements being made in presently used ones (e.g., with socially rejected children, examining those who are aggressive and those who are submissive) (Asher, Parkhurst, Hymel, & Williams, 1990). Development of new approaches for special populations is also needed (e.g., intellectually low-functioning clients). Agreement regarding a standard battery of measures and the points at which a clinical level of social incompetence is judged would allow for comparability in identifying samples for treatment, as well as allow for a determination of when "relapse" has occurred. Again, this should be done with attention to cultural diversity. Such work would help us to direct RP efforts at those most in need of services and allow us to evaluate the results of our efforts.

Second, efforts directed at identifying risk factors for relapse, both person based (e.g., demographic characteristics and beliefs) and situation based (e.g., high-risk situations) are needed. The work of Sanders and his colleagues provides some of the best examples of such work (Sanders, 1984). For instance, they have identified high-risk situations where negative parenting interactions occur (e.g., grocery stores), as well as the dimension within these situations that will present the most problems (e.g., the specific areas within such stores) (Sanders & Hunter, 1984). Utilizing such information, future research might identify the cognitive and behavioral skills utilized by newly "cured" clients or competent parents to get themselves through such high-risk situations. Parental cognitive schema regarding childrearing and children's behavior may also be important to examine (Azar, 1989). Unrealistic beliefs regarding appropriate child behavior have been shown to distinguish maltreating parents (Azar, Robinson, Hekimian, & Twentyman, 1984; Azar & Rohrbeck, 1986). There is some evidence that such expectations may guide parents' attributions about the causes of their children's behavior and the responses they choose (Barnes & Azar, 1990). They may also determine which parents are most responsive to the negative effects of contextual stress, a factor that has already been associated with risk for relapse. Failure to impact on such factors, therefore, may hinder maintenance. Third, improvements are needed in our knowledge base on the effectiveness of interventions. For example, it is clear that inadequate cognitive and behavioral assessment may produce less than optimal results in social skills training. Therefore, more individualized applications of social competency training should be undertaken, ensuring that subjects are in fact deficient in the skills being trained. Utilization of findings from basic research is crucial in determining which skills are targeted as well.

At the same time, more large-scale evaluations need to be undertaken. Much of what is known about the effectiveness of current techniques comes from single case studies. The largest efforts in the parenting area have included as few as 44 families. Currently, maintenance data in the two domains covered in this chapter have involved inadequately short follow-up periods. Since both parenting and peer skills are constantly evolving, long-term follow-ups are needed to see whether interventions have in fact impacted on the clients' trajectory of social development or merely produced a short period of respite from difficulties. In addition, few comparative outcome studies have been undertaken. Attention to these suggestions will provide studies that give us the clearest outcome data for determining the effectiveness of RP efforts (i.e., for which clients, over what period, and under which conditions are techniques effective).

Fourth, in the parenting area in particular, more research is needed regarding motivation and commitment for treatment, as well as during the posttreatment phase. Webster-Stratton (1982), for example, found that while mothers maintained improvement 1 year after parent training, they reported less confidence in their use of trained skills than at posttest. Decreases in perceptions of self-efficacy (or in the efficacy of techniques) may increase risk of relapse. In general, samples in this area have been highly motivated, middle-class volunteers. When efforts have veered from this group, success has been lower. Innovative approaches addressing the needs of less motivated and multistressed populations are needed. Systematic evaluations of the impact of "motivators" for such clients are needed. Consumer satisfaction in both peer interventions and parenting also need to be included as an indicator of outcome and as a predictor of relapse.

Finally, and probably most important, efforts need to be directed at theory development. Attempts at positing the determinants of parenting and childhood social competency, for example, are beginning to appear in the literature (Abidin, 1989; Azar, 1989; Belsky, 1983; Dodge, 1989; Ladd & Crick, 1989). Such models will guide treatment development, define successful outcome, and allow the identification of children and parents who are most at risk for relapse.

CONCLUSION

Evidence from the social competency literature to date suggests that behavioral and cognitive–behavioral approaches to training have produced positive changes in the interpersonal skills of both parents and children. Efforts directed at maintaining these effects, however, have not been made in any great number and are crucial for the long-term viability of such approaches. Efforts thus far have been hampered by a lack of definitional clarity, an inadequate knowledge base regarding the course of social skills problems and factors affecting relapse, and a lack of connection between the basic research findings available and intervention efforts. Once these issues are addressed, a more cohesive body of knowledge and effective RP efforts can be developed.

Acknowledgments

Completion of this chapter was supported by a First Independent Research Support and Transition Award (MH46940) from the National Institute of Mental Health to the first author.

REFERENCES

Abidin, R. R. (1989, August). *The determinants of parenting: What variables do we need to look at?* Paper presented at the annual meeting of the American Psychological Association, New Orleans, LA.

Asher, S. R., Oden, S. L., & Gottman, J. M. (1977). Children's friendships in school settings. In L. G. Katz (Ed.), *Current topics in early childhood education* (Vol. 1, pp. 33–61). Norwood, NJ: Ablex.

Asher, S. R., Parkhurst, J. T., Hymel, S., & Williams, G. A. (1990). Peer rejection and loneliness in childhood. In S. R. Asher, & J. D. Coie (Eds.), *Peer rejection in childhood* (pp. 253–273). New York: Cambridge University Press.

Azar, S. T. (1989). Training parents of abused children. In C. E. Schaefer & J. M. Briesmeister (Eds.), *Handbook of parent training* (pp. 414–441). New York: Wiley.

Azar, S. T., Robinson, D. R., Hekimian, E., & Twentyman, C. T. (1984). Unrealistic expectations and problem-solving ability in maltreating and comparison mothers. *Journal of Consulting and Clinical Psychology, 52,* 687–691.

Azar, S. T., & Rohrbeck, C. A. (1986). Child abuse and unrealistic expectations: Further validation of the Parent Opinion Questionnaire. *Journal of Consulting and Clinical Psychology, 54*, 867–868.

Azar, S. T., & Siegel, B. (1990). Behavioral treatment of child abuse: A developmental perspective. *Behavior Modification, 14*, 279–300.

Azar, S. T., & Twentyman, C. T. (1984, November). *An evaluation of the effectiveness of behaviorally versus insight oriented group treatments with maltreating mothers.* Paper presented at the annual meeting of the Association for the Advancement of Behavior Therapy, Philadelphia, PA.

Azar, S. A., & Wolfe, D A. (1989). Child abuse and neglect. In E. J. Mash & R. A. Barkley (Eds.), *Treatment of childhood disorders* (pp. 451–489). New York: Guilford Press.

Barnes, K. T., & Azar, S. T. (1990, August). *Maternal expectations and attributions in discipline situations: A test of a cognitive model of parenting.* Paper presented at the annual meeting of the American Psychological Association, Boston, MA.

Barth, R. P., Blythe, B., Schinke, S. P., Stevens, P., & Schilling, R. F. (1983). Self-control training with maltreating parents. *Child Welfare, 62*, 313–324.

Baum, C. G., & Forehand, R. (1981). Long-term follow-up assessment of parent training by use of multiple-outcome measures. *Behavior Therapy, 12*, 643–652.

Beck, S., & Forehand, R. (1984). Social skills training for children: A methodological and clinical review of behavior modification studies. *Behavioural Psychotherapy, 12*, 17–45.

Belsky, J. (1983). The determinants of parenting: Process model. *Child Development, 55*, 83–96.

Billings, D. C., & Wasik, B. H. (1985). Self-instructional training with a preschooler: An attempt to replicate. *Journal of Applied Behavior Analysis, 18*, 61–67.

Bolstad, O. D., & Johnson, S. M. (1972). Self-regulation in the modification of disruptive classroom behavior. *Journal of Applied Behavior Analysis, 5*, 443–454.

Brody, G. M., & Forehand, R. (1985). The efficacy of parent training with maritally distressed and non-distressed mothers: A multimethod assessment. *Behavior Research and Therapy, 23*, 291–296.

Burgdorf, K. (1988). *Study of national incidence and prevalence of child abuse and neglect, 1988.* Washington, DC: National Center on Child Abuse and Neglect.

Campbell, R. V., O'Brien, S., Bickett, A. D., & Lutzker, J. R. (1983). In-home parent training of migraine headaches and marital counseling as an ecobehavioral approach to prevent child abuse. *Journal of Behavior Therapy and Experimental Psychiatry, 14*, 147–154.

Chamberlain, P., Patterson, G., Reid, J., Kavanagh, K., & Forgatch, K. (1984). Observation of client resistance. *Behavior Therapy, 15*, 144–155.

Cohn, A. M. (1979). Essential elements of successful child abuse and neglect treatment. *Child Abuse and Neglect, 3*, 491–496.

Coie, J. D., & Dodge, K. A. (1983). Continuity of children's social status: A five-year longitudinal study. *Merrill-Palmer Quarterly, 29,* 261–282.

Coie, J. D., Dodge, K. A., & Coppotelli, H. (1982). Dimensions of social status: A cross-age perspective. *Developmental Psychology, 18,* 557–570.

Combs, M., & Slaby, D. (1977). Social skills training in children. In A. Kazdin & B. Lahey (Eds.), *Advances in clinical child psychology* (pp. 161–201). New York: Plenum Press.

Conger, R. D., Lahey, B. B., & Smith, S. S. (1981, July). *An intervention program for child abuse: Modifying maternal depression and behavior.* Paper presented at the Family Violence Research Conference, University of New Hampshire, Durham, NH.

Connolly, J. A. (1983). A review of sociometric procedures in the assessment of social competencies in children. *Applied Research in Mental Retardation, 4,* 315–327.

Crimmins, D. B., Bradlyn, A. S., St Lawrence, J. S., & Kelly, J. (1984). A training technique for improving the parent-child interaction skills of an abusive, neglectful mother. *Child Abuse and Neglect, 8,* 533–539.

Dadds, M. R., Sanders, M. R., Behrens, B. C., & James, J. E. (1987). Marital discord and child behavior problems: A description of family interactions during treatment. *Journal of Clinical Child Psychology, 16,* 192–203.

Dadds, M. R., Schwartz, S., & Sanders, M. R. (1987). Marital discord and treatment outcome in behavioral treatment of child conduct disorders. *Journal of Consulting and Clinical Psychology, 55,* 396–403.

Dawson, B., deArmas, A., McGrath, M. L., & Kelly, J. (1986). Cognitive problem-solving training to improve the child care judgement of child neglectful parents. *Journal of Family Violence, 1,* 209–221.

Denicola, J., & Sandler, J. (1980). Training abusive parents in cognitive–behavioral techniques. *Behavior Therapy, 11,* 263–270.

Dodge, K. A. (1989). Problems in social relationships. In E. J. Mash & R. A. Barkley (Eds.), *Treatment of childhood disorders* (pp. 222–224). New York: Guilford Press.

Dumas, J. E. (1984). Interactional correlates of treatment outcome in behavioral parent training. *Journal of Consulting and Clinical Psychology, 52,* 946–954.

Dumas, J. E., & Wahler, R. G. (1983). Predictors of treatment outcome in parent training: Mother insularity and socioeconomic disadvantage. *Behavioral Assessment, 5,* 301–313.

Dush, D. M., & Stacy, E. W. (1987). Pretesting enhancement of parent compliance in a prevention program for high-risk children. *Evaluation and the Health Profession, 10,* 201–205.

Elliott, S. N., Sheridan, S. M., & Gresham, F. M. (1989). Assessing and treating social skills deficits: A case study for the scientist-practitioner. *Journal of School Psychology, 27,* 197–222.

Fantuzzo, J. W., Wray, L., Hall, R., Goins, C., & Azar, S. T. (1986). Parent and social skills training for mentally retarded parents identified as child maltreaters. *American Journal of Mental Deficiency, 91,* 135–140.

Ferlinger, N., Glenwick, D. S., Gaines, R. R., & Green, A. (1988). Identifying correlates of re-abuse in maltreating parents. *Child Abuse and Neglect, 12,* 41–49.

Forehand, R., & McMahon, R. J. (1981). *Helping the noncompliant child: A clinician's guide to parent training.* New York: Guilford Press.

Forehand, R., Middlebrook, J., Rogers, T., & Steffe, M. (1983). Dropping out of parent training. *Behavioral Research & Therapy, 21,* 663–668.

Foster, S. L., DeLawyer, D. D., & Guevremont, D. L. (1985). Selecting targets for social skills training with children and adolescents. *Advances in Learning and Behavioral Disabilities, 4,* 77–132.

Gilbert, M. R. (1976). Behavioral approaches to treatment of child abuse. *Nursing Times, 72,* 140–143.

Giovannoni, J. M., & Becerra, R. M. (1970). *Defining child abuse.* New York: Free Press.

Gordon, S. B., & Davidson, N. (1981). Behavioral parent training. In A. F. Gurman & D. P. Kniskern (Eds.), *Handbook of family therapy* (pp. 517–555). New York: Bruner/Mazel.

Gottman, J. M. (1977). Toward a definition of social isolation in children. *Child Development, 48,* 513–517.

Greenwood, C. R., Walker, H. M., & Hops, H. (1977). Some issues in social interaction/withdrawal assessment. *Exceptional Children, 43,* 490–499.

Gresham, F. M. (1981). Validity of social skills measures for assessing social competence in low status children: A multivariate investigation. *Developmental Psychology, 17,* 390–398.

Gresham, F. M., & Lemanek, K. L. (1983). Social skills: A review of cognitive behavioral training procedures with children. *Journal of Applied Developmental Psychology, 4,* 239–261.

Griest, D. L., & Forehand, R. (1982). How can I get any parent training done with all these other problems going on? The role of family variables in child behavior therapy. *Child and Family Behavior Therapy, 4,* 73–80.

Gronlund, N. E. (1959). *Sociometry in the classroom.* New York: Harper.

Hart, B. M., Reynolds, N. J., Baer, D. M., Brawley, E. R., & Harris, F. R. (1968). Effect of contingent and noncontingent social reinforcement on the cooperative play of a preschool child. *Journal of Applied Behavior Analysis, 1,* 73–76.

Herbert, E. W., & Baer, D. M. (1972). Training parents as behavior modifiers: Self recording contingent attention. *Journal of Applied Behavior Analysis, 5,* 139–149.

Hops, H. (1983). Children's social competence and skill: Current research practices and future directions. *Behavior Therapy, 14,* 13–18.

Horton, L. (1984). The father's role in behavioral parent training: A review. *Journal of Clinical Child Psychology, 13,* 274–279.

Howes, C. (1987). Peer interaction of young children. *Monographs of the Society for Research in Child Development, 53* (Serial No. 217). Chicago: University of Chicago Press.

Hughes, J. N. (1986). Methods of skill selection in social skills training: A review. *Professional School Psychology, 1,* 235–248.

Hymel, S., & Asher, S. R. (1977, April). *Assessment and training of isolated children's social skills*. Paper presented at the biennial meeting of the Society for Research in Child Development, New Orleans, LA.

Irueste-Montes, A. M., & Montes, F. (1988). Court-ordered vs. voluntary treatment of abusive and neglectful parents. *Child Abuse and Neglect, 12,* 33–39.

Johnson, C. A., & Katz, R. C. (1973). Using parents as change agents for children. A review. *Journal of Child Clinical Psychology and Psychiatry, 14,* 181–200.

Knapp, P. A., & Deluty, R. H. (1989). Relative effectiveness of two behavioral parent training programs. *Journal of Clinical Child Psychology, 18,* 314–322.

Kohlberg, L., LaCrosse, J., & Ricks, D. (1972). The predictability of adult mental health from childhood behavior. In B. Wolman (Ed.), *Manual of child psychopathology* (pp. 1217–1283). New York: McGraw-Hill.

Kohler, F. W., & Fowler, S. A. (1985). Training pro-social behaviors to young children: An analysis of reciprocity with untrained peers. *Journal of Applied Behavior Analysis, 18,* 187–200.

Kupersmidt, J. B. (1983, April). *Predicting delinquency and academic problems from childhood peer status.* Paper presented at the biennual meeting of the Society for Research in Child Development, Detroit, MI.

Ladd, G. W., & Crick, N. R. (1989). Probing the psychological environment: Children's cognitions, perceptions, and feelings in the peer culture. *Advances in Motivation and Achievement, 6,* 1–44.

Li, A. (1985). Early rejected status and later social adjustment: A three-year follow-up. *Journal of Abnormal Child Psychology, 13,* 567–577.

Lutzker, J. R., & Rice, J. M. (1984). Project 12-Ways: Measuring outcome of a large in-home service for treatment and prevention of child abuse and neglect. *Child Abuse and Neglect, 8,* 519–524.

MacMillan, V. M., Guevremont, D. C., & Hansen, D. J. (1988). Problem-solving training with a multiply distressed abusive and neglectful mother. *Journal of Family Violence, 3,* 313–326.

Marlatt, G. A., & Gordon, J. R. (1985). *Relapse prevention: Maintenance strategies in the treatment of addictive behavior.* New York: Guilford Press.

McCrady, B. S. (1989). Extending relapse prevention models to couples. *Addictive Behavior, 14,* 69–174.

McFall, R. M. (1982). A review and reformulation of the concept of skills. *Behavioral Assessment, 4,* 1–33.

McMahon, R. J., Forehand, R., Griest, D. L., & Wells, K. C. (1981). Who drops out of treatment during parent behavioral training. *Behavior Counseling Quarterly, 1,* 79–85.

McMahon, R. J., & Wells, K. C. (1989). Conduct disorders. In E. J. Mash & R. A. Barkley (Eds.), *Treatment of childhood disorders* (pp. 73–132). New York: Guilford Press.

Mira, M. (1970). Results of a behavior modification training program for parents and teachers. *Behaviour Research and Therapy, 8,* 309–311.

Moreland, J. R., Schwebel, A. I., Beck, S., & Wells, R. (1982). Parents as therapists. A review of the behavior therapy parent training literature—1975 to 1981. *Behavior Modification, 6,* 250–276.

Nay, W. R. (1979). Parents as real life reinforcers: The enhancement of parent training effects across conditions other than training. In A. P. Goldstein & F.

H. Kanfer (Eds.), *Maximizing treatment gains: Transfer enhancement in psychotherapy* (pp. 249–302). New York: Academic Press.

Nomellini, S., & Katz, R. C. (1983). Effects of anger control training on abusive parents. *Cognitive Therapy and Research, 7*, 57–68.

Novaco, R. W. (1975). *Anger control: The development and evaluation of an experimental treatment*. Lexington, MA: Lexington Books.

O'Connor, R. D. (1969). Modification of social withdrawal through symbolic modeling. *Journal of Applied Behavior Analysis, 2*, 15–22.

O'Connor, R. D. (1972). Relative efficacy of modeling, shaping, and the combined procedures for modification of social withdrawal. *Journal of Abnormal Psychology, 79*, 327–334.

Oden, S. L., & Asher, S. R. (1977). Coaching children in social skills for friendship making. *Child Development, 48*, 495–506.

Oltmanns, T. F., Broderick, J. E., & O'Leary, K. D. (1977). Marital adjustment and the efficacy of behavior therapy with children. *Journal of Consulting and Clinical Psychology, 45*, 724–729.

Panaccione, V. F., & Wahler, R. G. (1986). Child behavior, maternal depression, and social coercion as factors in the quality of child care. *Journal of Abnormal Child Psychology, 14*, 263–278.

Parker, J. G., & Asher, S. R. (1987). Peer relations and later personal adjustment: Are low accepted children at risk? *Psychological Bulletin, 102*, 357–389.

Patterson, G. R. (1971). *Families: Application of social learning theory to family life*. Champaign, IL: Research Press.

Patterson, G. R. (1974). Interventions for boys with conduct problems. Multiple settings, treatments, and criteria. *Journal of Consulting and Clinical Psychology, 42*, 471–481.

Patterson, G. R., Cobb, J. A., & Ray, R. B. (1973). A social engineering technology for retraining the families of aggressive boys. In H. E. Adams & I. P. Unikel (Eds.), *Issues and trends in behavior therapy* (pp. 139–294). Springfield, IL: Charles C. Thomas.

Patterson, G. R., & Fleischman, M. J. (1979). Maintenance of treatment effects: Some considerations concerning family systems and follow-up data. *Behavior Therapy, 10*, 168–185.

Patterson, G. R., & Forgatch, M. S. (1985). Therapist behavior as a determinant for client noncompliance: A paradox for the behavior modifier. *Journal of Consulting and Clinical Psychology, 53*, 846–851.

Reid, J. B. (1985). Behavioral approaches to intervention and assessment with child abusive families. In P. H. Bornstein & A. Kazdin (Eds.), *Handbook of clinical behavior therapy with children* (pp. 772–802). Homewood, IL: Dorsey Press.

Reisinger, J. J., Frangia, G. W., & Hoffman, E. H. (1976). Toddler management training: Generalization and marital status. *Journal of Behavior Therapy and Experimental Psychology, 7*, 335–340.

Rhode, G., Morgan, D. P., & Young, K. R. (1983). Generalization and maintenance of treatment gains of behaviorally handicapped students from resource rooms to regular classrooms using self-evaluation procedures. *Journal of Applied Behavior Analysis, 16*, 171–188.

Rickel, A. V., Eshelman, A. K., & Loigman, G. A. (1983). Social problem-solving training. A follow-up study of cognitive and behavioral effects. *Journal of Abnormal Child Psychology, 11,* 15–28.

Robertson, S. J., Simon, S. J., Rachmann, J. S., & Drabman, R. S. (1979). Self-control generalization procedures in a classroom of disruptive retarded children. *Child Behavior Therapy, 1,* 347–362.

Rogers, T. R., Forehand, R., Griest, D. L., Wells, K. C., & McMahon, R. J. (1981). Socioeconomic status: Effects on parent and child behaviors and treatment outcome of parent training. *Journal of Clinical Child Psychology, 10,* 98–101.

Rubin, K. H., & Daniels-Bierness, T. (1983). Concurrent and predictive correlates of sociometric status in kindergarten and grade one children. *Merrill-Palmer Quarterly, 29,* 337–351.

Sallis, J. F. (1983). Aggressive behaviors of children: A review of behavioral interventions and future directions. *Education and Treatment of Children, 6,* 175–191.

Sameroff, A. J., & Chandler, M. J. (1975). Reproductive risk and the continuum of caretaking casualty. In F. D. Horowitz (Eds.), *Review of child development research (Vol. 4,* pp. 65–100). Chicago: University of Chicago Press.

Sanders, M. R. (1984). Clinical strategies for enhancing generalization in behavioural parent training: An overview. *Behaviour Change, 1,* 25–35.

Sanders, W. (1978). Systematic desensitization in the treatment of child abuse. *American Journal of Psychiatry, 135,* 483–484.

Sanders, M. R., & Christensen, A. P. (1985). A comparison of the effects of child management and planned activities training in five parenting environments. *Journal of Abnormal Psychology, 13,* 101–117.

Sanders, M. R., & Dadds, M. R. (1982). The effects of planned activities and child management procedures in parent training: An analysis of setting generality. *Behavior Therapy, 13,* 452–461.

Sanders, M. R., Dadds, M. R., & Bor, W. (1989). Contextual analysis of child oppositional and maternal aversive behaviors in families of conduct-disordered and nonproblem children. *Journal of Clinical Child Psychology, 18,* 72–83.

Sanders, M. R., & Hunter, A. C. (1984). An ecological analysis of children's behaviour in supermarkets. *Australian Journal of Psychology, 36,* 415–427.

Sanders, M. R., & James, J. E. (1983). The modification of parent behavior. A review of generalization and maintenance. *Behavior Modification, 7,* 3–27.

Schloss, P. J., Schloss, C. N., Wood, C. E., & Kiehl, W. S. (1986). A critical review of social skills research with behaviorally disordered students. *Behavioral Disorders, 12,* 1–14.

Sears, R. R., Maccoby, E. E., & Levin, H. (1957). *Patterns of childrearing.* Evanston, IL: Row, Peterson, & Co.

Shure, M. B., Spivack, G., & Jaeger, M. (1971). Problem-solving thinking and adjustment among disadvantaged preschool children. *Child Development, 42,* 1791–1803.

Stokes, T. F., & Baer, D. M. (1977). An implicit technology of generalization. *Journal of Applied Behavioral Analysis, 10,* 349–367.

Strain, P. S., Young, C. C., & Horowitz, J. (1981). Generalized behavior change during oppositional child training. *Behavior Modification, 5,* 15–26.

Straus, M. A., & Gelles, R. J. (1986). Societal change and change in family violence from 1975 to 1985 as revealed by two national surveys. *Journal of Marriage and the Family, 48,* 465–479.

Szykula, S. A., & Flesichman, M. J. (1985). Reducing out-of-home placements of abused children: Two controlled studies. *Child Abuse and Neglect, 9,* 277–284.

VanHasselt, V. B., Griest, D. L., Kazdin, A. E., Esveldt-Dawson, K., & Vries, A. S. (1984). Poor peer interactions and social isolation: A case report of successful in vivo social skills training on a child psychiatric inpatient unit. *Journal of Behavior Therapy & Experimental Psychiatry, 15,* 271–276.

Wahler, R. G. (1975). Some structural aspects of deviant child behavior. *Journal of Applied Behavior Analysis, 8,* 27–42.

Wahler, R. G. (1980). The insular mother: Her problems in parent–child treatment. *Journal of Applied Behavior Analysis, 13,* 207–220.

Waldrop, M. F., & Halverson, C. F. (1975). Intensive and extensive peer behavior: Longitudinal and cross-sectional analyses. *Child Development, 46,* 19–26.

Walker, H. M., & Buckley, N. K. (1974). *Token reinforcement techniques.* Eugene, OR: E-B Press.

Webster-Stratton, C. (1982). The long-term effects of a videotape modeling parent-training program: Comparison of immediate and a 1-year follow-up data. *Behavior Therapy, 13,* 702–714.

Webster-Stratton, C. (1984). Randomized trial of two parent-training programs for families with conduct-disordered children. *Journal of Consulting and Clinical Psychology, 52,* 666–678.

Weissberg, R. P., & Allen, J. P. (1986). Promoting children's social skills and adaptive interpersonal behavior. In B. A. Edelstein & L. Michelson (Eds.), *Handbook of prevention* (pp. 153–175). New York: Plenum Press.

Weissberg, R. P., Gesten, E. L., Carnrike, C. L., Toro, P. A., Rapkin, B. D., Davidson, E., & Cowen, E. L. (1981). Social problem-solving skills training: A competence building intervention with second- to fourth-grade children. *American Journal of Community Psychology, 9,* 411–423.

Wells, K. C., Griest, D. L., & Forehand, R. (1980). The use of a self-control package to enhance temporal generality of a parent training program. *Behavior Research and Therapy, 18,* 347–353.

West, D. J., & Farrington, D. P. (1973). *Who becomes delinquent?* London: Heineman.

Wiig, E. H., & Bray, C. M. (1983). *Let's talk for children.* Columbus, OH: Charles E. Merrill.

Williams, G. (1983). Child abuse reconsidered: The urgency of authentic prevention. *Journal of Clinical Child Psychology, 12,* 312–319.

Wolfe, D. A., Aragona, J., Kaufman, K., & Sandler, J. (1980). The importance of adjudication in the treatment of child abuse: Some preliminary findings. *Child Abuse and Neglect, 4,* 127–135.

Wolfe, D. A., Kaufman, D., Aragona, J., & Sandler, J. (1981). A competency based parent training program for abusive parents. *Journal of Consulting and Clinical Psychology, 49,* 633–640.

Wolfe, D. A., & Sandler, J. (1981). Training abusive parents in effective child management. *Behavior Modification, 5,* 135–148.

Wolfe, D. A., St. Lawrence, J., Graves, K., Brehony, K., Bradlyn, D., & Kelly, J. (1982). Intensive behavioral parent training for a child abusive mother. *Behavior Therapy, 13,* 438–451.

Worland, J., Carney, R. M., Weinberg, H., & Milich, R. (1982). Dropping out of group behavioral training. *Behavioral Counseling Quarterly, 2,* 37–41.

CHAPTER 14

STUTTERING

Gavin Andrews

UNIVERSITY OF NEW SOUTH WALES

T here is obvious clinical utility in being able to predict from pretreatment characteristics or from progress in treatment which patient is likely to respond best to a particular treatment. This becomes especially important when there is a treatment that is successful for a majority of patients, for then it would be even more valuable to be able to predict the few likely to relapse so that remedial action can be taken before the relapse occurs. This chapter is concerned with the prediction of relapse after successful treatment for stuttering.

Stuttering is an interesting disorder. In most classifications it is listed as a mental disorder, but it almost certainly differs from other emotional disorders of children (Andrews et al., 1983). Population studies of children show that stuttering does not cluster with other symptoms of emotional or behavioral disorder and that children who stutter are no more likely than normal-speaking children to show symptoms of the conventional emotional disorders. To further emphasize the difference between stutterers and other mental disorders of childhood, mothers of stutterers have been shown to have similar psychiatric histories and to score similarly on personality measures to mothers of normal-speaking children (Andrews & Harris, 1964). When stutterers grow up, they too show normal scores on most personality inventories and report that their parents were no less caring or more overprotective than matched normal speakers report their parents to have been (Andrews et al., 1983). Why, then, do so many believe in an association between stuttering and anxiety or nervousness? White and Collins (1984) have presented evidence that the stereotype may be formed by inference. Since normal speakers stumble and hesitate under conditions of emotional stress, stutterers, observed by others to be stumbling and hesitating, are inferred to be abnormally nervous.

Stuttering is characterized by involuntary repetitions or prolongations of sound or syllables that occur even though stutterers know precisely what they wish to say. As such, the symptoms are different from the stumbling and hesitancy associated with anxiety. Idiopathic stuttering begins between 2 and 14 years (median age 5) and affects 5% of children, but because of early remission or late onset, the prevalence seldom rises above 1%. Four out of five children seem to recover spontaneously, and as this recovery is especially pronounced in girls, the sex ratio rises with increasing age (Andrews, 1984a). Remission is rare after puberty. An increased familial incidence of stuttering is well established, and, as with other genetically determined conditions in which there is sex limitation, the risk varies by sex of proband and sex of relative. Estimates based on twin and family studies have suggested that genetic factors account for 50% to 80% of stuttering. A recent study on a population sample of twins confirmed these estimates, with 29% of the variance in ever stuttering being attributed to individual environment and 71% to additive genetic effects (Andrews, Morris-Yates, Howie, & Martin, 1991). Idiopathic stutterers appear to have a genetically determined reduction in their central cortical capacity for the efficient sensory motor integration of speech (Neilson & Neilson, 1987). Acquired cases are much rarer and usually follow some perinatal or later cerebral insult that presumably produces an analogous cortical deficit. There is much current interest in describing the nature of the neuroscientific deficit associated with stuttering.

TREATMENT OF STUTTERING

When population samples of stutterers are compared with nonstutterers, they are found to have been slower in developing speech, more likely to show other articulatory deficits, and more likely to perform less well on intelligence tests and measures of sensory motor skill. Temporary reduction in the frequency of stuttering, even to the extent of elimination of the disorder, occurs under a variety of conditions such as speaking slowly, shadowing another's speech, singing, chorus reading, whispering, or speaking with a masking tone. There is evidence that these conditions are effective because they reduce the complexity of the sensory motor integration tasks required for fluent speech, and hence performance is improved despite the cortical deficit (Andrews, Howie, Dozsa, & Guitar, 1982).

It is not surprising, therefore, that successful treatment of stuttering

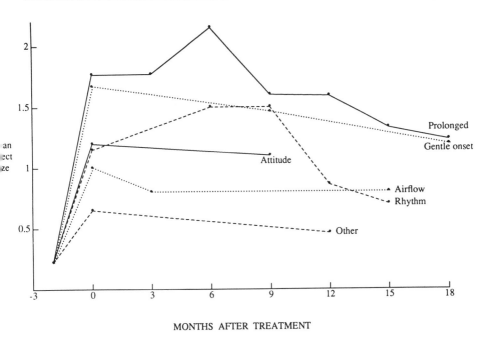

FIGURE 14.1. The average pre-/posttreatment effect sizes for six treatments from 0–18 months after the end of treatment. The pretreatment effect size of 0.22 allows for regression to the mean in stuttering severity while subjects waited for treatment. The average duration of treatment was two months. Redrawn from Andrews, Guitar, & Howie, 1980.

depends on many hours of speech retraining with an appropriate technique (Andrews, Guitar, & Howie, 1980). Relapse occurs but is not striking, averaging a quarter of a standard deviation per year across all treatments. The results of a meta-analysis of six different treatments are displayed in Figure 14.1 and demonstrate the stability of results.

In the treatment program for adult stutterers, which is the focus of this article, the technique used is "smooth speech," which involves emphasis on the gentle onset of each utterance and on continuous phonation between phrase junctures. At slow rates, this eliminates stuttering. Gradually, over the next 50 hours of treatment, this abnormal but stutter-free speech is systematically shaped to become normal-sounding speech in terms of both rate and prosody. Each subject then undertakes a series of graded assignments outside the clinic so that the new fluent speech skill is generalized to the outside world.

The treatment program was developed from that of Andrews and Harris (1964), with the original fluency-producing agent of syllable-timed speech being superseded in 1970 by the prolonged or smooth speech technique. The present treatment program has been repeatedly described and evaluated (Andrews & Feyer, 1985; Andrews, Neilson, & Cassar, 1987), and the description of the participant observer's report in the former paper is informative.

> In the first week subjects were instructed in the new speech pattern and then were required to use it at 50 syllables per minute (SPM), one-quarter of the normal rate, in the hourly rating sessions conducted throughout each day. At this rate, provided the smooth speech was used correctly, no stuttering was observed and all secondary symptoms disappeared. From 50 SPM, target speech rate was gradually increased to normal rates of 200 in steps of 5 SPM. Progress to beyond 50 SPM was contingent upon subjects producing a specified amount of stutter-free conversational speech in each rating session, at a rate within a specified range. Continuous feedback on the rate of speech was delivered via syllable counters in front of each subject, and stutters were immediately punished by erasure of credit for syllables already spoken in that session. In addition, money was the basis of contingent reward and punishment for performance of the required response—namely, stutter-free speech at the correct rate—in each rating session and in each evening's homework assignment. The reinforcer was delivered on an incremental scale: as the number of correct performances increased the amount of money also increased. This appeared to encourage a steady, high level of performance of the correct response. Failed sessions and homework assignments resulted in no reward for that session and a return to the bottom of the pay scale for the next session, and failed homework was repeated. Thus the cost of inappropriate responses, either stuttering or speaking at the incorrect rate, was high. Any stutters that occurred outside the assignments or rating sessions incurred immediate monetary fines, thereby reinforcing the use of the skill at all times.
>
> Several secondary reinforcers were also observed. First, there was reinforcement of social and conversational skills because in order to be listened to people had to be assertive and interesting as well as fluent. Second, progress to any syllable rate was contingent upon successful completion of the previous one. Therefore, progress toward normal rates indicated success, and this secondary reward was enhanced to varying degrees by group approval; continued exposure to this reinforcing event required continuous correct behavior. Social interaction with the therapists was also a source of reward and punishment. Because the program was not experimental, this interaction was not standardised, yet it appeared effective because correction of inaccurate speech patterns occurred via the therapist. Consequently, therapist praise and remonstrances appeared to acquire highly reinforcing properties. During the first week, increasing precision in speech skill was required as normal rates of speech were approximated. The contingencies became more stringent in order to shape the appropriate response. The clearest

instance of this was in the video sessions that occurred twice daily. During the replay, individuals were asked to assess the quality of their response, as compared to the therapist's assessment. At first only the most rudimentary characteristics came under scrutiny, but by the fifth day a broader spectrum of verbal behaviours was being assessed. Correct assessment accrued monetary rewards. There was an almost total absence of stutters during the first week of treatment, and this appeared to be facilitated by a continuity of therapist and co-patient observation outside the treatment setting. This continuous experience of success seemed to aid generalisation of the speech skills and extinction of avoidance responses.

In the second week, subjects worked at their own pace on a standard graded hierarchy of 15 speech assignments. For each assignment, 1400 syllables of stutter-free speech at the normal rate of 200 + 40 SPM were required. Completion of all 15 assignments within the week accrued a greater financial reward than if subjects took longer, whereas partial completion did not achieve any reward. This shift to an intermittent schedule of reinforcement in the latter stages of treatment, while capitalising on the well-known resistance to extinction of such schedules, also appeared to be designed to allow the reinforcement of complex goals rather than details. The successful and continuous exposure to increasingly difficult speaking situations appeared to allow increasingly elaborate stimulus and response generalisation of skills and extinction of fears and avoidances.

In the third week, the assignments, of which five were standard and five were tailored to the individual, accrued no monetary reward. It appeared that the aim in the third week was to maximize generalisation by allowing patients to move closer and closer to the fabric of their own lifestyle. All assignments were assessed by the subjects, but no reward was given for accuracy of assessment—assignments passed or failed on the basis of therapist assessment. (Andrews & Feyer, 1985, pp. 448–450)*

The smooth speech technique fulfills the criteria for a satisfactory treatment (Andrews, 1989). Data on more than 300 subjects have been reported since the prototype treatment was introduced by Curlee and Perkins (1971). Subjects, both adolescents and adults, have had their speech assessed by reliable and objective techniques on a number of occasions from the end of treatment to 18 months later. Speech attitudes have also been measured. Both speech and speech attitudes have been shown to improve significantly with treatment. Furthermore, evidence has been gathered by covert assessment (Andrews & Craig, 1982) and from independent judges (Craig & Calver, 1991) to show that real-life performance has improved. Evidence has been presented that neither spontaneous remission, regression to the mean, nor response to placebo

*Reprinted by permission of Sage Publications.

could account for these changes (Andrews & Harvey, 1981; Andrews et al., 1980). Since comparable reports have come from clinics in different countries, it is unlikely that the later reports of benefit are due to the halo that surrounds a new treatment or to the charisma associated with a particular clinician.

The principal goal of therapy has always been to produce stutter-free, normal-sounding speech and, as stuttering reduces communication efficiency, the focus of treatment has been the elimination of stuttering. In recent years, it has been realized that the acquisition of normal communication attitudes and an internalized locus of control are other important attributes of long-term fluent speech (Guitar & Bass, 1978; Craig, Franklin, & Andrews, 1984). After treatment, the majority of subjects are no longer handicapped by stuttering, and for many these gains are permanent. However, 1 year after treatment has concluded, one in seven will be stuttering on more than 3% of their syllables and one third will be stuttering on more than 2% of their syllables. The criterion for acceptance of stutterers for treatment is 3% syllables stuttered, because below this level the stutter is not conspicuous and the handicap to communication is minor. The criterion for relapse after successful treatment is 2% syllables spoken stuttered, for this level indicates that the subject no longer has control of stuttering and the speaker is, or will soon be, handicapped. One problem in improving the program further is that the low level of residual stuttering makes it difficult to obtain sufficient statistical power to warrant a randomized controlled trial. In fact, the 120 subjects required for a trial to have an 80% chance of detecting a reduction of half a standard deviation in residual stuttering as a result of improved treatment would be beyond the resources of most clinics.

FACTORS ASSOCIATED WITH RELAPSE

One strategy that would allow the treatment to be improved is to identify, on the basis of pretreatment characteristics or from progress in treatment, those most likely to relapse, and by providing additional treatment, reduce the number at risk prior to relapse occurring. This chapter is an expansion of an article by Andrews and Craig (1988) with additional descriptions of treatment and further data to elucidate the predictors of relapse. The progress of a large group of subjects was therefore analyzed to identify the pretreatment and posttreatment factors associated with relapse and then to confirm the results from a small replication sample. Prospective data were gathered on 62 subjects treated in 1981, and these data were supported with a replication sample of 22 subjects treated in 1983. In addition, data from clinical records on 36 stutterers treated in

1974 and 40 treated in 1976 were gathered retrospectively to strengthen the capacity to explore the relationship between pretreatment factors and long-term outcome.

The 160 patients were between 17 and 60 years of age, with a mean age of 30. All had been referred by general practitioners for treatment for chronic stuttering. Eighty-one percent were males. All were treated as previously described in groups of six for 10 to 12 hours a day, 5 days per week over 3 weeks. At the beginning of the first week, the patients were taught to speak in a slow form of smooth speech that completely inhibited stuttering. Once this was mastered, they conversed with each other for 10 hours per day over the next 4 days, systematically increasing their speech rate from 50 syllables per minute (SPM) to the normal rate of 200 SPM. The whole process was carefully measured and monitored by the therapist. In the second and third weeks, subjects continued with 4 hours of clinical practice each day and in addition spent 6 hours each day doing supervised and graded assignments (talking to strangers, telephoning, shopping) designed to systematically transfer fluent speech to contexts outside the clinic. Maintenance of the skill after therapy terminated was facilitated by periodic clinical review and by support from an aftercare organization conducted by recovered stutterers.

Severity of stuttering was assessed from 600-syllable telephone calls to strangers and measured as frequency of stuttering in percent syllables stuttered (%SS) and rate of speech (SPM). The interrater reliability of these measures for the 1981 group was 0.95 for %SS and 0.90 for SPM. For the 1983 replication group, it was 0.94 for %SS and 0.92 for SPM. For the 1974 and 1976 cohorts the interrater reliabilities were 0.99 and 0.98 for %SS and 0.92 and 0.90 for SPM, respectively. Other aspects of the stuttering syndrome were measured on scales of avoidance and reaction to speaking situations (Andrews, 1984b) and by the S24 Scale of Communication Attitudes (Andrews & Cutler, 1974). Personality traits were assessed by the Eysenck Personality Inventory (Eysenck & Eysenck, 1964), and locus of control of behavior (LCB) scale (Craig et al., 1984).

These measures were taken on the day prior to the beginning of treatment in all cohorts, but the immediate posttreatment measures of %SS, SPM, S24, and LCB were measured at the end of the 3-week treatment period for the 1981 and 1983 cohorts only. The dependent measure, the frequency of stuttering (%SS) at follow-up, was taken from a telephone call to a stranger 10 to 18 months after treatment concluded. This has been shown to be a valid and reliable measure of treatment outcome (Andrews & Craig, 1982). The validity of measuring before and after treatment (a pre–post design) for the evaluation of stuttering treatment in adolescents and adults is supported by the very small remission, regression to the mean, and placebo response that occurs with this disorder over such periods of time.

The pretreatment, posttreatment, and long-term follow-up scores for each cohort are presented in Table 14.1. Before treatment, the cohorts were comparable in terms of age, sex, personality, speech attitudes, locus of control, and severity of stuttering (grand mean = 12.3%SS at 150 SPM). At the end of treatment, the 1981 and 1983 cohorts had made similar progress (mean = 0.3%SS). Immediate posttreatment data were not available for the 1974 and 1976 cohorts. Ten to 18 months later, all four cohorts remained significantly improved (grand mean = 2.5%SS).

The correlations between pretreatment variables and the frequency of stuttering in the long term were examined and are presented in Table 14.2. As the distribution of the frequency of stuttering is heavily skewed (Kraemer & Andrews, 1981), and this is particularly marked in the long-term outcome data (skew 3.1, see Figure 14.2), all %SS scores were log transformed to partially normalize the distribution prior to the correlation's being calculated. The relationships between the nine variables measured when the stutterers were first interviewed, and the eventual long-term outcome was explored. The only pretreatment variables that were significantly associated with long-term outcome were the two pretreatment measures of severity of stuttering: frequency of stuttering and rate of speech. These associations were significant but modest ($r = 0.24$ and $r = -0.32$, respectively), but as these two measures were themselves intercorrelated, they accounted for only 10%–15% of the variance in long-term outcome. Thus, they provided little basis for identifying subjects at risk of relapse.

Measures were taken on the last day of treatment for the main (1981) and replication (1983) cohorts. Severity of stuttering (%SS and SPM), speech attitudes (S24 scale), and locus of control (LCB) scores were all significantly correlated with the long-term outcome measure of the frequency of stuttering (%SS $r = 0.37$, SPM $r = 0.26$, S24 $r = 0.35$, and LCB $r = 0.23$, $p < 0.05$). Together they accounted for only 25% of the variance in the long-term outcome, and so again they were of little use to predict individuals at risk of relapse.

The scores were therefore examined as to whether individuals had achieved each of three specified treatment goals at the end of treatment. These goals were absolutely no hint of stuttering on the telephone task, communication attitudes at or below the S24 population mean of 9 (the criterion used by Guitar & Bass, 1978), and the LCB score reduced by greater than 5% between pretreatment and posttreatment assessment, taken to be evidence of internalization of the LCB during treatment. Using the chi-squared and Fisher's exact tests, significant associations were obtained between long-term outcome and the achievement of each

TABLE 14.1. Means and Standard Deviations (in Parentheses) for Main and Replication Groups of Adult Stutterers

	Cohort				
	1974 n = 36	1976 n = 40	1981 n = 62	1983 n = 22	Total n = 160
Pretreatment					
Age in years	27 (6)	30 (7)	32 (9)	28 (6)	30 (8)
Percent male	83	88	81	64	81
EPI neuroticism score	12.4	13.2	12.6	13.3	12.8
Locus of control (LCB)	—	—	29.7 (10)	30.3 (10)	29.9 (10)*
Avoidance of stuttering	2.3 (0.8)	2.4 (0.7)	2.5 (0.7)	2.5 (0.7)	2.4 (0.7)
Reaction to stuttering	2.6 (0.6)	2.5 (0.6)	2.6 (0.6)	2.8 (0.5)	2.6 (0.6)
Communication attitudes (S24)	19.5 (5)	19.2 (4)	18.6 (4)	20.0 (5)	19.1 (4)
Frequency of stuttering (%SS)	9.5 (8)	11.8 (7)	12.4 (6)	17.2 (12)	12.3 (8)
Rate of speech (SPM)	128 (51)	142 (51)	171 (45)	142 (54)	150 (52)*
Posttreatment					
Locus of control (LCB)	—	—	23.3 (9)	22.8 (9)	23.1 (9)*
Communication attitudes (S24)	—	—	7.2 (5.5)	9.1 (6)	7.7 (6)*
Frequency of stuttering (%SS)	—	—	0.3 (1.6)	0.2 (0.3)	0.3 (1.4)*
Rate of speech (SPM)	—	—	217 (22)	208 (17)	214 (21)*
Long-term outcome					
Frequency of stuttering (%SS)	2.8 (5)	2.8 (3)	2.1 (3)	2.6 (6)	2.5 (4)

*Data from 84 subjects only.

TABLE 14.2. Prediction of Long-Term Outcome: Correlation of Pretreatment Variables with the Long-Term Frequency of Stuttering

Pretreatment variable	Cohort				
	1974 $n = 36$	1976 $n = 40$	1981 $n = 62$	1983 $n = 22$	*Total* $n = 160$
Demographic					
Age	–0.04	0.01	0.09	– 0.09	0.02
Sex	–0.39*	–0.15	0.05	–0.05	–0.10
Psychological					
EPI neuroticism score	0.44**	0.35*	–0.09	0.05	0.18*
Locus of control (LCB)	—	—	–0.35**	–0.08	–0.27**
Speech attitudes					
Avoidance of stuttering	0.45**	0.27	–0.2	0.21	0.21**
Reaction to stuttering	0.40*	0.23	0.03	0.23	0.19*
Communication attitudes	0.31*	0.02	–0.02	0.31	0.13
Severity of stuttering					
Frequency of stuttering (%SS[a])	0.31*	0.31*	0.18	0.22	0.24**
Rate of speech (SPM)	–0.46**	–0.30*	–0.22	–0.42*	–0.32**

*$p < .05$.
**$p < .01$.
[a]All measures of stuttering (%SS) were log-transformed prior to computation.

of these treatment goals in the 1981 cohort, and in two of the three goals in the replication cohort (see Table 14.3).

The cumulative effect of attaining these treatment goals is displayed in Table 14.4. In both cohorts there was a strong association between progress in treatment in terms of the number of goals attained and long-term maintenance of fluency. The data from both cohorts were combined and the results displayed in Figure 14.2. The frequency of stuttering is displayed on a logarithmic scale, with the criterion for relapse (stuttering at more than 2%SS) being represented by the bold horizontal line in the middle of the figure. The left section of the figure shows the distribution of frequency of stuttering on the telephone task immediately prior to treatment (median 12%SS, range 3%–56%, $n = 84$).

TABLE 14.3. Relationship between Attaining Treatment Goals by End of Treatment and Long-Term Outcome

Treatment goal	1981 cohort outcome ($n = 62$)		1983 cohort outcome ($n = 22$)	
	Maintained	Relapsed[a]	Maintained	Relapsed[a]
Speech				
Fluent	37	7	8	5
Not fluent	7	11	7	2
		$p < .01$		$p = $ NS
Attitudes				
Normal	35	9	12	2
Not normal	9	9	3	5
		$p < .05$		$p < .05$
Locus of control				
Internalized	40	4	15	2
Not internalized	4	14	0	5
		$p < .01$		$p < .01$

[a]Relapse is defined as greater than 2%SS at long-term (10-month) assessment.

The middle section shows the distribution at the end of treatment (median 0.0%SS, range 0-12%SS), when all but two of the subjects were below 2%SS and 57 of the 84 were not heard to stutter at all. In this section, the subjects are arranged in subgroups according to the number of treatment goals they had attained. The right section of the figure shows the distribution of stuttering frequency scores 10 months after the end of treatment (median 0.9%SS, range 0-24%SS) again with subjects arranged in groups according to the number of treatment goals achieved at the end of treatment. Twenty-five, or 30% of the 84 subjects, were stuttering at levels above 2%SS, the criterion for relapse. At 10 months there was a systematic decrease in the median values for each group, from those who had attained no treatment goals by the end of treatment to those who had attained all three goals. The data show that 10 months after treatment, all eight who had failed to achieve any of the three treatment goals during therapy had relapsed, 7/14 (50%) of those who had achieved one goal had relapsed, 9/25 (36%) of those who had achieved two goals had relapsed, and only 1/37 (3%) of those who had achieved all three goals at the end of treatment had relapsed 10 months later.

How independent are these goals? If the aim of treatment is to teach

TABLE 14.4. The Relationship Between Number of Treatment Goals Achieved and
Long-Term Fluency

Fluency at 10 months	N	Number of goals achieved at end of treatment[a]			
		0	1	2	3
1981 cohort	62				
Maintained	44	0	4	12	28
Relapsed	18	6	5	7	0
Percentage maintained		0%	44%	63%	100%
1983 cohort	22				
Maintained	15	0	3	4	8
Relapsed	7	2	2	2	1
Percentage maintained		0%	60%	67%	89%
Total	84	8	14	25	37
Percentage maintained		0%	50%	64%	97%

[a]Goals were no stuttering and normal communication attitudes at end of treatment, and internalization of locus of control during treatment. Fluency was deemed to be maintained if stuttering was 2% or less 10 months after treatment.

the skill of mastering stuttering and the desire of patients is to control their stuttering, could each of the treatment goals be but further measures of skill mastery? This is obviously so in regard to the measure of stuttering at the end of treatment, but the S24 scale of communication attitudes could also reflect stutterers' judgments of how good their skills are, and the LCB could reflect their awareness of how much control over their disorder they had really acquired. To elucidate this issue, we explored the importance of goal attainment within the groups that had achieved only one or two goals. There were 39 such subjects. Twenty of these achieved the goal of being stutter free by the end of treatment and 11/20 (45%) relapsed. Of the 19 who were not absolutely stutter free at the end of treatment, 5/19 (36%) relapsed. Twenty-one subjects achieved normal attitudes during treatment and 10/21 (48%) relapsed. Twenty-three internalized their LCB during treatment and 4/23 (17%) relapsed. Therefore, no single goal was either necessary or sufficient to guard against relapse, yet it is obvious that progressive achievement of all three goals during treatment did reduce the probability of relapse to very low levels (i.e., to 3%).

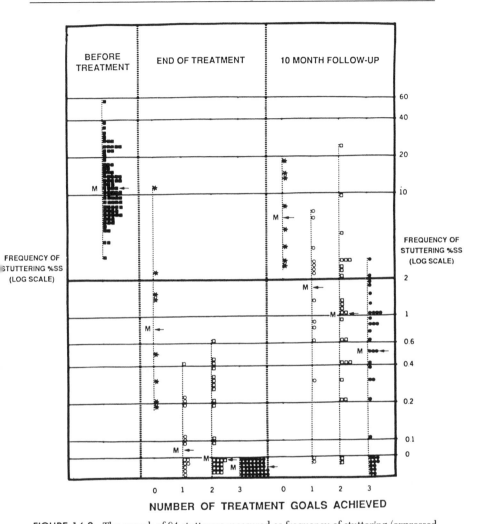

FIGURE 14.2. The speech of 84 stutterers measured as frequency of stuttering (expressed as %SS on a logarithmic scale) before treatment, at the end of treatment, and at 10-month follow-up by the number of treatment goals achieved at the end of treatment.

Note. Filled stars = no treatment goals; open circles = one treatment goal; open squares = two treatment goals; filled circles = three treatment goals achieved at the end of treatment. M = median for each group.

This chapter documents a search for predictors of the persons at risk of relapse so that preventive action can be taken before relapse occurs. Data were obtained on adult stutterers before, at the end, and 10 to 18 months after treatment. For the average stutterer, treatment eliminated stuttering, normalized communication attitudes, and internalized LCB scores. But 10 to 18 months later, 30% of the subjects were stuttering on more than 2% of their syllables and the mean frequency of stuttering, which was 12.3% prior to treatment and 0.3% posttreatment, had risen to 2½ %SS. Pretreatment severity of stuttering and measures of posttreatment fluency, communication attitudes, and LCB were correlated with outcome in the long term, but none to a sufficient extent to identify particular subjects at risk of relapse.

Stutter-free speech, normal communication attitudes, and internalized LCB on the last day of treatment all significantly predicted continued well-being at 10 months for the main group of 62 subjects, and these findings were partially replicated in a further 22 subjects. No single treatment goal was either necessary of sufficient to guarantee well-being in the long term. More important, the relationship between the number of these treatment goals achieved by the end of therapy and long-term outcome was highly significant in both cohorts. Ninety-seven percent of the subjects who achieved all three goals (stutter-free speech, normal communication attitudes, and internalized LCB) remained fluent in the long term, whereas all of the eight who failed to achieve any of the treatment goals relapsed, even though the speech of six of the eight at the end of treatment (%SS = 0.2, 0.2, 0.3, 0.5, 1.5, 1.6) would have been regarded by many as evidence of successful treatment.

The independent contribution that each of the three treatment goals made to the prediction of long-term outcome is pleasing, and one is tempted to believe that no stuttering on the last day of treatment is less important than changes in attitude or in LCB. But these data do not necessarily indicate that perceived speech skill mastery is more important than actual mastery in long-term outcome, for these subjects had already reduced their stuttering from a mean of 12.3% to 0.3%, so that even those who were not absolutely stutter free by the end of treatment had still attained a considerable degree of skill mastery. Treatments for stuttering that focus solely on improved attitudes to oneself and one's speech (see Andrews et al., 1980) have only shown small changes in the severity of stuttering. Learning skills to control stuttering are probably the most important factor in the treatment of the disorder, with the changes in attitude and LCB functioning as important maintaining variables once the capacity for fluency has been established.

This information has been utilized in two ways. First, the described treatment program has been revised so that the last 4 days of the program are predicated on the goal attainment of the subjects at that point. For instance, those who are still not reliably fluent are given additional speech retraining, those whose communication attitudes are still abnormal are required to do further assignments outside the clinic, and those whose LCB has not begun to internalize are placed on a self-control program.

We have no data concerning the effect of these changes to the program, but we do have data on the retreatment of six of the subjects who, despite attaining fluency at the end of treatment, did not manage to internalize their LCB and relapsed 10 months later (Craig & Andrews, 1985). After reinstating fluency, we instituted a 3-day self-control program in which the subjects learned and applied self-monitoring, self-evaluation, and self-reinforcement. They were taught to monitor stutters and by using a wrist counter keep count of any stutters that occurred. Goals as to the desired number of stutters were set each day. They also learned to monitor and evaluate the quality of their fluency skill. Agreement with the trained raters' evaluations averaged 84%. Every half hour they recorded the quality of their fluency using a visual analog scale. Goals for fluency quality were set by each individual each day. At the start of the program, the subjects had contributed some money out of which they specified contingent rewards if they maintained the level of freedom from stuttering and quality of speech set by themselves for that day. These self-control techniques were applied throughout the 3 days as subjects completed speech assignments outside the clinic. By the end of the 3-day self-control program, five of the subjects had internalized their LCB scores and four of these five subjects were fluent 10 months later. One subject did not internalize her LCB score during this program and she had relapsed when measured 10 months later. The self-control program was considered effective in internalizing LCB, and an internalized LCB was deemed instrumental in reducing the future prospect of relapse.

In most mental disorders, the advent of a drug that will suppress symptoms and not cause unwanted toxic effects seems to be all that is required, even if symptoms recur after the drug is stopped. With the nondrug behavioral treatments, we seem to ask more: evidence of stable symptom relief coupled with some change in underlying personality or vulnerability factors as well. The present results demonstrate that these goals can be achieved in the treatment of adults who stutter.

REFERENCES

Andrews, G. (1984a). The epidemiology of stuttering. In W. H. Perkins & R. F. Curlee (Eds.), *Nature and treatment of stuttering: New directions* (pp. 1–12). San Diego: College-Hill Press.

Andrews, G. (1984b). Stuttering: Evaluation of the benefits of treatment. In W. Perkins (Ed.), *Current therapy of communication disorders: Stuttering* (pp. 241–250). New York: Thieme-Stratton.

Andrews, G. (1989). Evaluating treatment effectiveness. *Australian and New Zealand Journal of Psychiatry, 23,* 181–186.

Andrews, G., & Craig, A. (1982). Stuttering: Overt and covert measurement of the speech of treated stutterers. *Journal of Speech and Hearing Disorders, 47,* 96–99.

Andrews, G., & Craig, A. (1988). Prediction of outcome after treatment for stuttering. *British Journal of Psychiatry, 153,* 236–240.

Andrews, G., Craig, A., Feyer, A-M., Hoddinott, S., Howie, P. M., & Neilson, M. (1983). Stuttering: A review of research findings and theories circa 1982. *Journal of Speech and Hearing Disorders, 48,* 226–246.

Andrews, G., & Cutler, J. (1974). Stuttering therapy: The relation between changes in symptom level and attitudes. *Journal of Speech and Hearing Disorders, 39,* 312–319.

Andrews, G., & Feyer, A-M. (1985). Does behavior therapy still work when the experimenters depart: An analysis of a behavioral treatment program for stuttering. *Behavior Modification, 9,* 443–457.

Andrews, G., Guitar, B., & Howie, P. (1980). Meta-analysis of the effects of stuttering treatment. *Journal of Speech and Hearing Disorders, 45,* 287–307.

Andrews, G., & Harris, M. (1964). *Syndrome of stuttering: Clinics in developmental medicine, no. 17.* London: Heinemann.

Andrews, G., & Harvey, R. (1981). Regression to the mean in pretreatment measures of stuttering severity. *Journal of Speech and Hearing Disorders, 46,* 204–207.

Andrews, G., Howie, P. M., Dozsa, M., & Guitar, B. E. (1982). Stuttering: Speech pattern characteristics under fluency inducing conditions. *Journal of Speech and Hearing Disorders, 25,* 208–216.

Andrews, G., Morris-Yates, A., Howie, P. M., & Martin, N. G. (1991). Genetic factors in stuttering confirmed. *Archives of General Psychiatry, 48,* 1034–1035.

Andrews, G., Neilson, M., & Cassar, M. (1987). Informing stutterers about treatment. In L. Rustin, H. Purser, & D. Rowley (Eds.), *Progress in the treatment of fluency disorders* (Progress in Clinical Science Series, pp. 213–232). London: Taylor and Francis.

Craig, A., & Andrews, G. (1985). The prediction and prevention of relapse in stuttering. The value of self-control techniques and locus of control measures. *Behavior Modification, 9,* 427–442.

Craig, A., & Calver, P. (1991). Following up on treated stutterers: Studies of perceptions of fluency and job status. *Journal of Speech and Hearing Research, 34,* 279–284.

Craig, A., Franklin, J., & Andrews, G. (1984). A scale to measure locus of control of behaviour. *British Journal of Medical Psychology, 57,* 173–180.

Curlee, R. F., & Perkins, W. H. (1971). Conversation rate control therapy for stuttering. *Journal of Speech and Hearing Disorders, 34,* 245–250.

Eysenck, H. J., & Eysenck, S. B. G. (1964). *Manual of the Eysenck Personality Inventory.* London: University of London Press.

Guitar, B., & Bass, C. (1978). Stuttering therapy: The relation between attitude change and long-term outcome. *Journal of Speech and Hearing Disorders, 43,* 392–400.

Kraemer, H. C., & Andrews, G. (1982). A non-parametric technique for meta-analysis effect size calculations. *Psychological Bulletin, 91,* 404–412.

Neilson, M., & Neilson, P. D. (1987). Speech motor control and stuttering: A computational model of adaptive sensory-motor processing. *Speech Communication, 6,* 325–333.

White, P. A., & Collins, S. R. (1984). Stereotype formation by inference: A possible explanation for the "stutterer" stereotype. *Journal of Speech and Hearing Research, 27,* 567–570.

CHAPTER 15

DIRECTIONS FOR FUTURE RESEARCH IN RELAPSE PREVENTION

Peter H. Wilson

THE FLINDERS UNIVERSITY OF SOUTH AUSTRALIA

T his book has surveyed the literature on the study of relapse and its prevention following cognitive and behavioral interventions for a broad range of psychological disorders. The problems covered have included some of the most common and debilitating conditions, such as excessive alcohol consumption, panic disorder, agoraphobia, obsessive–compulsive disorder, social and marital problems, stuttering, schizophrenia, depression, smoking, chronic pain, sexual deviations, obesity, anorexia, and bulimia. This final chapter draws together some of the general themes that have emerged in the preceding chapters and identifies the major directions in which research on relapse prevention (RP) should proceed. The authors have raised a number of methodological, conceptual, and practical problems in the study of relapse and in the development of RP strategies that deserve to be highlighted here.

METHODOLOGICAL PROBLEMS

Some of the general methodological problems of research in the relapse area were highlighted in Chapter 1. One of the most obvious problems that emerges from a perusal of the book is the length of the follow-up period itself. Remarkably few studies exist over long time spans, that is, in excess of even 3 years (e.g., Blanchard, Andrasik, Guarnieri, Neff, & Rodichok, 1987; Burns, Thorpe, & Cavallaro, 1986; Lisspers & Öst, 1990; Rychtarik, Foy, Scott, Lokey, & Pruse, 1987). The study of relapse is generally confined to periods of about 12 months, and in reality, most follow-up periods reported in the literature are even shorter. Undoubtedly, a number of social and economic factors led to this state of affairs. The conduct of treatment outcome studies is a lengthy and time-consuming process, even under ideal circumstances. The inclusion of a long follow-up necessitates periods of study that are unattractive to the agencies that provide research grants in the area and to researchers who wish to publish work quickly and regularly. In addition, there are problems that arise in longitudinal studies such as the retention of subjects over long periods in relatively mobile societies. The use of payments to subjects, deposit returns, or obtaining additional contact addresses could help to reduce the problem of attrition. Seeking opportunities to collect samples that are likely to be less mobile (e.g., for geographic or social reasons) might also be helpful. Most important, there is clearly a need for studies of the long-term effects of treatment.

A clear distinction needs to be made between long-, medium-, and short-term relapse. To define these time spans may be somewhat arbitrary, but I suggest that short term be regarded as 6 months or less, medium term as 7 to 24 months, and long term as beyond 2 years. The distinction between short-, medium-, and long-term maintenance could be particularly useful when studying predictors of relapse. As mentioned earlier, it is possible that different processes operate to initiate relapse at different stages of the posttreatment period. For example, some relapse in the short term may very well be a result of the operation of nonspecific factors during the intervention. Medium- and long-term relapse may be triggered by other processes, and there may even be important differences in causal processes between medium- and long-term relapse that await identification from researchers. The separation of time periods at least enables researchers to test predictions arising from these conjectures. Of course, whether the processes that initiate a relapse are related to the basic mechanisms that are responsible for the original onset of the disorder remains a contentious issue, but it represents an important and potentially fruitful area of study.

CONCEPTUAL PROBLEMS IN PREDICTION AND PROCESS STUDIES

There has been a relative lack of research into the mechanisms responsible for relapse, or its obverse, the maintenance of treatment effects. The approach of Marlatt and Gordon (1985) is one model that allows certain predictions to be made about the likely causes of relapse. At this stage, I would like to take a broader perspective on the study of relapse and suggest one possible direction in which research could proceed in a systematic way. Statistical prediction offers the best solution to many of the problems at this stage of the research on relapse. In particular, a general model that can be tested using multiple regression techniques has great appeal. One can consider several different sources that potentially contribute to the occurrence of relapse. These sources of variance are pretreatment factors (relatively enduring or permanent characteristics of the person, such as gender), factors related to the disorder itself (duration, types of symptoms, subclassification), factors related to the initial intervention (type of intervention, compliance with procedures, etc.), outcome of initial intervention (early response to treatment, posttreatment severity, overall change, presence of residual symptoms, self-efficacy about performance of certain therapy-related tasks), postintervention factors (adherence to procedures taught in therapy, social support), and variables proposed as specific relapse-inducing or RP agents for a given problem (e.g., certain types of life events, cognitive style, biochemical changes, specific social factors). Multiple regression analyses will assist in ascribing the proportion of variance in relapse that is associated with each of these broad classes of variables. An important feature of such analyses is the ability to control for posttreatment severity while other predictors are being examined.

The first task for those who are interested in the mechanisms involved in relapse is to improve our ability to predict its occurrence. Understanding and prediction go hand in hand, and I am certainly not advocating a theory-free approach. Presumably, our ability to predict will be informed by the growth in understanding of the processes involved. Likewise, our understanding of those processes will be enhanced by more accurate prediction. In turn, the development of RP strategies probably depends on a growth in knowledge that will occur as a result of prediction studies. Other research strategies that are needed include those that are capable of describing fine-grain analyses of the relapse process, such as the studies of factors that precede "lapses" in relation to different types of addictive behaviors (e.g., Shiffman, 1892). Similar detailed analyses of triggers of relapse in depression, the eating disorders, and other problems are needed.

Investigators need to make clear predictions about the causes of relapse and include measures that are capable of providing tests of such predictions. With few exceptions, notably the research stimulated by self-efficacy theory (Bandura, 1977), learned helplessness, and other cognitive accounts, or the hypotheses suggested by Marlatt and Gordon

(1985), predictors that have been selected for examination have often not been derived from any theoretical perspective or any clear conceptualization about likely mechanisms of change or maintenance. While the theory-driven predictions have had mixed results, they do offer the promise of a coherent and potentially useful way of proceeding. One area that has been relatively neglected is the measurement of adherence to the skills taught in therapy during the follow-up period. Methods for ensuring adequate use of techniques after treatment termination need to be developed and evaluated. As mentioned above, prediction from various prior points in time needs to considered (e.g., prediction made prior to treatment vs. prediction made posttreatment).

RP PROCEDURES

There are several conceptual and practical problems in the delivery of RP approaches that remain to be fully explicated. The rationale for the selection of procedures and the timing of the implementation of relapse interventions have often not been clearly stated. This problem has been particularly prominent in the evaluation of booster sessions (see Whisman, 1990, for a more extended discussion). As pointed out by Nicholas in his chapter on chronic pain (Chapter 11, this volume), a popular solution to this problem has been the use of shotgun approaches in which all viable techniques have been utilized in a possibly uneconomical fashion. Apart from the content, there has also been an arbitrariness about the scheduling of booster sessions. There may be particular points in time, either for the disorder as a whole or for certain individuals, when booster sessions have a greater potency than otherwise would be the case. Careful study of the natural history of relapse in each disorder is badly needed. While this type of research has already begun in the addictive disorders, it remains virtually ignored in most other problems areas. Studies of the natural history of relapse should have the potential to answer questions such as: What proportion of subjects relapse over each period in the total time span under investigation? Is there a point in time when new relapses become relatively rare? What differences are there between people who relapse and those who do not relapse? Are there differences between early, medium-, and long-term relapsers? Are there common triggers of lapses and relapse? What are the consequences of lapses and relapse? Answers to these questions will provide valuable information that will assist in the design of research on RP programs, the development of specific RP strategies, and the formulation of a theoretical framework with which to explain the occurrence of relapse.

The RP program for addictive problems proposed by Marlatt and

Gordon (1985) has been adapted for different problems within the addictive area. Still, it is surprising that the program has not been subjected to more evaluative research. Research on the relative effects of the different components of this type of RP program also needs to be conducted. The overall program is quite complex, and it is unclear precisely which components have been included in some studies. There is also a need to consider how some of these RP concepts might be into other areas such as depression, anxiety disorders, chronic pain, and schizophrenia. Admittedly, other approaches to RP have already begun to emerge in somes areas, such as schizophrenia in which attempts to reduce the impact of expressed emotion in families have been encouraging (see Kavanagh, Chapter 8, this volume). RP in depression has lagged behind both the addictions and schizophrenia, despite the acknowledgment of relapse as a significant problem in depression. Evaluations of a Marlatt and Gordon style of RP, booster sessions, and other techniques need to be conducted.

The relative efficacy of the different types of RP programs has also been the subject of little study. As suggested in Chapter 1, there are several different types of RP programs of which the most prominent are (1) RP, which is integrated into the initial treatment program, (2) booster sessions, which occur at some point in time after the termination of treatment, and (3) minimal-contact procedures, which can be provided through self-help support groups, telephone calls, or correspondence and through audio, video, or printed media. The comparative effects of these approaches warrant further study across the different problem areas. In particular, it is surprising that more use has not been made of the minimal-contact procedures. The development and evaluation of materials that might be useful for clinicians would seem to be relatively timely at this stage.

The evidence for the effectiveness of booster sessions is relatively mixed at this stage. Furthermore, some researchers have suggested that they simply delay the inevitable, at least for smoking cessation (Brandon, Zelman, & Baker, 1987). However, as Mermelstein, Kanartz, and Reichmann (Chapter 3, this volume) point out, low statistical power may have contributed to this problem, and they suggest that "more recent evaluations of booster or maintenance sessions suggest, though, that they should not be dismissed so readily" (p. 16). Similarly, Whisman (1990) concludes that there are numerous methodological or conceptual problems with many of the evaluations of booster sessions that need to be overcome before a more definitive conclusion can be reached. Some of these problems include low statistical power, attrition, short follow-up periods, and unclear rationale for the timing and content of the booster sessions. Clearly, these problems need to be addressed in future studies. There are other questions that remain to be answered in relation to boosters. Where are they successful and why are they successful? There are numerous factors that might influence the effects of booster sessions which need to be identified and utilized, such as the nonspecific components of attention from the therapist, regular appointments, social support from others when the boosters are delivered in a group format, and the specific elements of the booster program itself. The economics of RP also warrants further consideration. Is it cost effective? Do the various procedures differ in their cost effectiveness? Do booster sessions only delay eventual relapse for certain problems?

CONCLUSION

The authors of each chapter have attempted to provide an overview of the present status of research on relapse—its prediction and prevention and the processes that initiate it. Maintenance of treatment effects remains an important goal for researchers and clinicians. In some areas, this goal is a great deal closer to being reached than in others. Across all problem areas, however, there are many research questions waiting to be pursued. It is hoped that this book stimulates researchers to address some of the important questions raised throughout its pages. Those readers who are primarily clinicians, of course, cannot wait for all the answers, but it is envisaged that some of the suggestions expressed here will help to stimulate ideas for the implementation of RP techniques. The great value of the scientist–practitioner approach and of the empirical tradition is that we possess the skills and commitment to formulate theories and test hypotheses that will serve to enhance both our understanding of behavioral problems and our ability to deliver more effective treatments. Like the seismologists who attempt to predict and control earthquakes, those researchers who are interested in the RP need to further develop our knowledge of the nature of each disorder, the factors that trigger relapse, and the processes by which durable maintenance is achieved.

REFERENCES

Bandura, A. (1977). Self-efficacy: Toward a unifying theory of behavioral change. *Psychological Review, 84,* 191–215.

Blanchard, E. B., Andrasik, F., Guarnieri, P., Neff, D. F., & Rodichok, L. D. (1987). Two-, three-, and four-year follow-up on the self-regulatory treatment of chronic headache. *Journal of Consulting and Clinical Psychology, 55,* 257–259.

Brandon, T. H., Zelman, D. C., & Baker, T. B. (1987). Effects of maintenance sessions on smoking relapse: Delaying the inevitable? *Journal of Consulting and Clinical Psychology, 55,* 780–782.

Burns, L. E., Thorpe, G. L., & Cavallaro, L. A. (1986). Agoraphobia 8 years after behavioral treatment: A follow-up study with interview, self-report, and behavioral data. *Behavior Therapy, 17,* 580–591.

Lisspers, J., & Öst, L.-G. (1990). Long-term follow-up of migraine treatment: Do the effects remain up to six years? *Behaviour Research and Therapy, 28,* 313–322.

Marlatt, G. A., & Gordon, J. R. (1985). *Relapse prevention: Maintenance strategies in the treatment of addictive behaviors.* New York: Guilford Press.

Rychtarik, R. G., Foy, D. W., Scott, T., Lokey, L., & Pruse, D. M. (1987). Five-six year follow-up of broad-spectrum behavioral treatment for alcoholism: Effects of training controlled drinking skills. *Journal of Consulting and Clinical Psychology, 55,* 106–108.

Whisman, M. A. (1990). The efficacy of booster maintenance sessions in behavior therapy: Review and methodological critique. *Clinical Psychology Review, 10,* 155–170.

INDEX